The Developing Brain

The Developing Brain

Neurobiology and the Role of Information Preschool – PhD

ATINA A.

To order additional copies of this book, contact:
Xlibris
844-714-8691
www.Xlibris.com
Orders@Xlibris.com
760109

CONTENTS

The Developing Brain
Neurobiology and New-Century

Preschool-PhD

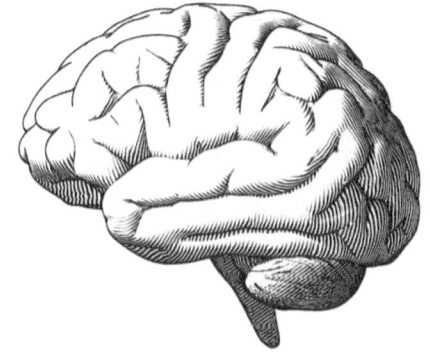

A Journey to the
Heart of Brain
Mind, Conscience, and
Information

Acknowledgments

To my life coach, my experience: because I owe it all through life lessons.

My *forever love*, interested, encouraging, and always enthusiastic: my wonderful, intelligent, educated, well-mannered, beautiful four kids. The greatest gift I can give to my four kids is my time, my attention, and my love. The love for my kids is what gives me strength and that is the reason I am here and alive today.

A very special gratitude goes out to all down at research: science, physics, theories, authors, educational information updates, for the foundation and for helping and providing the information we all have out there for the work.

And last but by no means least, to everyone in my life: it was great sharing love and interests with all of you throughout my life journey.

Introduction

Truth becomes obviously stranger than fiction when it comes to self-deception. Fiction at least is obliged to stick to possibilities. However, truth in this matter won't. I was gazing through decades of research beyond life-and-death stories, especially the question of how it was that a patient with terminal cancer or serious infection could so courageously fight to stay alive against all odds. Could it be that the patient and the physician were actually denying the reality of what they were up against? Optimistic thinking that helps us understand to go on despite the odds isn't just in life or death, but it's part of what makes us human. How this mental awareness of one's own personhood could aware the personhood of others—gaining useful ability and consequently awareness of the deaths of others of our own kind—mortality and evolutionary dead end. Despite brain process information, human higher-level awareness, the fullest abilities to mental state to others, and the realization of one's own life and mortality is the mind. You may say what a piece of work is human; how aristocratic in reason.

Hello, welcome to the fascinating, informational, integrated, interconnected neweuro century of new science, the interpersonal neurobiology. It is beyond the nature and nurture divisions that traditionally have forced much of our understanding about development, exploring the role of interpersonal experience and information in shaping the integration with the brain. Since the publication of many editions of *Developing Brain, Mind, Consciousness, and Human Evolution* (evolutionary psychology) over a period of dozen years, much has emerged (time brings changes) from the objective study of science, theories, physics, economy, society, politics, pandemic, human power, and the subjective understanding of interpersonal knowledge. This book synthesizes information as flow of energy from a range of scientific disciplines (*updated* researchers, professors, books, etc.) to explore all ideas that the brain, mind, or consciousness emerges at the interface of interpersonal experience throughout human evolutionary development (how evolution changes implemented in the embryonic development of organisms) under the structure and function of the *integration system as a whole*. Fifty years ago, critics reported that the twentieth century was the era of the "psychological man" in many ways. Despite the fallacy in this logic might be, today modern human whose ancestors have already crossed the barrier, thus already capable. It might be mistaken the psychological human of today with psychoanalysis of then. It might have been an error assumption if we could nothing grow ourselves in terms of brain, mind, and consciousness in the natural world and interplay with the content of culture and civilization. Unfortunately, today we examine the three spheres of life at the laboratory that defined the earliest stage of our life concept as a manifestation of human nature.

The human mind is one of the last frontiers of great science, which is a significant organ of the brain. It allowed us to walk on the moon as addition to discover the secret of the universe and life on earth. However, because of its powerful nature, it raises many paradox and concerns. For example, how we know certain things, like eating dirt is disgusting or something similar. It can be the goal of the mind to explain these patterns through its brain processing information systems. The one aspect to look at is just as the heart's responsibility is to pump blood flow, so is the brain to process the information flow. How we know eating dirt is disgusting is examining mind via our thoughts (consciousness). It's clear that our mind and thoughts have no physical property nor weight test, sound, or smell system, as much as our spoken language and information within our head daily. However, we can determine the physical aspect of such social behavior through its process, way of computational brain experiences, and evolution psychology. This brings some degree of understanding the body and mind process of *awareness* and development.

The exploration of such nature of understanding is one aspect of information system through belief and desire. We are in one part recycled information networking systems of patterns, matters, and energy systems to correlate the states of the world, just like the school teaches children about the rings of tree describing the age of the tree. It is the information of such tree to its biology. Also, with this high level of knowledge—awareness and intersubjectivity—comes awareness of death and mortality. Thus, far from being a useful being, the resulting overwhelming fear would be a dead-end evolutionary barrier and restrain activities and cognitive functions necessary for survival and reproductive fitness. However, human mechanisms allowed us to delude the mind by denying (unconscious defense) to deal with such terror of knowing. Depending on the context, denying reality can become a problematic behavior, such as smoking, gaining weight, and not exercising, despite our full awareness that these habits are exceptional.

Truth to reality can be stubborn; whatever may be our inclination, hopes, passions, they cannot alter the state of evidence. As we mentioned, one aspect of human development can be humans are the products of biological evolution (biological evolution by natural selection). Although science raises more questions than answers, we accepted the earth is round and that it orbits a minor star called the sun. future resource might still be limited to understand our full fundamental nature, but what we can say no is that human organisms are *unique genetically.* Despite having good or less fortunate genes, traits are passed on to one's progeny, which might be heritable better traits. Therefore, this leads to the changes of human organisms. Looking back forty years ago, I too became filled with a particular intellectual passion of the brain-mind and the nature of human that I think is superseding psychoanalysis as the ideal behind psychology human of today.

Our development journey and our mind are complex systems integrated with this information (to mind neural information) that process and build mental models of the physical and social world and follow the goals that are essential to survival and reproduction in modern society. Despite much attempts on many theories and practices, nature has shown us in ingenious solutions that human engineers *cannot* yet be duplicated. We cannot duplicate mind, awareness, or consciousness as psychologically is reverse engineering of mind. We can only define its reverse engineering system by its processing system of its integration to information. Studies cannot define and frame something that has a *continuum journey.*

Likewise, everyone has a mind of their own. Even the mind has its own mind. Hence, every minute of every day one can change their mind. Further, the mind is a complex system that gives us insight to many mental and engineering programs that have many tools and devices for solving such activities. Just knowing our mental abilities to movement of arms to seeing a three-dimensional world, or finding love, and so on.

Through a series of journeys, I eventually worked with children of all ages and their families most of my life. Alongside, I have encountered a variety of people and the stories of their lives. I have read and explored many updates, research, and books and have gained experiences. Therefore, I found myself naturally trying to understand the process of human development—how people become who they are—by investigating what was known from new research and getting as close as possible to the subjective experiences at the core of people's lives that I hope would stand the test of time. Over the course of time, am still yearning for clarity which I am only now aware—this book presents the integration of this effort to gain insight into our interconnected lives and the development journey of the brain, mind, and consciousness.

The brain is complex also self-organize and self-processor. I also trust enough to say the brain has an open-ended definition. If I could ever give the brain an explanation over definition it would be "the self-regulated continuum information processor, yet through its consciousness trusts its mind." With modern technology and much updated research, humans have no issues opening up under a microscope, exploring deeper secrets and possibilities to what might be possible. However, dissecting our DNA or brain structure has not shown us its definition. Also, this living system is an open system that is capable of responding based on its development and can adopt new things in any given moment.

Brain development is an unstoppable journey from childhood to adulthood. Therefore, the brain represented as symbols of whole cannot be defined by any boundaries nor any given definition. It might take another forty years of my life—maybe then, sitting on my old desk like a Zen master, I shall finish a final book, but it will have no words. After all, if we continually don't attempt to define and refine our relationship (how to communicate) with brain stimulation and our mind, how can we define well-being? The structure and function of our developing brain is intent on how much experience and interpersonal relationship architecture the genetically coded maturation of our nervous system.

To microscope human relationship (attachment) shapes neural connections, and each contributes to brain and mind development, even right now as you are trying to communicate with me through this book. How we perceive the world and see the nature of reality depends much on how we have experienced the world. For instance, these often-used words, "make me care" or "when I see it, I believe it" or perhaps "never mind," make the brain curious about its mind and its *relation*. Let's not forget the complexity of our brain and mind is still challenging the embedded brain and humans. That might have taken us longer to figure ourselves out. Let's go back to our sentence with a more open mind, instead of a "never mind." It seems there is a connection between the eyes ("when I see it") and to our brain ("I believe it").

Seemingly, there's a sense of relationship between the brain to the body-mind (eyes as retina to the brain as processing the information to the mind) as opposed to just the brain as form of neurons be enskulled in our head alone. In the point of psychology, the dimmer the patch of light at the retina, the steeper the angle of the surface of the world.

Therefore, the brain reconstructs the shape from the angle of the layer of thousands of the fastest neurons that collectively defines the three dimensions of surfaces. That might be another reason why television and computers give us an illusion in understanding the three-dimensional world and hold our intellect to the interest. Either way, if our brain tells us what to see or our eye sends information to the thalamus for interrupting the information, it shows equal *integration*. All right, we get that; our brain lives inside our whole body, but what about the "make me care" phrase?

What is the correlation between others' input *(brain relationship)* and our neurons' stimulation for adaptation or refusal of any decision-making? *This is where our neuron networking and the function of mind integration (communication) begin.* How can this be possible for the rational mind to be embedded (enskulled) and at the same time be relational (with others)? Does this mean interpersonal communication advances with internal neural integration, which only means that neural integration is the basis of our healthy self-regulation system? So when we come to a conclusion for making any discussion, this means we achieve a "balanced self-regulation" by integrating neural systems and interpersonal relationships. Can it be then, attachment relationships work to create the central basis from which the mind of the brain develops?

Therefore, any narrative life events we create with others will begin to narrate such event to ourselves (recycle information flow) that will be driven by explicit (later memory) and implicit (early memory) recollections of repeated experience. Also, where does this knowledge of knowing beyond sense of me or "make me care" and sense of self, when "I" see it, "I" believe it, come from? Who's this "I" who "knows" it? Can't these implicit memory (early memory) encodings shape the architecture of our self from childhood, or is it the continuum mind of our ancestors as a way of psychological evolution and biology? Aside, explicit memories (late memory) are what refer to generic ideas of memory when their recollections are retrieved, they will have the initial sensation of "I am"—remembering. Well, human memory is not steady or fixed, but it's pretty much an active set of processes.

Remembering is not the sole responsibility of reactivation of just our old engram (the impact of experiences on the brain), but actually, it's the construction of a new neural net profile with the futures of the old engram, elements of memory from other (past) experiences, and influences from the now moments of state of mind (mental or emotional). Memory and our consciousness, depending on their integrative processes (relationship and communication) inside the brain for their creation as much as information and energy flow, are shared within relationships with others in our interconnected world as a whole.

The *conscious experience* we might have about ourselves is formed in part by how our synapses are shaped through social experiences within society. *Consciousness* is the window through which we understand ourselves and others. In other words, experience (personal information) shapes the structure of the brain. Can't then be possible evolution also been proven track for our brain development? Everything is a contributor to brain development. Based on our relationships, communication *can create an information-processing brain.*

How experience affects our brain is happens by the increased probability of firing similar patterns so the neural networks will remember. Our brain is composed of spiderweb-like neural networks. These networks have the potential to fire in a multitude of patterns, which are called neural net profiles. Therefore, this neural network structure allows it to learn through an encoding process that initially activates a specific set of linked neuronal firing patterns dispensed throughout our brain. The interconnectedness and the balance of such neuronal network process is how learning takes place. Any disconnection is a brain abnormality, such as autism. Therefore, can't be fact that our development and memories process based on similar neural and molecular mechanisms underlying synapse formation, which changes in these synaptic connections would alter the way our brain would function?

What's important here to keep in mind is our development does not only complete before birth as processing of evolution or during childhood, but throughout our lifetime. We are in lifelong development as our experience shapes us through our life span. Being ten years old has much developmental experience and stages as much as being sixty years old. Thus, being part of whole patterns is essential over what we discover as a single structure to stages—bodily self. These developmental interdisciplinary patterns of our psychology have occupied our brain-mind-consciousness stimulation for the past decades.

Various scientific disciplines come close enough to definition, but are many on description of psychology (mental activities). Odd, we may think, but true enough. We may shed light on the important role of the mind of the brain—at least for academic purposes, as we may hold a spot to "unknowns" when it comes to its definition. Wouldn't this mean majority of our health professionals perceive health without the definition (well explanation) of the mind? If who we are—both in our personal identity and in our personal experiences of life journey—appears as a mental process and the function of the brain to mind, then isn't who are we is who our mind is?

Bearing in mind the issue of *causality*, we might ask ourselves, why do we think the past causes the present? Indeed, we might search what is with the past which we remember the most and the future which we don't. Can it be the answer, the fundamental laws of physics, is completely neutral with regard to the direction of the time? They are unchanged if we change the direction of the time variable. What separates the past from the present is now time that does not have a natural place in the laws of physics.

Parapsychology deals with the interaction between our mental and physical. It straddles the boundaries between psychology and physics as it studies the interaction of the mind and matters.

Therefore, it's best to know for now that psychology is not the parent discipline of psi, that is, one that does not include key references to purely mental concepts such as intent, meaning, or belief. The psi phenomenon can be problematic because they involve events in reality and require exploration, yet they are pretty much bound with certain states of mind. Therefore, they cross the dividing line between objectivity and subjectivity which normal mental phenomena do not. Science is still not at that level of developing psi, for example, like chemistry was born out of alchemy or astronomy out of astrology, later to develop from science. When it comes to understanding psi, it's best to know the physical theories and psychological theories.

The physical theories attempt to deal with the environment. The psychological theories deal with the problem of how psi comes to manifest itself in the human consciousness in ways that it does. The realization of intentions is the essential property of psi. However, the mind's relationship with the brain is of authentic interest. For instance, if we can be conscious just now by what is just said or read, is the *focus*; we use the condition of enters into this *focus* to gain insight into mind jurisdictions, and role in relation to the brain subsystem.

What make the brain and the mind aware of its information and its processing can also be intuitively physic. As well, we are aware of the world's existence, even if we look or close our eyes.

We are opening the dialogue in a scientific way, inviting inquiry into mind, brain, consciousness, for all, including academicians, clinicians, educators, students, parents, and anyone with an interest in brain development and mental health while leaving belief systems for this book journey. Focusing on the brain in the head as a main source of mind, consciousness, or our fundamental development has been profoundly important in our lives for full understanding, mental health, well-being, our challenges and who we are on this planet Earth.

We may consider the brain central to understanding not just the mind of the brain, but our consciousness. Therefore, is no argument for the importance of our brain to health, especially when it comes to lesion, cancer, etc. Nevertheless, these views of our mental abilities (psychology) or perhaps our mind coming from the brain are two thousand five hundred years old. Yet these findings and research do not logically or scientifically mean that only the brain creates the human mind, consciousness, or even sense of self. Even perhaps these bodily parts might not be the same, the influential relationship among them is an essential part of this book. Could it be the brain is an important component, yet a bigger story of our well-being hasn't been explored well enough?

We can say at minimum, beyond the head and our relationship with others—and even with the universe maybe there is other contextual factors influence our mental (psychological) awareness, experience, and development than the brain between our shoulders.

Nothing in my life—formal training, whether in medical schools, as teaching professors, pediatric, psychiatry—had prepared me for the situation I learned and faced in the treatment room with my patients. This is a new science of personal transformation *(interpersonal neurobiology)* that has said by so many well-known neuroscientists, neurologists, and psychologists. The area behind the forehead is a part of the frontal lobe of the cerebral cortex, which is the outermost part of the brain. This is the location responsible and is associated with the majority of our complexities of how we think and how we plan. Activating this part of our brain fires neurons in patterns which enable us to form a neural representation to understand various parts of our world. The image that is created from the clusters' neuronal activities will serve to create an understanding or a map for our mind. This process also determines our subjective experiences (personal experiences) to some point.

Just gazing at a tree, our eyes send this signal to the brain where there our neurons fire patterns which enable us to have the visual picture of this tree we are gazing. This neuronal activity has changed our subjective experiences to a degree. For instance, each time we come across a tree, we might feel what we felt at that point—who were there; what we were thinking; whether we were in pain or pleasure; whether we were scared, dry, or wet; what we heard, tasted, or said; etc. This frontal cortex is responsible for the neuronal representations which enable us to make images of the mind.

What the *past images* we have as our personal subjective experiences, we build images based on the future. Next time when we gaze at a tree, we might not just trust our vision alone—which realizes that tree but includes the mind's vision—but experience everything that happened at that time. Therefore, our physical brain is a broadly integrated social organ, but not internal compass; it leaves experience to the mind, which might be fine to say the phenomenological feature of such is allowed to be given a physical account.

The way our brain-mind-consciousness develops depends much on its communication and its relationship. That creates a "whole brain" development and our well-being. Science is not the combination to understand human experience and its events. How a colorful sensitive neuron gives rise to the subjective feel of brightness is not a whit less mysterious, overall, how the whole brain gives rise to the entire stream of consciousness is even more impressive. The "I" is not a combination of body parts, brain states, and bits of information alone, but an *integration of selfness* over time, a single point that is nowhere in particular. The idea of this framework is organized around these fundamental principles in general to its relationships as such:

Brain and its structure of development (embedded). Our genes. Brain stimulation to body parts (our organs) embodied. The mind-to-brain or brain-to-mind integration as a whole. Our consciousness, sense of awareness, and the brain. The personal subjective experience of our life journey. The relationship with others, our memory, and our attachment—including our culture. The *relationship with the universe* (physics and metaphysics) and *spiritual belief systems*. The relationship with our ancestors and evolutionary biology—psychology.

The conscious mind knows its objectivity and physiological and psychological mechanisms by which experiences are conveyed. *The brain-mind regulates this flow of energy information with a sense of consciousness (awareness) as a form of interconnectedness (integration).* There is no approach to the mind might be a cynical view of human nature that will be a dark place, which bring us that the mind might be a system of computer design by natural selection to permute survival and reproduction alone. What might have motivated such information is that a rational human knowing about *modern* brain science *(new neuron century / neweurocentury)* can deny that the mind is the product of the brain, the brain produces of evolution, and evolution does not depend on smooth sailing. Let's be *open-minded* and start our research further.

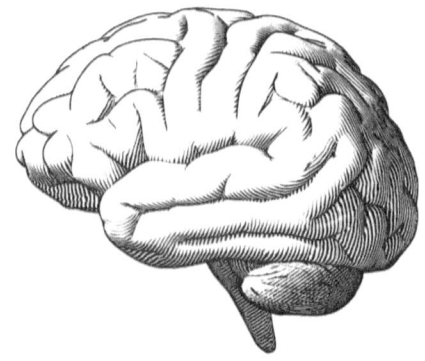

The Interconnected Mind Consciousness: The Role of Education (Information) on Developing Brain

Managing life is unquestionably the primary function of the human brain, and it's the most distinctive feature of being. If the human brain were too simple that we could understand it easily, we would be "simpler" to not understand. Therefore, the theory of evolution continues over two hundred years—from waking up to growing up journey, from nature and nurture perspective, from science to physics, from religion to spirituality, and so on. The key to the answer still remains to improve for the education that lies in understanding on how the human brain works: "Since that is where the knowledge take place."

Likewise, this is one of the most important education and discussion human could ever had, because it deals with the human interior. Virtually all the human problems or approach to the problems we hear are nothing but based on exteriors, whether it's global warming, war, economy crisis, infection crisis, power and politics, addiction, suicide, mental health, fail marriages, abuse, or other concerns. Much of the answer to many these problems is coming from interior development. The eyes see only what the mind is compared to comprehend. The same as language tells us, when a point is unclear, for instance, it's dark now.

The brain exclaims at the moment of clarity, "I see it!" We trust our vision of what we see to be a true representation of the external world.

However, the brain, working with the nerve cells of the eyes, constructs the outside world inside our heads. This work is the combination of the eye-and-brain activity, not passively. We see what the brain tells us to see. What is beneficial is being open to experience that leads us into success. Meaning just to be open to any stages of awareness awakens. Psychology perhaps is a discipline that cries out for scientists to engage with people beyond the walls of academe. Even better is cognitive psychology that is the branch of psychology which focuses on the way humans process information.

It deals in a way —how humans process information they receive and how the treatment of this information leads to others' responses. In other words, cognitive psychology is interested in what is happening within human minds that links stimulus (input) and response (output). Just about everyone we know has a mind, and almost nobody knows very much about how it actually works, which is odd. Just for the purpose of this book, I have explored many books, research, and updates from the best practices of psychology, cognitive science, neuroscience, and professors of famous universities such as Harvard, UCLA, and McGill and each research has shown some degree of intellect integration and much deeper—different understanding.

Some points put me in a hard problem of consciousness and mind development as we all share a different mind but some brain stimulation and different experiences yet the same processing. We would not allow anyone to build a bridge without learning some physics or practice medicine without learning biology at first, would we? Thus, wouldn't it be to everyone's advantage to learn about how the brain actually functions before we develop an opening, make a thought or decision, or create a curriculum? What is fascinating is we have much research, map, and heritage on interior development, from ignorance to great librarians to supreme enlightenment that is a greater part of human growth and evolution, but less applied to the education system.

If we were to have a global change in human behavior in order to handle our problems, then I think we have to look into human interiors in a larger picture to the human brain, mind, consciousness, experiences, spirituality, awareness, science, physics, and educational systems that tie all as forms of interconnectedness (the frame of well-being). From any development of interconnectedness or integral evolutions of practice two hundred years ago, the new growth that emerged did not exist in the cosmos prior to that time. Thus, evolution becomes conscious itself. What some studies have shown is that despite many types of intelligence, they typically develop through six basic stages of development. People like Howard Gardner and several developmental psychologists believe that we have multiple intelligences.

For instance, if we mention these six multiple intelligences as cognitive, emotional, moral, musical somatic, aesthetic, and spiritual intelligences.

The growing-up journey will take place in these six basic levels: archaic, magical, mythical, rational, pluralistic, and integral levels. These levels have different names. However, they generally point to the same ideas. If education were about to include all development stages of growing up, then we might include all the stages, as development has no partial stage in any study. This is the sum total of one hundred years of researching modern, Western, and developmental psychology. This is relatively recent where the waking-up stages go back; we said several thousand years.

Likewise, the growing-up stages weren't really discovered until about one hundred fifty years ago. Human development is not necessarily the examination of human brains, but *overall* development which requires further understanding of developmental practices. To take a look at significance issue in developmental psychology is the *relationship* between innateness and environmental influence in regard to any particular aspect of development. This is often referred to as *nature and nurture*. A nativist account of development would reason that the processes in question are inherent, that is, they are specified by the organism's *genes*.

Today developmental psychologists rarely take such polarized positions with regard to most aspects of development; rather, they investigate, among many other things, the *relationship* between *innate* and *environmental* influences. One of the ways this *relationship* has been explored in recent years is through the emerging field of evolutionary developmental psychology. These levels can also be simplified. For example, sense of *identity* has these four levels of development: egocentric, ethnocentric, world-centric, and cosmos-centric. Aside from growing up, waking up is the first part of development and has five basic to advanced stages: waking, dreaming, deep dreaming, witnessing or pure awareness, and having unity consciousness or nonduality.

Some theorists trust that development is a *smooth, continuous process*, and individuals gradually add more of the same types of skills throughout their lives. Other theorists, however, think that development takes place in a discontinuous pattern. People change rapidly and step up to a new level, and then no change or very less for a while. With each of these new steps, the person shows interest and responds to the world qualitatively. Most life span developmentalists recognize that extreme positions are unwise.

Therefore, the key to a comprehensive understanding of development at any stage requires the *interaction of different factors* and not only one. For example, *cognitive* development is primarily concerned with the ways that newborns and children acquire, develop, and use internal mental forces such as solving problems, the memory, and their language. *Language* is the window of the human mind and is also a fundamental topic of human science. This ability has distinguished human species. It's essential to our communication and cooperation, and it is still a mystery how language evolves and develops in humans.

The beauty of making sound, from the sound of bubbling and hissing, to the ears of human to understand the purpose of information given. Linguistics is one aspect of understanding the brain. There are six thousand languages spoken on earth that are complex. Still, humans have the instinct to speak. The idea of linguistic language and its studies, on how language works, perhaps the grammar (the word to sentence structure—phrases, nouns, verbs, etc.); phonology, the study of sound; semantics, the study of meaning; pragmatic, the usage of conversations. Aside, the process of this according to time, meaning how language developed, how it acquired by children from young age that is the study of language acquisition and how that computed to our brain as study of neurolinguistics.

Written language is not the same as spoken language, so let's not confuse our abilities. *Writing* is unlike spoken word; children, however, have no tendency unless guided by school and instruction. Also, how we *speak* in nonformal language is different from what we read or write as formal. *Language forms in thought. However, it's not necessary to function as written, but as a form of* information processing *in our memory in the form of gist or meaning to the context of thoughts over the form of the exact words. It has a great contribution to our brain development in general.*

How would we discipline language without language? Language is a bottom-up phenomenon and the contribution of evolution from people creating slangs, jargon, which shaped the language of today. Language is also the idea behind our thoughts, emotions, interpersonal relationships, and experiences but not necessarily into words or perhaps reciting sentences as forms of language. To distinguish such discipline, language has three components: words (the basic component of words, sentences), rules (how we use these words into more complex), and syntax, morphology, and phenology.

In addition, the *integration* of such knowledge with the word that brings us the understanding self and others. If we look into *integration language* and such discipline, it will shape such diagram:

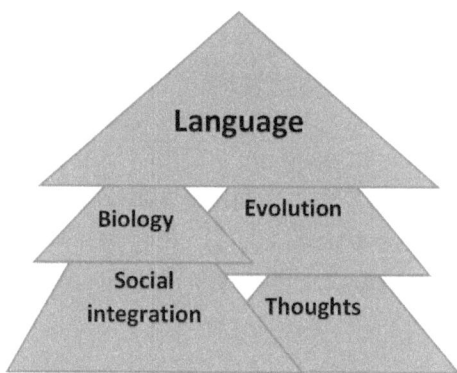

The biggest topics in *cognitive development* are the study of language acquisition and the development of perceptual and motor skills. If we look into the theory of Piaget, he was one of the influential early psychologists to study the development of cognitive abilities. His theory suggests that development proceeds through a set of stages that is from infancy to adulthood and that there is an end point.

Other theories, such as that of Lev Vygotsky, have viewed that development does not progress through stages (the six stages mentioned above) but rather that the *developmental process that begins at birth and continues until death* is too complex for such structure and finality. From this viewpoint, developmental processes proceed more continuously. Therefore, development is best examined instead of treated as a product to acquire. This is sounds more like the process of development counts over the products of what's take development there.

Similarly, other theories, such as that of K. Warner Schaie, have expanded the study of cognitive development into *adulthood*. Rather than being stable from adolescence, K. Warner Schaie sees adults as progressing in the application of their cognitive abilities. One thing can be true: adults understand when it comes to children's development. What might be needed for adults' development is adulthood education. For instance, there are cultures whose development is equal to a grade 8 level. The world-acknowledged level of education is till grade 12, where individuals can participate in modern democracy. What is essential is that these levels not only teach the skill to grade, but also identifies what development interior that brings forth. For example, when a child is in grade 8, it's continuance education, which is good. However, when an adult who dropped school at grade 8 might be the continuation of issues. Would this mean that maybe adults need education of development as our society might not be united to teach since the big bang? So far, education has lightened much of civilization's darker ages' stages of development, yet still up to date, we have places where people are heading toward one another.

Accordingly, we have learned enough about our journey of the brain to: its mind, function to its embedded system, our overall development journey from psychology—milestone and from theory to practice. One thing did add well: either one of these practices and research projects has explored one aspect of human development if we *combine them with whole* other practices. Therefore, as much as we cannot skip over cognitive development and all other developments, we cannot skip over consciousness, human mind, and experiences. As much as our bio depends on molecular cells and atoms, as much as we are connected to our mental health and awareness in whole that shapes our daily life, we remain the *sum* of our development if we don't consider the *whole stages* of development.

Today modern cognitive development has *integrated* the considerations of cognitive psychology and the psychology of individual differences into the interpretation and modeling of development. This is interesting and new experience for science education and psychology of independent studies of development. For instance, children who grow up in the same household with the same parents do not always necessarily develop the same. For instance, given the study of genes, nature and nurture, evolution, awareness, and also how the child has been treated by parents and society as a whole.

This leads to the uniqueness of personal experiences and integration of parenting with social networking. Piaget's development showed that the successive levels or stages of cognitive development are associated with increasing processing efficiency and working memory capacity. These have explained the differences between the stages, progression to higher stages, and the differences. Regardless, other theories have moved away from the Piagetian *stage theories* and are influenced by the theory of domain-specific *information processing*, which forwards that development is guided by *innate evolutionarily specified* and *content-specific information processing* mechanisms.

Developmental psychologists have a number of methods to study changes in individuals over time. These research methods include systematic observation, including naturalistic observation or structured observation, as well as self-reports, which could be clinical interviews or structured interviews. It can be a clinical or case study method and ethnography or participant observation.

Each of these developmental investigations is characterized in terms of whether its underlying strategy involves the experimental, correlational, or case study approach. This method involves actual manipulation of different treatments, circumstances, and events to which the subject is exposed the experimental design points to *cause-and-effect relationships*. The advantage of using this research method is that it permits the determination of cause-and-effect relationships among variables.

On the other hand, the limitation is that data obtained in an artificial environment may lack generalizability. There are a number of theories and practices of human nature and human development. It's the best way to explore and understand human nature in many dimensional patterns and anticipate the behavior of others. There are many theories we explored that guide us through children's development, manage our relationships, and continue to control our behavior.

Therefore, the theory of human nature ties us with intellectual learning about our well-being, guides, policies, laws, regulations, and religion. Although there are many other case studies that are arguable, modern science has challenged three "linked ethics" that constitute the dominant view of human nature in intellectual life. For instance, the mind has no innate traits. This roughly equates to the English term "blank slate," which refers to emptiness, meaning that we were born a blank book, ready to be written by the process of evolution—according to our development.

We will look into the brain function further into our book journey. At this point we can say psychologists and neurobiologists have shown evidence that initially the entire cerebral cortex is programmed and organized to process sensory input, control motor actions, regulate emotion, and respond reflexively. These programmed mechanisms in the brain afterward act to learn and refine the ability of the organism. For example, in contrast to written language, our brain is programmed to pick up the spoken language voluntarily.

Also, the meaning in life or human purpose doesn't require that the process (interpersonal experience) that shaped the brain must have a purpose alone or only that the brain itself must have purposes. If the human mind is a blank slate completely formed by the environment, then wouldn't entirely controlling every aspect of the environment create perfect minds? In this integration, wouldn't the excessive blame of parents if their children do not turn out well be assumed to be entirely environmentally caused? Similarly, how can we create laws knowing dangerous psychopaths who commit new crimes are environmentally appropriated?

On the other hand, some studies show that the brain is tabula rasa only for certain behaviors. The evidence against the tabula rasa model of the mind comes from behavioral genetics, for example, the study development of twins and their adoptions. These patterns shape strong genetic influences on personal characteristics such as human IQ, gender identity, and other traits. Multiple studies show that the distinct faculties of the mind, the memory and reason mixture, aside to genetic boundaries. In the point of view of computer science, tabula rasa refers to the development of autonomous agents with a mechanism to reason and plan toward their goal.

However, there is no built-in knowledge base of their environment, which means they truly are a blank slate. Second, the noble savage meaning, people are born good and corrupted by society. A noble savage was a literary stock character who embodies the concept of the indigene, outsider, wild human, another who has not been corrupted by the civilization. Thus, it symbolizes humanity's innate goodness. On the other view, the ghost in the machine is done by others. The phrase was referred to in the book *The Concept of Mind* to highlight the view of dualist systems. For instance, mental activity carries on in parallel to physical action. However, their means of interaction are unknown. The British philosopher Ryle's *Concept of Mind* is a critique of the notion that the mind is distinct from the body, and a rejection of the theory that mental states are separable from physical states.

In this book was the idea of a fundamental distinction between mind and matter as the ghost in the machine. As we are getting further in our book journey, we can see there is a belief about the nature and place of the mind, which is prevalent among theorists. The philosophical arguments lay out the notion of the mistaken foundations of mind-body dualism conceptions, comprising a suggestion that to speak of mind and body as a substance, as a dualist does, is to commit a category error. It is particularly critical of B. F. Skinner's behaviorist theory.

One of the book's central concepts is that as the human brain has grown, it has built upon earlier, more primitive brain structures and that this is the "ghost in the machine" of the title.

Other theories, including Koestler's concept, show that at times these structures can overpower higher logical functions and are responsible for hate, anger, and other such destructive impulses. All the integration of theories and information is surely fine; indeed, we will explore much of it. We can look into how to understand the nature of human so that we can learn it again. We can also study three lifelines: the new sciences of the mind, the new research on cognitive science and behavioral genetics, and the importance of evolutionary psychology. These might shed light and provide free education on the age-long ignorance.

From the *earliest* 1950s, the cognitive revolution has changed a lot. With the new century, it's possible to make sense of mental processes and even to study them literally at the lab. Much studies review the brain function and the development of the mind, so we now can conclude one another's aspect that the mind might not a homogeneous ring invested with unitary powers or across-the-board traits. The mind can be a single integrator helping people into the study of human's nature.

However, there are major dimensions of human experience—beauty, morality, cooperation, parenting, sexuality, love, and violence—in which evolutionary psychology can educate and provide individuals the only coherent theory to vibrant new areas of logic research. In addition, human mental experience can be grounded in the physical world by the notion of information, computation, and learning experiences. However, studies on cognitive science and evolutionary psychology are not physical sciences that could claim the benefit.

On the other hand, the state of behavioral genetics is compelling. Genetics is part of science indeed. Nonetheless, integrating it to human behavior is a complex process that requires a better understanding of selection. With *integration* of interpersonal relationships and experiences, *the gene* has now become a community word. What has brought the understanding to this public notice is the metaphor integrated with it—egotism as the metaphor that resolves some debates about motivation. Self-interest is indeed the best solution to human motive. Unfortunately, we are open to the debate and notion of information served to fulfill mending the mind-body gap. We can determine some conclusions based on evolutionary psychology, but not all. Our emotional nature is indeed not a balanced system but a generally evolved balanced system.

Moreover, with new generation comes new live in crowded, artifact-filled conditions, which is not the same as when it was formed. It's an important learning process that if we could discover the details of our prior nature by referencing them from the social conditions accomplishment, then it was formed in the Stone Age. Afterward, we could have converted such and divided it into separate representations which determine recognizable articles of behaviors. The method fails because we don't have Stone Age sociology, and similarly the mind is not the sum of the whole, but the whole and no amount of splitting will disclose their general structure.

However, gradually we need a notion of human nature. This isn't the way in which we are going to find it. We humans have long records of history of pursuing neural enhancements and ways to improve the brain that evolution creates for us. From centuries ago till now, all of these and other innovations are designed either to improve the brain we carry on today or to off-load some of its functions to external sources. Although our genes haven't fully caught up with the human demand of modern civilization, fortunately human's knowledge has—we know better understanding how to overcome evolutionary *limitations*. That's how humans have coped with a *world of information* and organization from the beginning of civilization.

From the *first development* of the brain to five thousand years ago, humans have figured out how to write things down trying to increase the capacity of the hippocampus, part of the brain's memory system. From that point, they have effectively extended the natural limits of human memory by preserving some of their memories on the clay table or walls that are today's books and computer software. Therefore, these external memory mechanisms are generally of two types: either they follow the human brain's own nature of organizational systems or they reinvent it, which sometimes overcomes its limitations. How we cope with *the flow of energy and information system* is an essential part of brain design of *memory*.

The richness and associative access sorts our lives and experiences. From the beginning of our memory, the large number of things humans ever experienced throughout is still there inside our brain by stimulation of richness access. Associative access manages thoughts a bit different by semantic or perceptual association—memories can be triggered by related words or name, touch, smell, pictures, or neural firing that brings them up to our daily consciousness. Throughout this book, we will explore many venues of human brain and mind development and its connection between ourselves, history, and relationships. The brain is much self-regulatory and self-organizing organization (information processor). It's important to understand, it doesn't organize things the way we might want to.

The *evolved architecture* of the brain is haphazard and disjointed, and it's incorporated multiple systems that each of which has a mind of its own, so to speak. It's important aspect of reading any books or learning new things *to learn how our brain organizes* information *so that we can use what we have rather than fight against it.* The two key ways we can control and improve the process are to pay special attention to the way we engage with information flow into our memory (system encoding) and to pay attention to the way we pull it out (retrieval).

Our brain has the capacity to process information systems. However, it has its cost. We can have trouble separating the trivial from the important. This process requires energy stream, and therefore, it makes individuals lose interest due to the tiring process. Neurons are living cells with a metabolism which requires oxygen, glucose, and time to survive while they are in working process. One way to look at this is the processing capacity of the human conscious mind is 120 bits per second, which gives us a window to traffic stream of information at any given time.

For generations, cognitive science, neuroscience, and psychology focus primarily on localization of the brain function and neural mapping, from the ways we think, speak, or do any physical activity to what part of the brain becomes active in such performance. However, with the stream of recent information come chances to change the old system of understanding development. For instance, neuroscientists have concluded that mental operations may not always be occurring in one specific brain region but rather are carried out by circuits, an integration of networks of *relationships* with neuron groups.

If we were to explore the electrical system within our house, soon we might understand it's not necessarily the plugs or electrical box that runs our light fixture or our stoves, but the *networks* of ingredient systems of signals and wires outside of the house as a whole. The same as human: cognitive function, our neural stimulation, brain regions as to our mental abilities, language . . . isn't raised in a specific region of the brain; rather, its complexity of compromise a distribution of networks. Also, to the mind-wandering mode, the central executive, and the attentional filter, there's another attentional system which allows us to switch between ourselves (mind-wandering) and the central executive mode, which allows us to shift from one task to another and to multitask.

This can be viewed as a neural switchboard that directs and redirects our attention flows. This switch in the region of the brain is called the insula, which is located an inch beneath the surface of where the temporal lobes and frontal lobes are joined.

A switch between two external objects involves the temporal-parietal junction. The insula has bidirectional communication to the important brain regions called the anterior cingulate cortex. When it comes to mind-wandering, the relationship between the central executive system and the mind-wandering system is more like zigzags; and with the insula, the attentional switch is like an organization of one-sided zigzag up while other side can stay down.

Since we understood the concept of *living in the information world requires* education *to navigate through attention and memory systems.* Aside it's a guidance through learning, perhaps understanding the aim of this book. To recap, there are four components in the human attentional filter and its switch which we explored. It directs neural and metabolic systems. These components are the mind-wandering mode, the attentional filter, the central executive mode, and the attentional switch. The mind-wandering network recruiting the neurons within the prefrontal cortex as addition to cingulate integrate them to the hippocampus, the center of our memory consolidation.

This happens through the activity of noradrenaline located deep inside our skull that has evolved a dense mass of fibers linking to the prefrontal cortex. Dopamine and serotonin are chemicals and components of brain networking. Although noradrenaline and adrenaline might sound similar to our ears, they are much different chemically. Noradrenaline is similar to dopamine which is synthesized by the brain. Balance is the essential aspect of staying connected to the mind-wandering mode between the excitatory neurotransmitter glutamate and the inhibitory neurotransmitter gamma aminobutyric acid.

Sustainable attention also depending on noradrenaline and acetylcholine which is much important in distracting environment that is an essential part of our chemistry underlying the concentration it takes to focus. When focusing our attention on a given task, acetylcholine in the right prefrontal cortex helps to improve the quality of the work done by our attentional filter. The acetylcholine density inside our brain changes quickly at the subsecond level, and its release is tied to the detection of task we are searching for. The attentional filter comprises a network in the frontal lobes and sensory cortices, the auditory and visual cortex.

Therefore, when we try to look for something, the filter can retune neurons to match the characteristics of the things we are looking for, like browsing through your pictures or finding your house keys. One other aspect of the attentional filter is that it *communicates closely* (how-to relationship) with the insula to activate the switch there in order to pull us out of the mind-wandering system and create an appropriate behavioral response such as shield when flying objects are thrown at us. These are lifesaving and warning systems that are governed by noradrenaline in the frontal and parietal lobes.

Therefore, each step of the research reveals the key opponent to our whole development is not just integration alone, yet the relationship to how neurons communicate. What's so astonishing is how much knowledge we actually have right now versus how much of that knowledge is generally available to most people or, for that matter, generally available to most educators and professors which this book aims for exploration of learning and educational programs to some degree for all-age readers. Let's break it down more to understand; we have come to another realization: life is normal when it's balanced—between education, health, home, relationship, and importantly love. If the world creates out of business, then we made survival important over life.

To be educated intellectually, it's easy ten or more years requires to study. However, to remain uneducated of human intelligence and its potential is the hardest lesson of all. The important success of life is well-being before well intellect. Some have no opportunity to go to school. Some believe information isn't knowing alone. Information is an essential part of interpersonal experience. However, *knowing* can only *define* this function. Knowledge comes from human potential that is interconnected to well-development-brain and mindfulness as information (intellect) gives names to what might be relevant for our survival alone. Human potential is an essential part of our growing-up journey and depends on how we experience life, which again ties us up to *relevant information* flow. Let's keep in mind—that how the world be tomorrow is much depending on how parent you are today—which is the best contributing aspect.

Chapter 1

General Introduction

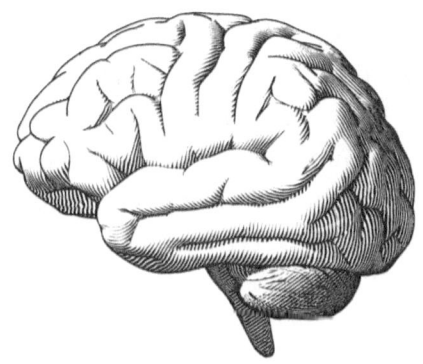

Hello, and welcome to the fascinating journey of interdisciplinary thinking, growing, and developing. It's the new face of theories, including practice and science (physics, metaphysics, and consciousness of interpersonal neurobiology). I invite you to join me on this interconnectedness journey to explore the complex intertwining of *mind, brain, consciousnesses, and relationships.* This book honors and explores how past and recent findings from a range of developmental theories and practices (science, physics, metaphysics, spirituality, and personal experiences) can bring us to a new understanding of the developing brain and the collation of our educational system.

The findings give us many views of how the mind, brain, and consciousness function, providing in-depth but distinct perceptions of *human experience* from past to present and years to come. The book can be a complete educational source to guide one through the triangle of what fine, healthy brain, mind, and consciousness might be and as a result to who we are today while eliminating the *overflow of information*. From personal experiences that shape the brain structures and, what's in the mind that brain can be that's how who we become therefore. An example is the science and neuroscience point of view on how the brain gives rise to *mental processes*, such as memory and perception. Physical anthropology gives us insight into how relational experiences and *communication* with different cultures directly affect the development of the human brain and mind, which is the *overall development* to some point.

The greatest psychology findings give us a view of how humans may suffer from emotional patterns of stress that weave behavioral disturbances into our daily lives and how the changing mind moves from a changed brain to a changed life. On the other hand, the exploration of top metaphysics gives us a view of consciousness as part of a natural state of awareness and the last surviving mystery that is the fundamental reality. This gives us the answer to consciousness that is the essential of "I am" a true identity. The dimension that exists within that cannot be hepatized by reality or break the barrier of self from others and the universe. This gives us the findings that each person's life represents a unique world of its own thus in a countless world which universe and consciousness experiencing itself.

Modern developmental psychologists have identified numerous features of an individual's consciousness, such as *cognition* (what one is aware of), values (what one considers most important), and self-identity (what one identifies with). Up-to-date consciousness explanations gain much popularity among the people of all nations and is written well by many philosophical theories and practices like Ken Wilber among a million others who left its door open for human growing up journey of development. The majority of consciousness theory features consciousness developed through recognizable stages, each stage revealing a markedly different understanding of the world. It shows there are eight stages of consciousness as understood through research about the unfolding development of values and *self-identity*.

Correspondingly, some studies show there are at least two very different types of things that have been called religion in humankind's history. One of them occurs in the waking-up dimension. Another occurs in the growing-up dimension. Waking up has to do with states of consciousness. Waking up has to do with general practices of things like meditation, contemplation, and centering prayer. These are paths that humans have had a fairly good understanding of for at least a couple of thousand years. Some versions of these interior paths of growth—these paths of meditation, contemplation, shamanic origin go back possibly thousand years.

If you take all of the really sophisticated meditation systems worldwide—these include everything from Zen Buddhism to Hinduism and Daoism and certainly from Tibetan Buddhism to Sikhism and Islam—education might start to see some family resemblances to the stages that they outline. If a study takes all of the great reflective systems, puts them all on a table, and looks at the stages they described that the human being in their own school goes through as they move from a very narrow, separate self-sense, they expand their space of consciousness all the way up to an identity with a ground of all being and a sense of unity with the entire universe *in their own way*. In growing up, what most developmental psychologists study are direct states. They are more than interpretative structures or frameworks that human beings use after they have intelligence in a particular line.

I'm expecting things that I've found as I began my writing of trying to view a whole lot of different knowledge areas together is how rarely all of the different types of knowledge that I was looking at were acknowledged and are actually utilized. One of the things that I did, for example, was look at ways that human beings over the centuries have developed in order for what studies call *self-improvement* (development). The explanation of self-improvement is self-explanatory, meaning it is the improvement of one's knowledge, status, or character by one's own efforts.

Self-improvement can be distinct as *an integral development process* that *evolves* throughout life, by which one learns to have self-awareness, improve one's personal abilities, and pursue one's life goals. Self-improvement consists of self-realization, doing what one really wants to do and living more fully. Furthermore, formal education is great for living a good life, yet if individuals want to live an extraordinary life and the life they dream about, they need to self-educate.

Self-education is important for success and growth in life, not just academics alone. The *neural basis of self* is the knowledge of using modern concepts of neuroscience to designate and understand the biological procedures that underlie humans' perception of self-understanding. The neural basis of self is closely related to the psychology of self with a deeper foundation in neurobiology. Two areas of the brain that are significant in retrieving *self-knowledge* are the medial prefrontal cortex and the medial posterior parietal cortex. The posterior cingulate cortex, the anterior cingulate cortex, and the medial prefrontal cortex are believed, in association, to deliver people with the aptitude to *self-reflect*.

The insular cortex is likewise alleged to be tangled in the development of self-reference. In command to comprehend how the human mind makes the human *perception of self*, there are diverse experimental techniques. One of the more common approaches of influential brain areas that pertain to different mental processes is by using functional magnetic resonance imaging (fMRI). The information individuals remember as autobiographical memory is vital to their perception of self. These memories form the way individuals feel about themselves. The left dorsolateral prefrontal cortex and posterior cingulate cortex are *tangled* in the *memory of autobiographical information.*

Looking over the world at large, research can find that there are— depending on exactly how narrowly the study defines self-improvement— anywhere from two major groups of growing up and waking up and so on. How can a study formulate an approach to psychology that honors and embraces every legitimate aspect of human consciousness and pulls these multiple aspects together into a single coherent model of the human mind? Interconnectedness of past enlightenment to today's modern education is one of the finest and most complete summaries of an integral approach to psychology, while suggesting how a more comprehensive understanding of human consciousness can help shape a better, kinder, and more sustainable future.

There is a strong drive for psychology to be more inclusive, more comprehensive, and more embracing. Thus, there is a strong sense that the psychology of the new generation will be one that does indeed cover many areas that are so noticeably absent or just inefficiently addressed today. Above all, it's fascinating to imagine a feeling full of gratitude for this gift of being here, for being human, and for *being alive.* These words pale in contrast to the sensation of *love* I feel for the many individuals with whom I've been given the privilege of sharing this life journey. Also, this is the feeling of connection to each of us here, now, including whom we live on this planet with, our collective home, and this place we've named Earth.

The sun is rising now as I write these words, and the planet Earth is doing its great work of daily turning. I live in Calgary, Alberta, Canada, where the sky is bluer and bigger to appreciate sunny days like today. And I thank the mind and consciousness for being the fundamental essence of this nature, the deepest sense of being alive in this moment. Yet beyond consciousness and its knowledge of knowing within awareness of our subjective sense of being alive, the mind may also include a large process that *connects* us to each other and our world.

The feeling of interconnectedness includes the *integration* of brain, mind, and consciousness within the bodily system and outside of our life experiences with others and the *universe.* This is an important process of the mind that is hard to scope, despite *modern study* however, it is a crucial aspect of our lives we'll explore in depth in this book journey.

Often much research and many disciplines and findings function in isolation from one another. However, when one explores, an incredible convergence of many independent fields of study is revealed. The presumption from such exploration for now might be that brain, mind, consciousness, evolutionary biology, and so forth offer an additional understanding of human experience (interpersonal and informational development) and might be the sum of the parts (the bigger picture to the unknown) or split intellect to the unknown. If a study identifies the mind as the *physical mind* and conscious as the *electrical signal* and neural as the *networking system* and the brain's neuronal activities with mind to consciousness as the *integration system,* wouldn't it be apparent that the neurons that *fire together* perhaps are *wired together?* Consequently, *relationship* is the other main key, not just *communication,* which generates desire, intent, intuition, goal, personal development, and so on that differentiate people.

Each neuron signal is a *bit of information* that gives individuals knowledge and awareness. With that said, *education* plays a bigger role in the formation of this *information* that feeds the story of *nature needs nurture.* These findings also shed light on how the mind emerges from the brain, its connection with consciousness, and its communication with daily interpersonal experiences. Since the publication of many educational editions of brain, mind, and consciousness over a dozen *years ago,* much has emerged from the objective study of science, physics and subjective of internal reflection.

My goal in thoroughly updating the important information and findings and revising my knowledge into this textbook is to make the idea of brain, mind, and consciousness and its role in development as clear as possible. Importantly create a relevant education for the *current nation* and to provide an overview of these integrations and how humans can evolve from these educational findings and experiences. More specifically, to help individuals to understand the developing mind, brain, and consciousness. *I provide an integration of brain health, brain development knowledge from birth to adulthood and educational systems from preschool to university levels.*

I had the good fortune of having a curious brain to explore and search and having the opportunity of over forty bright books that are written by a combination of many professors, neuroscientists, neurologists, directors of universities, and education psychologists, and the findings from neuroscientists, professors of psychology, psychiatrists, professors of cognitive neuroscience who worked for years at top universities (UCLA, Harvard, Yale, who are *New York Time* best authors, so that we could *discard any proposals that were outdated or unfounded.* Also, I have included myself because of my own forty years' case study of human knowledge and *realistic life experience.* The natural study of human development trials not on guinea pigs nor for making profit. The education I hope to have thirty years ago when I was in elementary level of brain development education. However, with brain and human evolution come technology and social media that made this journey enjoyable and healthy to a billion others who are at the infant level—giving them access to this book of mine and so many similar today.

As a result, I tried to include many backgrounds as to way of reference for anyone who has less education in this area, or are parents, students, teachers, patients, doctors, politicians, etc. The materials support the educational system and brain health from classrooms to real-life journey. Classrooms are not only cogitative places but also emotional, social, motivational, and so on grounds. Second, the educational level of *cognitive science* is useful boundaries to practice. For example, from the physics point of view, how to build a bridge comes not from the exact prescription but how to predict if one builds.

This book hopefully guides classes and teachers to not predict how to teach or what to teach, but *how much the student can learn* (from the perspective of brain, mind, experience *development).* Theoretically speaking, we have many educational programs that are exciting to teach students, from top-down models and generationally existing curriculums up to this point. Much has changed, and the education system could balance the learning through brain evolution, for example, focusing on working memory and the ability to think well and concentrate, keeping the *relevant information* in mind while ignoring the overflow of information.

This is the important tools we need to inheret prior to entering into education to prevent and making sense of chaos. Additionally, it's a great book to our political system of creating educational programs for students and teachers. And an eye-opener might be, why students don't like school or studying is a basic primer for everyone, especially teachers who want to know how the brain and students work and how that knowledge can shape their teaching experience. Education is a passing on torch of wisdom for new generation that holds a promising life. At first, I tried to write a book for preschool to high school students titled *The Educated Brain Then Meditative Brain*.

Since, my education and background covers more information from birth to young adult. *I spent more than half of my life's work with children of all ages* and at some point *with the parents, despite being a mother of four healthy, well-behaved, intelligent children.* However, based on this experience, the adult on the children's life plays a bigger part to which I have to include. I learned throughout of my life the important role of parents and caregivers on developing children. And then the important part of teachers, society, family, growing-up journey to work environment, and so on. Thus, the goal of writing about brain, mind, and consciousness and the responsibility for the education system comes to life. Writing on such book was an easy choice and for concluding brain health education a direct discussion of important issues of children and adults' experiences as a result of not being able to recognize their own mental health experiences and having less resources available to them.

I had research on brain abnormalities: brain tumor, post-traumatic stress disorder (PTSD), weight issues, mental health awareness, learning disabilities, cancer-related concerns, bullying, and suicide as part of life issues. In addition, my own family and friends who dealt with cancer issues, and I am a survivor of benign brain tumor over the past twelve years. I gather information into this book and weave it together with true stories of actual people. So the information in this book has science, physics, theories and practices, real-life stories, and practical life-empowering knowledge while learning brain-developing skills that could be taken in any order and it will work its best.

One of the things I hassle about often are *words*, yes, the very simple words, in fact. Should it say "hello" or "hi"? Should it be "cheers" or "thanks"? There are several occasions when I sit over one line and change it many times, until it feels it actually sits right. Words are moved over to the left temporal lobe of our brain for processing, while the melody is channeled to the right side of the brain, a district more stimulated by music. The brain uses two different parts to recognize the disposition and then the actual meaning of the words.

On the other hand, I wonder why we can even distinguish *language* so distinctly from any other sounds. Some study played the speech sounds and then the nonspeech sounds, that still sounded similar to speech to the people. While exploring further into the brain activity speech singled out for special treatment near the primary auditory cortex. In short, the brain can single out language from any other sounds and port it to the right subdivision in the brain to give it meaning. A single word has the influence to impact the expression of genes that regulate physical and emotional stress. Positive words, such as "love," can alter the expression of genes, strengthening areas in our frontal lobes and endorsing the brain's cognitive functioning.

Likewise, it drives the motivational centers of the brain into action. Nevertheless, a single negative word can upsurge the activity in the amygdala (known as the fear center of the brain). This releases masses of stress-creating hormones and neurotransmitters that in turn interject the brain's operational system. (This is particularly with regard to sense, aim, and language.) Irritating words send alarm communications through the brain, and they somewhat close down the logic-and-reasoning centers positioned in the frontal lobes. *As we hinted, the brain takes speech and separates it into* words *and melody, the changing intonation in speech that discloses attitude, gender, and so on.*

Words are then shunted over to the left temporal lobe for processing while the melody is channeled to the right side of the brain, a region more stimulated by music. Through words, we express what's on our mind. The way that individuals refer to themselves and others is highly diagnostic of their mental state. Words, whether they are vocalized or remain unspoken as thoughts, can cast a spell on the mind. Things gain their names through words either at school or in the workplace and lose their identity by labeling. The importance of words becomes clear to our life journey and mind. Unfortunately, words from greater books or researchers can't explain everything at some point. Up to this point, the two big topics, "brain and universe," are rarely defined. This avoidance maybe due to several considerations. There are philosophical underpinnings that definitions may restrain the full notion of future characteristics of this mystery. In some ground, the words "universe," "consciousness," and "mind" remain our own inner-life mysteries. How exactly relevant are all the research and information still infancy to this point.

Nevertheless, if we don't attempt to explain the core aspect of brain, mind, and consciousness through education, how else can we define what healthy living might be? Thus, what can be more relevant than brain research to begin our journey? However, it does remind me of what comes first, the egg or the chicken. Is it the human in search of the explanation of the brain, or is it the brain guiding us through life slowly? Once a question like this has entered one's mind, it's not easy to cast aside. History has shown the close relationship between *human and education.*

Looking back one hundred years from now, the evolution of the human brain, life on earth, and knowledge is clear. Not only physical characteristics change but the mantle of evidence is evolving. Now, one hundred years from now, it only brings us back to the infancy point of development again. If humans begin to learn how to control global warming and adapt to better life cycles, life will experience considerable growth and history will be the witness of such changes *each decade.*

Former president Barack Obama's speech to American students, called "My Education, My Future," shed a good light on the responsibility each of us has for education, the responsibility we have for ourselves nation-wise and globally. Everyone has something that they're good at, and that's we will discover and offer. Almost everyone's knowledge teaches something. Sometimes we know this by definition of our purpose in life. That's the opportunity an education can provide. Any career path we choose, we need a good education for that. What we make of our education will decide nothing less than the future of our country.

What we are learning in school, college, or university each day will determine whether we as a nation can meet our greatest challenges in the future. We need the insight and critical-thinking skills we gain from science, physics, and math to cure cancer, brain cancer, and mental illnesses in the future. If we stop learning, we are not only quitting on ourselves but are quitting on the country's future generation that depends on us. I know it is not easy to challenge ourselves, complete school, and meet the educational grade requirements. I have graduated from college, so have my three kids, and one is still on the path of learning. I know the many challenges I faced in the school system that many of you and my kids have not witness.

I have studied in third world countries where there were more poverty and wars than there was an opportunity for education. Especially education for women was near to impossible. I had less opportunities as a young kid than many of you ever have. I studied under the waves of a candlelight, under the sound of tanks and pistols. Nonetheless, I graduated with much high honors in two countries in two languages. In the end of the day, our life less depending on the circumstances of our lives, what we look like, where we come from, how much money we have. None of it is an excuse to neglect our homework or have a bad attitude in school or toward education.

Simply there is no excuse for not trying. I needed a great deal of support for writing in English. Not only do I publish books, I write about the two important subjects of our lives: education and brain development. The significant aspect of our life journey to success and to surviving skill.

Some of the most successful people in the world are the ones who've had the most failures. Michael Jordan was cut from basketball teams over and over. Now we all know his contribution to his teams. Prior to this book, I have sent much encouraging messages—email for improvement of education and brain health (consciousness)—to each famous television program such as *Oprah*, *Dr. Oz*, and *The Doctors*, and to news channels, as well as to the well-known individuals in our society such as President Justin Trudeau and the former first lady Michelle Obama, to name just a few. The importance of education and brain health is a bigger part of those sent emails.

Despite many unresponsive emails, I am not hopeless nor am I stopping. Being an *advocate* of education and *brain health* is a long and sometimes lonely road. Sometimes it's not fun or pleasant. I have learned to excepted from the eye of billion others who left the door open to grow. Even if I struggle, even if I feel others might give up on the subject and feel discouraged, giving up means giving up on our country (planet Earth). The only thing giving me the motivation is the future of our nation, the future of our children, especially my four wonderful kids.

The story of education and evolution isn't about quitting when things get tough. It's about keeping going. It's the educational journey of *two hundred fifty years ago* that taught us what we learned today. It's the foundation of this revolution. It's the importance of their contribution that put men on the moon. It's the contribution of that *educational journey* to guide us through today's brain research, technology, teaching, and universe. What programs and discovery we are going to create depends on how much education we consider and how we learn.

The important question to think is to "think with an educated brain, then meditative brain," which brought me back to this chosen title. Today we are getting more information than ever, emails, seminars, open houses about what schools are teaching the best and which college is taking place in our future. The education system offers much support to students' next goals and the direction to reach those goals. From preschool to university students get their guides from teachers, principals, education ministers, and so on. The education system teaches many different programs to support learning.

However, the important key to education is our brain health and how can humans accumulate knowledge. It has been proven that humans are curious learning organisms. Thus, giving structure on what to learn or how to learn might be less convincing than learning how the brain actually learns. Majority of students are not aware of what a healthy brain, mind, or consciousness is. For instance, how can one learn about everything outside the self when they have not experienced the self first? *The brain is the only important organism that guides humans to knowledge in the form of information processor. However, it is the sum of the whole.*

Brain health education is not just for schooling purposes but a relevant education for today's nation of evolution that led human knowledge to understand biopsychology aside. Although biopsychology might seem like a fairly recent development thanks to the introduction of advanced tools and technology for examining the brain, the roots of the field date back thousands of years to the time of the early philosophers.

Biopsychology is a branch of psychology that analyzes how the brain, neurotransmitters, and other aspects of our biology influence our behaviors, thoughts, and feelings. This field of psychology is often referred to by a variety of names including biopsychology, physiological psychology, behavioral neuroscience, and psychobiology. Biopsychologists often look at how biological processes interact with human emotions, cognitions, and other mental processes. While we now consider the mind and brain synonymous, philosophers and psychologists long debated what were known as the mind/body concerns. In other words, philosophers wondered what the relationship was between the mental (psych) world and the physical world.

The field of biopsychology is related to several other areas, including evolutionary psychology that ties this book to its many chapters. One important thing to remember is that it is only fairly recently in human history that people have come to understand the actual location of the mind *(physical mind)*. Aristotle, for example, taught that our thoughts, emotions, and feelings arose from the heart. In this book journey, I narrow the location of the mind so close to the brain as I call it the physical mind. However, the idea that certain parts of the brain were responsible for certain functions played an important role in the development of future brain research and human development. If you are interested in the field of biopsychology, well-being, and general brain health education, then it is important to have an understanding of biological processes as well as basic anatomy and physiology.

Three of the most important components to understand areas of the brain are, the nervous system, and neurotransmitters. Research on evolution, the localization of brain function, neurons, and neurotransmitters has advanced our understanding about how biological processes impact thoughts, emotions, and human behaviors— something we deal with every day. Admittedly, I honor these positions, and I've *accepted the hundred old and new* books and research putting such knowledge into this work. With that said, we know all learning is about something happening in the brain.

Let's move on in depth to the next topic to create more understanding of our brain and the importance of education *(learning information)* into our journey.

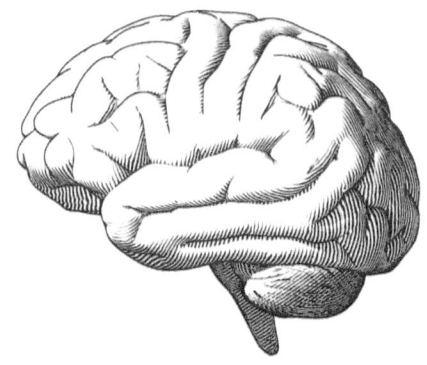

Integration of Education and Brain Development

One conclusion that arises from researchers is that the human development system is not sudden. The awareness of development has been a lifelong journey. However, how much past relationships with self, mind, or brain play a role depends on how much the mind/brain cares to remember, reclaim, and understand the benefit of this *change-learn-apply*. In the same token, our past plays a role for developing brain that create who we are today. For example, from the scientific masterpiece of the physicist Albert Einstein's theory of relativity and today's physics theories. Physicists reveal that the detection of gravitational waves has the capacity to generate its own application of acute importance that can be a new approach to observational astronomy. Furthermore, Newtonian physics was consigned in 2016 to the history book, to be replaced by Einstein's physics. Why aren't Newton's theories supplemented with Einstein's more general ones to give students insight into our present best understanding of our universe? Since the time of Galileo, education has turned telescopes skyward to gather light waves emitted by distant objects. The next phase of astronomy may very well center on gathering gravitational waves produced by distant cosmic disruption, allowing us to examine the universe in a whole new way. Maybe someday we could use gravity, not light, as our most penetrating probe of the universe's earliest time. As a result of human and *education evolution*, we must celebrate Einstein's theory during Einstein's year.

Today the human mind stretches to Mars for colonization. As we gaze into the future, we see that the event that took place thousands of years ago may actually be a rehearsal for future catastrophes. The advanced technology one day be discovering a new planet, imagining a civilization on such planet. It is as inescapable as the law of physics that humanity will one day confront some type of extinction event. If we will scan all the life-forms that have existed on our planet Earth with microscopic then from bacteria to plants, dinosaurs, and human organisms, we would find that majority will become extinct. Would this bring extinction to a normal format? Maybe. We are already witnessing such and such norms. Many species have appeared on Earth and have become extinct, such as dinosaurs.

No matter how much we treasure our planet, its higher mountains, the ocean sea, the sunrise, and our own colonies one day will all end.

Modern technology and education are not only important parts of human knowledge from the past and today's world of learning, but a great source of survival skills to predictable result. From Professor Michio Kaku and his book *The Future of Humanity*, the history of life on earth shows that faced with a hostile environment, organisms inevitably meet one of three fates: they leave the environment, adapt to a new environment, or die as a last resort.

For human looking to the future, results might remain the same. There is no between-the-line answer. What history shows happened in the past eventually will happen again. The beautiful atmosphere that we call home rooftop one day will turn against us. For example, with the knowledge of global warming so as the awareness of modern warfare, as nuclear weapons, weaponized microbes like Ebola, AIDS on to of natural disasters to which we have no control.

Can it be we all shared the same vision that we owe it to our future generations to teach our best understanding of the nature of our universe, rather than the obsolete nineteenth-century science that might still influence the school curriculum? Because the awareness of observing the mind is greater than the awareness of experience. The important aspect of education is not how the brain needs to learn but how the brain learns at any given moment. That's the important aspect of our education when it comes to teaching and learning the definition of brain and universe to what make us human.

What I have learned yesterday has not much influenced today's lesson of learning. The past is gone, leaving us its experience. What has not arrived is the future, and it is mysterious with less control. However, what creates change is the now. A lesson to become part of a teacher's daily evaluation. War, addiction, and bad behavior are not parts of continuum ancestry genes—generation, but part of evolutionary lesson. The one-world education serves one purpose to one tribe if the translation is made clear.

From the pen of the world's expert on education and brain health comes a comprehensive and compelling statement of why learning matters for human beings. Let's look at what might be fundamentally not there yet with our education systems and correspondingly show what and how could be differently. While writing this book, I paused to each chapter thinking, *Can such book be useful or even hopefully a wake-up call to the emerging global human resources?*

Would it be beneficial for boredom, disengagement, class daydreaming, learning disabilities, bullying, suicide, sexting, drugs, LGBT concerns, weight issues, mental health concerns, diseases, and school dropouts among students that might have become chronic aspects of many school and college systems around the world? Brain/mind education is a must-learn tool for anyone who is interested in critique, vision, and theory of change for the new course of brain health education system and development of brain not just in school grounds as we learned alone. Education is personal and acts as the other brain to speak, because education is only about the people.

To shed light on education, it's also about economy, getting the best job and paving the path for our children. We should teach our family the importance of education and balanced lifestyle. It's best to learn education tied with economy, creativity, adaptivity, and culture, in addition to brain health that defines well-being. Education helps reduce poverty by preparing individuals to contribute productively in work environments. A minimum level of completed education is often required for obtaining a job.

People who are more highly educated tend to earn more money on average than those with lower levels of education. Learning about real-world transactions, such as investments and retirement planning, helps people avoid financial struggles and poverty. Disease prevention is a benefit of education that affects humanity. Teaching people how to avoid the dangers and risks of contracting diseases is important for halting the spread of diseases. Health is also impacted by education through the knowledge of dietary requirements. Consuming recommended amounts of nutrients is beneficial for maintaining and improving health. Knowing what to do in accidents or emergency situations is another way that education contributes to health.

For many years, women were not allowed to attend school or obtain an education. Because of this, there is a large gender gap, which only creates further problems. Women who gain an education are working toward minimizing the gap to further the abilities of women around the world. An education often prevents young girls from being married off into a potentially limiting, harmful situation. Additionally, women with an education are able to make better, informed decisions for themselves. They often wait longer to have children than those who do not have an education. This ensures that the woman is ready to have children, rather than just being pressured into it by her husband or society.

Women with an education have on average three children, while uneducated women have on average seven children. Education promotes peace and diplomacy, and understanding people with cultural differences has positive effects socially. Learning about various countries and cultures gives many people a greater appreciation for life. The ability to understand multiple perspectives improves problem-solving and decision-making skills.

Through contributing to personal development and growth, education helps to build character. In addition, *intelligence* is not always a matter of formal education. It is a matter of the capacity of the brain to process, represent, and surpass information through inference for the sake of current problem-solving needs.

But the capacity to process, represent, and surpass information changes with age (reflected in cognitive developmental levels) and with experience (including education) as the brain is an experience-handling tool. However, intellect can definitely be raised by education, especially education that is focused on increasing and challenging intelligence. When we read or listen to something, our intelligence is automatically put to work. As we go on using the various facets of learning centers in our brain, our IQ level increases. This is not the only way of raising intelligence, but cognitive abilities can be sharpened by continuously using all capabilities given to us.

Psychologists have long debated how to best conceptualize and measure intelligence These questions include how many types of intelligence there are, the role of nature versus nurture in intelligence, how intelligence is represented in the brain, and the meaning of group differences in intelligence. The mission to human development is to understand human development as characterized by different development orbits over the typical and atypical through a life span. It will be useful to look into biological evolution in order to understand the sequence of our development well.

Education is one of the main crucial aspects toward human development. This means it is important in shaping human life and development. Human development is the science that seeks to understand how and why people of all ages and circumstances change or remain the same over time. It involves studies of the human condition with its core being the capability approach. The inequality-adjusted Human Development Index is used as a way of measuring actual progress in human development by the United Nations. It is an alternative approach to a single focus on economic growth and focuses more on social justice as a way of understanding progress.

The term "human development" may be defined as an expansion of human capabilities, a widening of choices, an enhancement of freedom, and a fulfillment of human rights. This also simply means developing mentally and socially through growing and experiencing things in life and learning new things. When the world is busy getting equipped with deadly weapons and machinery, it is very important to understand that education is the real asset that can develop an individual as well as a nation. People across the world should join hands to make education not only a fundamental right for all, but also the guiding light which can take mankind ahead through any phase of darkness. As a matter of fact, let's take a look into human *biological evolution*.

The trend that education has printed on as form of blue print in our development at some point, for instance, although natural selection acts on individuals, it eventually shapes populations of organisms, which are made up of a collection of traits encoded in genes. What we are made up from is our genes too. How genetic information is copied when each cell divides and how these institutions are translated into specific proteins, whose activities are eventually manifested as traits. There are many genetic variabilities that evolutionary selection can choose to add to our current knowledge of life that evolution by *natural selection* may not be avoidable.

For example, fossil records or the battle of infection against bacteria to antibiotics, the emergence of new influenza strains or other viruses such as HIV, changes and causes of AIDS, to name few. Can it be true that species is just a concept invented by humans themselves in order to come to grips with the majority of biological diversity generated by the evolutionary process? Nature through nurture plays a great role in learning about human development as we cannot attribute anything to single genes alone.

Our *genes* are not alone the *blueprint* for what we may become but a simple entry to what we might do. Nurture interaction affects the chances that nurture will make it into the next generation but who is not what we become by single force. As we will learn deeper into this book, we'll discover the possibilities of environment and how we were brought up and therefore our mind. We can put a name to this *integration*, perhaps the "big bang of the mind." The full understanding of what might be personality and what is behavior which clearly defines the role of nature and nurture relationships.

After almost what differentiates human from other animals is our unusual mental abilities perhaps our mind which our brain might not be much different from other mammals. It's the mind that made humans capable of self-awareness and understanding of others. Can't this be a reason for evolution of human animals over other creatures on earth? Maybe. On the other hand, natural selection during human evolution also seems to have benefited from changes in the timing of some growth events. For example, our brain development much depends on environment, nature, and nurture.

Most of brain development occurs outside the womb under the influence of the environment and experiences of other humans (culture, languages, education, therapies, ideas, etc.). Humans and animals are more likely to be cooperative breeds that made survival continuum. This would require not only to be self-aware, but also to attribute the mental state to others. Therefore, such have created the ability of *networking* or integration so we call it mind. Being aware of self and others is one other aspect of the human mind and its capabilities. It seems this intelligence of humans has contributed to the requirements for taking over the planet Earth from other species. Individuals are aware of self, how they look, feel . . . owns body. Mimicking is a self-awareness, taking the role of someone's act. Second, be aware of others' personhood that they too have a mind of their own. Getting emotional in situations where blushing appears on are face as a result of this behavior. The second person must know how that feels prior to understanding the blushing behavior which might be the result of happiness or shamefulness. Third, awareness of the second person's mind while understanding the third person exists despite spearing or not.

Caring for others, perhaps hearing the children cry or painful stories, is another example of this. The fourth state might be the ability of being aware of everyone who is present or of only sharing the mental state. Death or concern about a family or group as social attention, by knowing the person among us is gone, can be another example. Healing or praying for sick patients or loved ones is a well-understood reason. Is self-awareness or mind related to consciousness? Well, conscious means being aware and has many cases. We might continue to that through the book.

In animals, such awareness is seen less. For example, a dog has the ability to follow its owner by its cues. However, it might not recognize itself in the mirror. Likewise, human brought up by ancestors as way of biological evolution, where dog might be belonging to wolf's pack while much involve with human—especially today. Also, it's very clear that much of humans' great uniqueness—self-awareness and other things beyond our attention—is the result of integration experiences of shared attention to cooperation. From enlightenment to ancestors to culture and music to laws and regulation to modern society. This genetic polishing over time has contributed to our intelligent experience of being here. The study of developmental genetics has shown that the extreme complicated web of genes and protein interactions turn the simple early embryo to the well-elaborated organisms we see today. Is it a time for gathering reliable databases for the sum of all integrations to form a whole? Or is it still impossible for a single brain to fully understand to commend more than its jelly ball protein? I think humans might not escape from this dilemma fully but must embark onto some facts, theories, and scientific views as secondhand knowledge to hopefully not create fools of ourselves in the future which our blueprint has shown us so far, we have not. However, let's not forget, the human race is the only race that knows life and death through its own experiences. It's much intelligent to not sow blind hope to future generations. Therefore, it will be inappropriate to document, stating the human development is not considering integration of the whole system over its sum part such as the brain, mind, or even some theories alone.

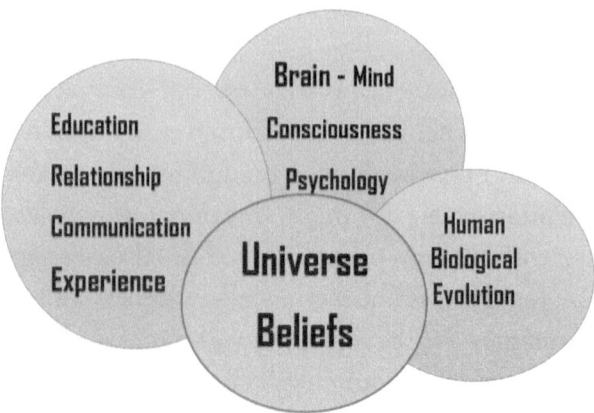

The Integration of Interpersonal Neurobiology and Role of Education (Information)

To the ancient Greek philosopher awareness was once the written word was on allowed to roam about everywhere, the world would never be the same again. Education provides people with access to different views and ideas about their predicament and fosters an attitude that encourages readers to view their world in new ways. It is through learning that a consciousness oriented toward change emerges and a sensibility toward originality gains definition. The act of education always contains the potential for subverting taken-for-granted assumptions. It also offers the promise of giving meaning to human experience. But since the written text invites its own critique, the meaning gained through reading often proves to be a temporary one. This book is not written to read only as we did that already, but to out into practice. The *history of reading for meaning* has shown that this arose more questions than answers, which bring us to the next topic.

The Grass Roots of Education

At some point, we have understood the role of education on human development. Also, education is a human *right*. It is a right for girls, just as it is for boys. It is a right for disabled children, just as it is for everyone else. It is a right for the million out-of-school children and youth in countries affected by crises and conflicts. Education is a right regardless of where individuals were born or where they grow up. And like other human rights, it cannot be taken for granted. Hence, as one nation, we have a responsibility to make sure we fulfill the promise we made at the beginning of the millennium, to ensure that boys and girls everywhere complete a full course of primary schooling.

It's possible to refer *education philosophy* either to the application of philosophy or to the problem of education This is the examining definitions goals, and chains of meaning that used in education by teachers, and administrators. Studying involves the philosophical study of education and its problems. The philosophy of education may be either the philosophy of the *process* of education or the philosophy of discipline of education. It can be part of the discipline in the sense of being anxious with the goals, forms, and methods of educating or being educated.

Also, it can be part of multidisciplinary system in the sense of being worried with the concepts, goals, and methods of the discipline. Thus, it is both part of the field of education and part of applied philosophy that branches off from fields of metaphysics, epistemology, axiology, and the philosophical approaches. Hence, to address questions in and about pedagogy, education policy, and curriculum, as well as the process of learning, to name a few.

Can education be transpersonal? "Transpersonal" is a term used by different schools of *philosophy and psychology* in order to describe experiences and worldviews that extend beyond the personal level of the psyche and beyond what's not understood well. It has been defined as experiences in which the sense of human identity (I am) or self extends beyond the individual. The wider aspects of humankind can be our life, psyche, and universe.

The field of transpersonal psychiatry has defined this term as human development beyond the conventional. It is related to the terminology of human peak experience, perhaps altered states of consciousness and spiritual experiences. This term has an early start in the writing of many philosophers. However, originally it comes with the *human potential* movement of the 1960s. Also, the founders of the field of transpersonal psychology are, such as Anthony Sutich, Abraham Maslow, and Stanislav Grof.

What has been considered in transpersonal psychology includes spiritual, self-development, pure self (beyond the ego), peak experiences, mystical experiences, systemic trance, spiritual crises, spiritual evolution, religious conversion, altered states of consciousness, spiritual practices, and other sublime and/or unusually expanded experiences of living. This practice makes an effort to *integrate* spiritual experience within modern psychological theory and to express new theory to encompass such experience. Transpersonal psychology has made several contributions to the academic field and the studies of human development, consciousness and spirituality, and the fields of psychotherapy and psychiatry.

When individuals are trying to understand education and developmental history, it's best to explore *all venues* in research from *as early as the Enlightenment experience to the twenty-first century.* The most fundamental question we might ask is, what is education for, and what is education in general? Our answers may provide insights that get to the heart of what matters for twenty-first-century children and adults alike. It is important to step back from divisive debates, politics, and top-down models to understand the *meaning of education* alone.

Looking for wisdom from some of the greatest philosophers, poets, educators, historians, theologians, politicians, and world leaders, I realized the answers that should not only exist in our history books, but also remain at the core of the current education dialogue. Just because human potential is not defined enough doesn't mean we did not evolve. For example, can it be true to this time of our journey to knowledge, we are still using 10 percent of our whole brain? This was urban legend, the 10-percent-of-the-brain myth, that most or all humans only use 10 percent of their brains. It has been misattributed to many people, including Albert Einstein.

By extrapolation, it is suggested that a human may harness this unused potential and increase intelligence. The change in the gray-and-white matter following new experiences and learnings has been shown, but we might not know yet what these changes are. Would it be true to our human experience that the large parts of the brain remain unused, and could it subsequently be activated? Might it be popular folklore and not science? Mysteries regarding brain function remain unsolved. However, all parts of our brain—memory, consciousness—and the physiology of brain mapping have a function. Along with academic skills, the educational journey from kindergarten through college is a time when young people develop many interconnected abilities.

As you read through the chapters, you'll discover common threads that unite the intellectual, social, emotional, and physical aspects of education. It is another way of saying the collaboration of the education system with *brain development.* In addition, a good education also facilitates the development of an internal essence that guides us through life. Parent engagement with children's education matters.

Study after study has shown us that student achievement improves when parents play an active role in their children's education and that good schools become even better schools when *parents are involved.* It is recognized that parent engagement is a key factor in the enhancement of student achievement and well-being. Students are more likely to be motivated, to earn higher grades, to have better behavior and social skills, and to continue their education to a higher level when their parents are actively engaged in supporting their success at school. There are ways parents can still balance work and home, and their children's education.

What makes the difference is the contribution of all parents toward the education system itself. For example, school bullying is a type of bullying that occurs in any educational setting. According to many studies, school-age children experience bullying at some point during their studies. Also, low self-confidence, weight and health conditions, cultural differences, GLB concerns, and drugs, in addition to family and divorce concerns, are contributing factors to children's overall well-being and education.

What can be done to ease the pain and raise awareness is to simply place *awareness education* as part of the daily curriculum of mathematics and science. *This book would hopefully be a better guide to students, parents, and educators as way of* learning experience *to some degree on overall brain-mind understanding.* Education means learning, and learning is more essential when it's natural. Humans are highly curious learning organisms. That's how many developmental facts gives human animal a recognition of relational being. To learn, it requires new knowledge and skills. From infancy to adulthood, we never stopped learning. School is not the only ground barrier to human knowledge and education. Schooling means learning with any group of community to any facilities who come together.

As we mentioned first, education is personal, and it means different things to different individuals depending on their culture, values, ethnicity, and opinion on how one views life. Education is not considered the only value in its own right. It is praised for its potential contribution to economic development and as an accessible instrument for encouraging social inclusion and mobility. What economy ties with *adaptivity* is a fine art. For example, the growing graduate students from university add up to new technology and new resources then new performance. The companies that can't adapt these new products, programs, and technologies are likely closing down their system. A good example is Kodak.

Many famous photography company of twenty-first century has gone bankrupt. Such companies invented photography. It seems like everyone's cellphone alone carries a camera. The accessibility of taking photos is extremely rising. Technology allows these photos to be posted on Facebook, Twitter, or Instagram. That's not the reason why they closed their business but adaptation to new technology. This is also an example of personal adaptation to education and anything new comes to learning.

Adaptation and creativity go hand in hand. Therefore, if there is a need to meet the education economic system, it's best to have a system to permute the *adaptivity* and *creativity* system in place. The small planet Earth can become a populated class setting. We could form an education to enable people to understand how they come to think as they do, why the patent of life is as they are, and why people are different as they are. We could create programs to teach the different cultures and different values of each ethnicity as they are. As addition learning about their rights and how they get alongside with other cultures and beliefs. For this, we need a broader education system that teaches humanity, a social study that brings more of this awareness in the class. Playing piano has made me realize how learning infuses with self, how soothing, personal, and unique music can become. Class study can be implemented in a degree that means something to self and helps students learn mindfulness *(think with an educated brain)*.

Also, *social integration* is a bigger place in the education system to engage this generation in the process in which our community is organized, like learning how to take part in voting. We mentioned education is more personal journey and how unique each of us are. is. We know how different talented individuals we are, how passionate and gritty we can be. One of the signature features of humanity is best known as diversity. Thus, it's important to know the different elements of different talents in different individuals always.

As learners, we have students (children) who were already born with the curiosity to learn. Till a certain age, we cooperate, scaffold, and guide their natural ability to learn, meaning schooling them as if we left them alone; they might not do or might do well. That is the point of the school and education system, to help children learn better. There are far too many children who have the talent of mature individuals. With diverse cultures and modern technology come these greater talents. Therefore, this is a bigger role of education to refine and cultures these talents amount culture diversity. Associating schools with particular types of characteristics, forms of structures that really are not aligned with the principles of learning but principles of organizations and efficiency; that might result in children losing their natural talents by the time we teach them.

The most effective forms of education are collective in characteristics. Schools that teach education in groups are less superior than as groups. Teaching is much more an art form to perform well. The more motivational characteristics of the class, the more successful the students. The less delivered curriculum, the more students participate. It's much on teaching each other and learning from experience.

The important aspect of education is the *student–teacher relationship* which can change the system for the better, because school is not the body or structure of the learning zone but the community of living, breathing entities. It's much more than making a difference to the life of education to understand education as ground up and the climate control system, meaning what is happening at the ground level.

We could go on talking about building, materials, field trips, curriculum, salaries, holidays, and so on; but if we don't talk about *students and teachers*, we won't improve education. Humans are creative beings. One can understand the notion as young as age two. However, the most creative people on earth have discovered their creativity after school. Creativity only needs reflection, much affordable natural human knowledge put on use at any system of learning.

Understanding the human brain, mind, or consciousness means understanding how human nature is and how we do things as we do and don't. Teachers are especially required to upgrade *with this development from time to time as we cannot define the human brain as we grow, but we are in much better experience, technology, and imaging than we ever were.* For instance, we don't teach an eighteen-month-old child to sit, yet we have to teach the child how to talk. However, we don't give a list of vocabulary words and their pronunciation to a child saying by the end of next month we will go over how this goes. Meanwhile, creativity is an essential part of the learning experience. It's almost the same as fixing a table without any sort of tools for that screw that requires one. Many intelligent accrue in mind in form of taught prior comes to knowledge. How to build a house for instance start with triangle of natural understanding of connection to dots through life experience.

Could it be true that if individuals who believe in definite growth on education, physics, or universe, either they're mad or they're economists? As we seek to refine and reform today's life system, we would do well to ask, how did we get this far? Our answers may provide insights that get to the heart of what matters for twenty-first-century adults and children. It is important to step back from divisive debates on power, fame, education, war, cancer, economy, family friends, diet, beauty, sex, evaluations—and really look at the *meaning of life itself.* This might bring our attention closer to educational psychology, which is concerned with the *scientific study of human learning*. It is the study of learning processes, from both cognitive and behavioral perspectives, that allows researchers to understand individual differences in intelligence, cognitive development, affect, motivation, self-regulation, and self-concept, as well as their role in learning.

The field of educational psychology relies heavily on quantitative methods, including testing and measurement, to enhance educational activities related to instructional design, classroom management, and assessment, which serve to facilitate learning processes in various educational settings across the life span. Educational psychology can in part be understood through its *relationship with other disciplines*. It is informed primarily by psychology bearing a relationship to that discipline analogous to the relationship between medicine and biology. It is also informed by neuroscience. Educational psychology in turn informs a wide range of specialties within educational studies, including instructional design, educational technology, curriculum development, organizational learning, special education, classroom management, and student motivation. Educational psychology both draws from and contributes to cognitive science and the learning sciences. In universities, departments of educational psychology are usually housed within faculties of education, possibly accounting for the lack of representation of educational psychology content in introductory psychology textbooks. The field of educational psychology involves the study of memory, conceptual processes, and individual differences (via cognitive psychology) in conceptualizing new strategies for learning processes in humans. Educational psychology has been built upon theories of operant conditioning, functionalism, structuralism, constructivism, humanistic psychology, Gestalt psychology, and information processing.

Psychology is the science of *behavior and mind*, including conscious and unconscious phenomena, as well as feeling and thought. It is an academic discipline of immense scope and diverse interests that, when taken together, seek an understanding of the emergent properties of brains and all the variety of epiphenomena they manifest. As a social science, it aims to understand individuals and groups by establishing general principles and researching specific cases. In this field, a professional practitioner or researcher is called a psychologist and can be classified as a social, behavioral, or cognitive scientist.

Psychologists attempt to understand the role of *mental functions* in individual and social behavior, while also exploring the physiological and biological processes that underlie cognitive functions and behaviors. Psychologists explore behavior and mental processes, including perception, cognition, attention, emotion (affect), intelligence, phenomenology, motivation (conation), brain functioning, and personality. This extends to interaction between people, such as interpersonal relationships, including psychological resilience, family resilience, and other areas. Psychologists of diverse orientations also consider the unconscious mind. Psychologists employ empirical methods to infer causal and correlational relationships between psychosocial variables.

In addition, or in opposition, to employing empirical and deductive methods, some—especially clinical and counseling psychologists—at times rely upon symbolic interpretation and other inductive techniques. Psychology has been described as a "hub science" in that medicine tends to draw psychological research via neurology and psychiatry, whereas social sciences most commonly draw directly from subdisciplines within psychology.

While psychological knowledge is often applied to the assessment and treatment of mental health problems, it is also directed toward understanding and solving problems in several spheres of human activity. By many accounts, psychology ultimately aims to benefit society. The majority of psychologists are involved in some kind of therapeutic role, practicing in clinical, counseling, or school settings. Many do scientific research on a wide range of topics related to mental processes and behavior and typically work in university psychology departments or teach in other academic settings, like schools and medical and hospital setting. This is where the word of psychology roots its meaning. The word "psychology" has Greek roots, meaning study of the psyche, or soul, breath, spirit, soul.

With the change of society toward modern life and experiences, it defined psychology as the *science of mental life*, both of its phenomena and their conditions. This definition enjoyed widespread currency for decades. However, this meaning was contested, notably by radical behaviorists, the discipline of psychology noted as the acquisition of information useful to the control of behavior. Also, they defined the term more strongly, connoting techniques of scientific experimentation. Folk psychology refers to the understanding of ordinary people, as contrasted with that of psychology professionals. It makes more sense to learn how human experiences and nature can become grounds for educational psychology. Where there is mind, there is knowledge of practice.

Educational psychology is new, so it is a growing field of study. Though it can date back as early as the days of Plato and Aristotle, it was not identified as a specific practice. It was unknown that everyday teaching and learning in which individuals had to think about individual differences, assessment, development, the nature of a subject being taught, problem-solving, and transfer of learning was the beginning of the field of educational psychology. These topics are important to education; and as a result, it is important in understanding human cognition, learning, and social perception.

Plato and Aristotle researched individual differences in the field of education, training of the body and the cultivation of psychomotor skills, the formation of good character, the possibilities and limits of moral education. Some other educational topics they spoke about were the effects of music, poetry, and the other arts on the development of individual, the role of the teacher, and the relations between teacher and student. Plato saw *knowledge as an innate* ability, which *evolves through experience and understanding of the world.* Such a statement has evolved into a continuing argument of *nature vs. nurture* in understanding conditioning and learning today. Aristotle observed the *phenomenon of association.* His four laws of association are succession, contiguity, similarity, and contrast. His studies examined recall and facilitated learning processes.

Well, psychology is a science, but *teaching is an art.* There is a connection between science and education, but the sciences never produce arts directly out of themselves. William James is the father of psychology in America, but he likewise made contributions to educational psychology. In his famous series of lectures *Talks to Teachers on Psychology*, he outlines education as the organization of acquired habits of conduct and tendencies to behave. Similarly, teachers must also realize the importance of habit and instinct to present information that is clear and interesting and relate this new information and material to things the student already knows about. Likewise, teachers should address important issues such as attention, memory, and association of ideas. Jean Piaget developed the theory of cognitive development. The theory states that intelligence develops in four different stages: the sensorimotor stage from birth to two years old, the proportional stage from two years old to seven years old, the concrete operational stage from seven years old to ten years old, and the formal operational stage from eleven years old and up. He also believed that learning was constrained to the child's cognitive development.

Piaget influenced educational psychology because he was the first to believe that cognitive development was important and something that should be paid attention to in education. Most of the research on Piagetian theory was carried out by American educational psychologists. Since education is global, schools, students, and teachers have taught most philosophical theories during Piaget's term and research explored in America or Europe. One thing is clear: individuals of all walks of life have similar characteristics, brain, awareness, and mind development, depending on their education, opportunities, learning, and life experience. Therefore, cognitive learning ability does play a role in global education.

Among current educational psychologists, the cognitive perspective is more widely held than the behavioral perspective, perhaps because it admits causally related mental constructs such as traits, beliefs, memories, motivations, and emotions. *Cognitive concepts* explain that memory structures determine how information is perceived, processed, stored, retrieved, and forgotten. In addition, problem-solving, according to prominent cognitive psychologists, is fundamental to learning. It is considered an important research topic in educational psychology.

A student is thought to interpret a problem by assigning it to a schema retrieved from long-term memory. A problem students run into while reading is called *activation*. This is when the student's representations of the text are present *during working memory*. This causes the student to read through the material without absorbing the information and being able to retain it. When working memory is absent from the reader's representations of the working memory, they experience something called *deactivation*. When deactivation occurs, the student has an understanding of the material and is able to retain information.

If deactivation occurs during the first reading, the reader does not need to undergo deactivation in the second reading. The reader will only need to reread to get a *gist* of the text to spark their memory. When the problem is assigned to the wrong schema, the student's attention is subsequently directed away from features of the problem that are inconsistent with the assigned schema. The critical step of finding a mapping between the problem and a preexisting schema is often cited as supporting the centrality of analogical thinking to problem-solving.

Cognition is the mental action or process of acquiring knowledge and understanding through thought, experience, and the senses. It encompasses processes such as attention, the formation of knowledge, memory and working memory, judgment and evaluation, reasoning and *computation*, problem-solving and decision-making, comprehension and production of language. Cognitive processes use existing knowledge and generate new knowledge. The processes are analyzed from different perspectives within different contexts, notably in the fields of linguistics, anesthesia, neuroscience, psychiatry, psychology, education, philosophy, anthropology, biology, systemics, logic, and computer science.

These and other different approaches to the analysis of cognition are synthesized in the developing field of cognitive science, a progressively autonomous academic discipline. The word "cognition" comes from the Latin verb *meaning I know*, perceive, meaning to conceptualize or "to recognize." "Cognition" is a word that dates back to the fifteenth century, when it meant thinking and awareness. Attention to the cognitive process came about more than eighteen centuries ago, beginning with

Aristotle and his interest in the inner workings of the mind and how they affect the human experience. Today with many technologies, we can go through the mind in better imaging. Aristotle focused on cognitive areas pertaining to memory, perception, and mental imagery.

The Greek philosopher found great importance in ensuring that his studies were based on empirical evidence, scientific information that is gathered through observation, and conscientious experimentation. And centuries later, as psychology became a burgeoning field of study in Europe and then gained a following in America.

Each person has *an individual profile* of characteristics, abilities, and challenges that result from predisposition, learning, and development. These manifest as individual differences in intelligence, creativity, cognitive style, motivation, and the capacity to process information, communicate, and relate to others. Therefore, *defining the brain* has much to do with everything we have explored including its own physical organ.

Furthermore, the most prevalent disabilities found among school-age children are attention-deficit hyperactivity disorder (ADHD), learning disability, dyslexia, and speech disorder. We shed light on it already. The less common disabilities include *intellectual disability*, hearing impairment, cerebral palsy, epilepsy, and blindness. It's important to mention no other time in the recent past has there been a greater focus on schools and educational process. Like involved parents, teachers, caregivers, and to some degree politicians, we might've read a great deal about the overscheduled children, underachievers, and children with learning disabilities such as ADHD. Some of us are aware of testing, the tutoring mania, the pros and cons of homework, and the pressure on children to excel. Can it be possible to look into learning disabilities and disorders in more relevant to *recent* brain-mind and subject experiences?

It's not easy to understand how the mind coordinates information processing in order to construct reality. We learned our brain is composed of billions of neurons; trillions of other integrated regions with much unique structures and functions become activities in such self-regulatory, self-organizing patterns that influence *our daily life*. How does this flow of energy within interconnected neurons regulate? Can it be the state of mind allows the brain to achieve cohesion in its function? Many questions come to mind, such as *what is the state of mind?* We can say state of mind is mostly patterns of our activities in the brain at a particular moment. These patterns of activities inside connected regions are the neural networks that disclose different circuits and arbitrate the process of information. These circuits are in distribution with all other interconnected webs with complex input and output connections and various clusters of cells that carry out specific functions. Our *state of mind is our mental state* and our moods in a particular time.

For instance, the state of mind for focal attention, caution, behavioral hypervigilance, past experiences of fear, replica of the self as victim in time of self-defense, and emotional arousal notifying the body and mind to get ready for harm are all processes that become functionally prepared for activity. A state of mind involves a group of functionally synergistic processes that allows the mind as a whole to form a connected state of activity.

Within each of us is the *notion of development*, either nature or nurture, from simplicity to complexity. From crying at birth to crawling, from sounding words to speaking, each effort took place in our life journey. If it's successful, the behavior is reinforced. This system maximizes its complexity and as a result its abilities by moving behavior forward and applying other patterns in different situations. From birth to death, each moment is the emergence of a unique pattern of activity in our life that is similar but never the same.

Only those parents engrained with the system, that had more value or it was by *repeated experiences*. It's safer to make a point for our state of mind can be attracted by our history, our value of the context, and our environmental conditions. For example, each day of school is not sorted in our memory, but only those that carry ' value of embarrassing moments, places, or funny situations. Therefore, our *brain's emotional responses constitute a primary value system that engrains patterns of neuronal firings and shapes the emergent states of activation of the system.* As states become *engrained throughout* life experiences and emotional severity (extreme happiness or sorrow), they become more activated.

Well then, can it be possible the integration of emotion with perception is channel specific? Do the temporal poles play a role in social and emotional processing? Or do the temporal pole ties compound, strong processed perceptual inputs to visceral emotional responses? The perceptual (interpretation of our senses) inputs remain into the dorsal (auditory/hearing), medial (olfactory/smell), and ventral (visual/see) streams; the integration of emotion with perception can be channel specific. *Emotions and interpersonal relationships are fundamental aspects of learning and memory. One thing is understandable, which is the goal of memory is not just to store information exactly, but to refine decision-making.*

Let's make room for *forgetfulness* in our memory. Forgetting is also an evolutionary procedure and a determined process that runs in the background of our memory. This process evaluates and discards information that doesn't promote the survival of the species. This answers the phrase we come across often—*never mind*. From this learning, forgetting should not look as a failure of memory, but it represents an investment in a more favorable mnemonic principle. The processes that support human emotional intelligence are the *integration* of interpersonal neurons and biology. This understanding provides a picture of human mental development and the possibility for transformation that exists in changing thinking and processing of our emotions, thoughts, and behaviors. The notion of emotional intelligence is *interrelated* with our interpersonal neurons and our biology in addition to the development of mindful awareness as a way of strategy for achieving well-being integration of emotional, psychological, physiological, and cognitive functioning.

For example, *neuroplasticity* plays a role in our neurons—the brain's ability to reorganize itself by creating new neural links through a life span. Neuroplasticity allows the neurons (nerve cells) inside our brain to compensate for injury and disease, as well as to maintain their activities in response to new situations given.

This recognition (of the brain) is done by mechanisms such as axonal sprouting. The undamaged axons grow new nerve endings for the purpose of reconnecting neurons whose links were injured. This integration of undamaged axons can sprout nerve endings then connect with other undamaged nerve cells, therefore creating new neural pathways which help to accomplish a needed function. For example, if one hemisphere of the brain is damaged, the intact hemisphere may take over some of its functions. The brain compensates for damage in effect by reorganizing and forming new connections between intact neurons.

In order to reconnect, the neurons need to be stimulated through activity. Neuroplasticity sometimes may also contribute to impairment. For example, people who are deaf may suffer from a continual ringing in their ears (tinnitus), the result of the rewiring of brain cells starved for sound. For neurons to form beneficial connections, they must be correctly stimulated. Therefore, neuroplasticity is brain plasticity, the brain's abilities to change (molded). On the other hand, neuroplasticity is the brain's size to rewire. This is beneficial for strengthening pathways between the neurons that are exercised and used while weakening connections between the cellular pathways that are not used.

As we learned, *rewiring our brain* circuits is based on our *daily experience.* We can change our synapses or connections that are firing when changing our perception and our behavior. Neuroplasticity reviews an experience or event that we observe and experience a different outcome. What we become conscious of and look for is what we get. It's simple, our brain sees and responds to our perception, not the reality. It's important to put the individual as the center of treatment, not the health care to many points. How a child views self is integrated with how the child is treated. Special program plans and special schools or activities are adding to some point in children's awareness of being different. Therefore, any negative lasting brain states (repeatedly experiences) can become neural traits that are hardwired into the child's circuitry. Hence, it's best for children to pathologies more, to clear if the health care system is designed disease (overall health concerns) center or its people.

The child should be brought up not *just by parents but society* such as schools, teachers, caregivers, classmates, and the community as a whole. This book explores more fully what is known about the *relationship* between parents, caregivers, teachers *(integration of relationships)*, and the child, enabling the child's brain to develop the circuits responsible for healthy emotion regulation. The aim of integration is to review what is known about the emotional connection inherent in *attachment* to understand and guide our emotion regulation within interpersonal relationships. This, such as our experiences, allows us to look into which our mind directly shapes the development and function of our neurons just by the essence of others' connections.

Our mental life is composed of the movement of energy and information as we learned which shapes our brain activities and development. Also, it might be safer to say our memory is the important contributor combined with imagination to daily experiences, well-being, and overall development. After learning this, we may *redirect, redefine, and rely on the integration of the brain to mind to consciousness to relationships within and others to bigger circles as far as the universe.*

Let's not forget *memory* is the recorder, the lens which one sees through experience (interpersonal relationships), love and hate, and importantly self-identification. As a result, it's essential to knowledge to remind our self, after all, we might not be what we accumulate from recycled patterns of information and flows of energy distribution to *some point.* For many with mental health concerns, this is a true medical treatment for understanding, to leave space between self (I am) and accumulated flow of *recycled information.*

To create the brain and mind barrier is a commitment to master oneself at all levels of integration, who develops the courage to do the right patterns not just for self but for interconnectedness. The understanding of such discipline must start from *preschool* for teachers who teach and for learners. The building blocks of neural stimulation and brain or mind development begins its journey of integration from birth to death. Although we explored many theories of practices, cognitive development, brain activities and its functions, neurologists and neuroscience research, etc., development covers not just this part or that, but it's an essential part of a whole. For instance, the information stream of energy we accumulate also comes through books, social environment, therapies, and media, to name a few.

The fundamental premise about the brain is that it's working—what we can safely call "mind" is a consequence of its anatomy and physiology. As we explore the *remembering mind* (relationship—what matters the most), try to keep an eye on the everyday basis assumptions about memory. The common misconception about memory is we are aware of what we have experienced. We might not be conscious of what mind *photograph of experience*. The structure of memory is complex. Recollections are often seen as the presentation of information, independent of the time of recall. Memory is more than what we can consciously recall about events from the past.

A good definition of memory then might be that memory is the way *past experiences* (integration of events and its relationship) *affect the future function* of being. In this manner, the brain (we) experiences the world (our lives) and encodes this interconnected interaction in ways to alter the future of responding. Just as we can receive information in various forms, our mind (working brain) can be relayed by different means. In addition, the electric action potentials of single neuronal axons and the patterned release of neurotransmitters . . . and hrence the complex neuronal activation of the neural network. Would it be possible to refuse our memory to see the reality or perhaps the true nature of being? When humans disengage with memory totally, the mind or brain is in a state of higher *consciousness*. When we speak of consciousness, it means awareness, being awake.

However, higher consciousness is when individual no longer awake by memory's awareness, but that "space" we talked about "between self and the memory." When we identify self or others, we become aware of our memory. Who am I and who are you are part of the learning experiences (interpersonal relationships) and information stream of energy within our brain-mind. This is also a good point for exploring what *consciousness really* is aside from being known as awareness or being awake.

Can it be consciousness is the boundary between life itself and life experiences? Life has many dimensions to explore, and mostly death is not spoken as one. From birth, humans gain and loses much of bodily weight, neurons change our brain stimulation and structure by daily experiences, and so as our well-being changes. We can't feel to say *a part of me died*, although we are familiar with this phrase. The transition is life, not death, at the same token this referred in some point to might be after death. Would it be better if we make room in our memory for nonacademic skills that are just as important to long-term student success as academic skills? I would say definitely life is a better lesson. Let's go one further step toward memory.

We are introduced to *core memories*. All of us are constantly creating memories, but what make them core or significant are the emotions that we attach to these past events, experiences, and *relationships*. Emotions drive our attention and perception. We form positive and negative core memories because of the emotional intensity that we've attached to the event or experience. The same neural circuitry appears to be involved in forgetting and remembering. If that is properly understood, students and teachers can adopt strategies to reduce memory leaks and reinforce learning.

Therefore, education becomes an essential part of schools for the development of brain-and-mind integration. This is a much deeper core of interpersonal experience and its *relationship with intellect* to bring up to the knowledge. As if numbing (antistatic) the pain be the solution to fix any pain or use as a form of treatment, one to ask. Neuroplasticity is the best news from neuroscience in recent years, interpersonal skills, in particular, conscientiousness and self-management. It turns out that just as we would have expected, these measures predicted the outcomes you would expect. For instance, kids who rated themselves lower in school at self-management had higher absentee rates, suspensions, and the like. Kids who rated themselves higher in growth mindset had higher GPAs. Some reports also find that students' mindsets about their intelligence can predict academic achievement.

Research shows that students who have a growth mindset—meaning they believe intelligence can increase through practice and effort—do better at school than students who think their intelligence is fixed at a certain level. The story of Jack reminds me of this, which we will explore more in further pages, to introduce us to the emotions lingering in a beautiful young brain. His joyful core memories are represented by friendship. At the beginning of his life, the sadness interferes with the relationship of joy-filled memories. When a core memory is touched by sorrow, the happiness fades to sadness, and joy becomes frustration.

Later, I learned through his various experiences that sadness and joy can work well together, therefore weaving a beautiful contrast to create a lasting core memory. These core memories are stored in his long-term memory and eventually become a part of his personality or what I have labeled as the self (I am), which individual can call such understanding as definition of interpersonal brain.

When neurons are frequently fired, synaptic *connections* are strengthened. For this purpose, knowing as synaptic plasticity explains why some memories persist while others fade away. Repeatedly accessing (communication relationship) a stored but fading memory—like a rule of crucial historical *information* system—reframes the neural networking system that contains the memory and encodes it more into the deeper structure. Researchers have also learned that not all new memories are created equal. For example, here are two sets of letters to remember: one will be random "APMSTSCA" and another "sky."

For those of us who speak English, the second set of letters is more memorable—the more connections neurons have to other neurons, the stronger the memory. The eight letters in the first appear to be random and incoherent. On the other hand, "sky" benefits from its existence of being known. Thus, it's a deeply encoded linguistic context. The word "sky" also brings up sensory memory, from the image of warm feeling of the sun, fresh air, to its smell, and perhaps even conjures other memories of sky in our picture, season, camping, stars, etc. As a result, we remember by patterns of new memories on the puzzle foundations of older ones.

A few years ago, I was working with a group of children in a professional development preschool, and I said, "We're always innovating and trying new things each day. For once, maybe we just need to stay the same." Even the children nodded—the group felt an overwhelming sense of initiative fatigue. Too often in education, change is presented as another new idea or as a new debate. It made me realize about these controversies of *teacher-directed* or *student-centered* traditional instruction or project-based learning system. Whole language or phonemic awareness? When this happens, teachers and students can feel like they are swinging from one end to the other.

Thus, teachers might find it difficult to begin new initiatives so teachers resist changes or just wait to swing back the other way. This initiative fatigue can lead to burnout. The balance in mapping helps identify interdependent pairs, which means that both sides have a purpose and a necessity. We've always had *balance* such as in education from individual work and collaboration, whole-group and individual instruction, individual responsibility, and teacher support. Consider traditional, teacher-directed instruction and student-centered learning. When a curriculum is teacher-directed, the students may not be as engaged or may not have opportunities for independent critical thinking. Similarly, when students have too much autonomy, they may feel unfocused or may miss key components of the daily curriculum. By identifying warning signs, the teacher can take steps to keep the system in balance. Instead of viewing change as either or, the teacher should suggest looking at it as a combination and balance. To meet this challenge, the teacher might use a lecture and guided reading to increase content knowledge.

These methods were designed for promoting student class discussion, self-reflection, and self-awareness. Can it be possible that neither the brain nor the mind could simply create the memories?

Or would it be possible if instead we gathered the organic sensory data information from the outside world which is around our body, nerves, and the first reptilian brain stem. Also, the primitive brain stem doesn't think for itself nor does it have conscious memories. For human's real permanent memory, the *explicit memory*, we need the hippocampus. This is located above the brain stem, in the limbic emotional lobe (thumb). The responsibility of the hippocampus is to integrate the essential sensory information into a coherent picture, then put a usage of time on it so it can be transferred into the long-term permanent memory, which can be retrieved later in life.

This is one way to get into human conscious thought that occurs in our frontal cortex. Explicit memory is referred to as thinking memory or our cognitive memory. However, there are few ways in which the hippocampus may not be available. This means we easily may not remember traumatic experiences in our life. During brain development from conception to thirty-six months, the hippocampus isn't ready to function. At this time of development, the hippocampus doesn't have enough myelin to fire. For this purpose, any experiences that happen by the first forty-five months of life do not automatically become part of conscious memories. For example, my son when he was nine months was bitten by a bee, then he got bitten again at age two years old at the same hand.

As a result of which, he feels fear when he sees bees. He has many memories, all implicit feelings of bee fear—feeling of pain in his hand, visual (what do bees look like), sound (what does a bee make), and the feeling that he is getting ready to run away. These implicit memories, once they are encoded and stay in that organic form into storage, those memories change in synaptic *connections*. Basically, it's a natural set of unconscious memory patterns. Without a functioning hippocampus, the collective information sits scattered throughout the body. Also, it's not necessary to neither of these two bee bites incidents at younger age would ever get integrated into a coherent conscious memory or perhaps they ever get a time capsule put on them. However, later in life, in fifteen years, let's say, when he sees a bee, his brain goes to retrieve whatever memory it has of the bees. Although retrieval of a memory is the same as firing of neural patterns, it is not identical to what was encoded the first time this past experience happened.

The important part of education on brain development is to understand the fundamental nature of mental abilities and our memory (relationship of the experience). Thus, knowing the implicit memory does not feel like it's coming from the past. When he hears a bee, he just feels fear and emotions ready to run. Also, during the development process of young-age children, the hippocampus itself might be damaged as a form of developmental trauma. If children *repeatedly (strong communication)* have traumatic experiences, the neurology of the primitive brain stem gets enough damage that it can harm the developmental of the higher brain lobes of the child. The hippocampus can be damaged enough to where when children feel scared, at some point, they cannot think their way out of a situation.

Trauma after the age of three throughout life overwhelms the body with stress hormones which result in turning off the hippocampus itself. What damages the hippocampus is too much of the cortisol stress hormone, which at the same time produces adrenaline, cortisol, in higher levels, shuts off the hippocampus first temporarily. However, in the long run, it might kill hippocampus cells permanently.

This is the experience of *PTSD disorder*—explaining the flashback of this journey. This happens when an implicit memory is reactivated without any given explicit elements. The hippocampus hasn't been *attached to experience* these things in full awareness. We cannot say this is more relevant than unconscious memory, but they are elements which are encoded and stored that are retrieving into mindfulness.

Unfortunately, there are types of trauma where children age preschool and older with a functional hippocampus can hardly, during a traumatic event, disconnect themselves to avoid such harsh experience when it's brought up to their mind, so they won't remember it later. There are ways for changing mind in ways of dividing our attention into something different. For example, if you are being hurtful of such memory, you can focus on a beautiful sunlight, so you've taken your hippocampus out of that momentary picture. Unfortunately, we cannot block the implicit coding of those raw separate bodily memories of what actually happened to the mind.

Socializing is an essential part of our developing brain to mind. This is crucial for infants till age six. The brain is a social organ, and our interactions create the neural connections from which our mind emerges. Thus, for young children, *relationships* are a very crucial system of development. When children are deprived of caregivers and parents' relationships in these critical early years of childhood experiences, it can deeply affect the way the brain develops. The brain is an interpersonal, conscious, and information processing system that self-regulates. It turns out the parts—the hippocampus is the narrator to the left hemisphere, then it has to draw on the hippocampus in the right hemisphere for all collective storage of autobiographical information gathered.

Despite deciding to divide the attention elsewhere, the consciousness of being sick or having nervous feelings is there. The scientific point of understanding human memory is to recall events and facts. Therefore, we commit them to our memory. This process involves *encoding*, storing, retaining, and subsequently recalling the information and our interpersonal experiences. Can it be possible we are our memory then? Memory is the process of retaining information over time. With that said, are we recycled information therefore? Obviously not; we do tend to use our memory as the ability to use our past experiences (interpersonal experience) to determine our future lives ahead of us. What majority recognize memory is either an essential part of school, learning, or remembering—where my keys are . . . unfortunately, memory is essential in our everyday lives.

We would not be able to continue to function or move forward without relying on our memory. Can it be possible that our brain is three times as large as those of our early australopithecine ancestors who lived 4 million, 2 million years ago? It's possible that for years, scientists have explored how our *brain got bigger*. Studies have discovered that social competition could be behind the increase in brain size. Are we saying our brain size depends on what we have gathered as a form of information? Maybe not; let's take one more look at how our memory system has been formed. For instance, the process of encoding to form a memory begins when we are born. That's explain slowly, and occurs *continuously*. What becomes a memory? For anything to become part of a memory, it must first be picked up by one or more of our senses. It begins in short-term storage, such as learning how to zip our jacket or put our boots on. Once we have the process down by repeated action, then it goes into our long-term memory. From there, we can do it without consciously thinking about the steps involved or recognizing its process.

Important memories typically move from *short-term memory to long-term memory*. The transfer of information to long-term memory for more permanent storage can happen in several steps. *Information* that has more *emotions* and has more *meaning* is stored from short memory to long memory easier *(the relationship experience)*. Also, data can be committed to long-term memory through repetition. One good example can be studying for an exam. Another way to store information from short memory to long will be individuals' *interpersonal interest,* motivation, and dedication. This is also a consideration, in that information relating to something individuals like is more likely to be stored in long-term memory. That's why someone might be able to recall the stats of a favorite hockey player even after years passed by.

Consequently, if we have much information or data savings inside of our memory system, how can we navigate the valley to explore—what is there to benefit from? We might not be conscious of everything. Every time, we might not typically know of what is in our memory, until we need to use a bit of its information. As they say, we might not be aware of our capabilities till we try ourselves. Hence, the memory uses the process of *retrieval* to bring it to the forefront when we need to use it to see what our capabilities are. Some of this recall comes up to surface without having to concentrate on it.

As we mentioned with common tasks we do each day, such as zipping our jackets. However, there are other types of memories that take much deeper awareness to bring to the forefront. So what we call our *unconscious memory* or *automatic memory system is our implicit memory.* We use past experiences to remember things without thinking about them with the help of implicit memory. When we are trying to sort information for long-term memory is procedural memory. This is a subset of implicit memory which is a part of the long-term memory system and responsible for knowing how to do our things. One good example is we don't have to think to recall how to walk each time we take a step forward or how to take steps climbing stairs. Moreover, semantic memory is not connected to interpersonal experience.

Semantic memory contains things that are common in daily use, such as the names of countries, alphabets, knowing whether clouds are dark or white, and knowing that flowers smell nice. On the other hand, episodic memory is a person's interpersonal recollection of a specific experience in life. This memory is usually able to associate particular details with an experience, such as how they felt at that time, the location, who was involved, what they heard, etc. It is clear why some memories of events in our lives are committed to memory and some don't get recorded. This might point out to our emotions in what we can remember permanently. This brings us back to the importance of children's development and interpersonal relationships with parents and caregivers throughout the community. It is a beautiful and important part of relationships to see how the internal world of an infant is actually seen by the parents, caregivers, and teachers; and that experience is a contingency, which basically means give and take, starting with a simple smile and recognition of smiling back.

A reciprocal signal of *communication and trust (relationship)* which is a building block for developing a sense of a coherent mind, a solid foundation, and that's what we call a secure form of attachment. This is an absolutely essential part of the development of the brain in a healthy manner. It really is, and you know everything we're learning about the brain—that the brain is the only social organ of the human body; and for this purpose of healthy development, we need interpersonal experiences that are that *integration of connection.*

In psychology, attachment refers to the psychological model attempting to describe the dynamics of long- and short-term interpersonal relationships between self and others. It's an important point for this book to understand that attachment, integration, experience, and communication are not formulated as forms of relationships, but how human beings respond within relationships. In the same token, *love is an internal process*, not necessarily relationships and how two individuals share this experience between them. Attachment can place us with our emotions when we are hurt, are separated from those we love, or feel fear when perceiving a threat.

Correspondingly, the tendency for infants to develop attachments to parents s and caregivers can be the result of evolutionary pressures. Strong *attachment behavior* would facilitate the infant's survival in the face of trust and dangerous situations. This directs the child to seek proximity with a familiar caregiver when they are uncertain. With higher expectations, they will receive protection and emotional support.

This communication allows them to have relationships where they can perceive the internal world of other people. From this point, we can see the other person's mind and/or empathy. Therefore, this will build an internal sense of themselves that's quite coherent, which they can make sense of the internal world and their interpersonal relationships that they will have in the world. This leads us to a thorough understanding of the brain to mind and overall human development again. This is about the mechanisms of that groundwork. The brain appears to have a built-in mechanism to create the neurobiological foundation of a developing mind.

As we learned, interpersonal experiences such as traumatic experiences interact with genetics to change the structure and function of our brain development. Children's early life experiences can change the number of specific communication cells within their brain the neurons. *Hence, these interpersonal experiences can then increase or decrease the* entanglement *of the neurons which are the dendritic branches and the number of communication sites between the synapses. From this point to sculpturing of the brain experience-based plays a big part has on how the brain functions hereafter.* To be more relevant, this can determine how the *emotional centers of the brain communicate with the cortex* and with its next to developing functioning to determine our personality and our choices.

Generally speaking, we learned that our brains have a hundred billion neurons. *Genes* are very important when babies are in the uterus as a fetus. This is important to separate the connection among neurons, and such connections in the brain are an essential part of development as they shape our mind, our thoughts, and our feelings through which we understand the world.

During birth, these connections are not developed well; and therefore, it is the relationship *between the experiences that begins to promote the activation of neurons.* For example, if a child is teething, she is in pain and cries out in discomfort; and when the parent of the child hears the cry, she comes to her child and maybe tries to put her to bed because she thinks the child might be sleepy.

However, she then realizes that the child is still crying, so then she gives her some milk, and still she does not figure out what's going on inside of her child. That experience will give the child a connection that if I cry in discomfort, I will be connected and understood by my parents, and ultimately my needs will be met. Hence, the child's brain will develop a coherence in its structural organization system in which the *communication of internal states* to parents or caregivers will be met with a possibility of response that then allows the child's needs to be met. That's how overall the brain gets its organizational structure and will be an integrated system of development.

However, if this attentional communication becomes an essential part of children's needs, its servers its purpose well. On the other hand, if the parents and caregivers mislead the child's needs to its behavior, then the purpose of trusting gets confused. What it means is that the children learn what I experienced internally and what I expressed externally by crying met the response of communication but didn't make any sense to what I needed. As a result, the organization of that child's brain will be different, because neurons which fire together as we learned wired together. In that case, it sends different signals such as what I learned as a child doesn't really matter or what I feel doesn't matter since my parents or perhaps the world doesn't really get me anyway.

Children, therefore, become quite disconnected not only from other people, but even from their own internal bodily self and their emotional experiences, so to speak. This sense leads hereafter to grown to adolescence and then adulthood which they've experienced life in a way where they are very disconnected from an awareness of the internal world of themselves or others and the absence of understanding the integrated mind.

One important aspect of attachment is to use caregivers and parents to the soothing experience. This eventually forms the development of the limbic areas of the brain to allow the child to learn to soothe themselves while using other people in communication first and next to learn to self-soothe.

The *limbic system* of the brain is genetically built from evolution to require a caregiver around. Unfortunately, as they grow beyond the first year, the capacity of the brain to adapt to relationships and attachment appears to become less and less dense. Also, children who have no attachment have all sorts of self-regulatory processes such as that are not interesting or they are *isolated*.

Children's *first three years of development* is an essential part of the whole brain development and who they would become as adults. The brain develop circuits by age two years old and the prefrontal circuits which are going to allow for things like empathy, self-regulation, having a narrative of yourself that allows the child to see their mind—all these begin. And the roots of such discipline begin with attachment and relationships (how relationship), then by around age three years old, these prefrontal circuits are ready for children to become social and prepared for the preschool system.

Children who deprived of relationships, this has ongoing impacts on many realms of the child's development. This places the child in cognitive realms as this is how we process information. In some, the ability to have balance attention means paying attention, aside from the ability to regulate their emotions. It's not that children won't function well throughout adulthood; it's just that they seem to have pretty significant interpersonal experiences which impact those early years when there've been no relationships.

During brain development, being deprived of such sensitive relationships has also an emotional impact that can affect the cognitive function's ability to think well. Often extreme traumas go beyond the normal processing of the child's brain and cause a pathway to pathology. This places the child to have a delayed expression until the child approaches preadolescence. *As a result, abuse at early interpersonal life experiences can be associated with brain damage from prenatal and postnatal.*

Unfortunately, years ago, such deficits were attributed to psychological problems alone not understanding there was a physical manifestation of these problems. However, with modern medicine and technology systems, today there is much knowledge that the structure and functioning of the human brain contribute to these behavioral traits. Another aspect of child abuse and neglect based on neuroscience is presented within the framework of attachment as though most abuses start at some point from caregivers.

It is important to look into *attachment* itself to understand its *definition*, which has two basic functions. First, attachments ensure the child remains in proximity of the caregiver (parent or other caretakers). Second, *attachment is capable of programming the lifelong structure and function of the brain.* It's important to understand how within this framework the effects of early childhood abuse can be a contributor differently at different ages. It has short- and long-term effects and brings up distinct patterns, and the most dramatic effects are delayed until later in life. This places attachment as another important implication for research that is possible to develop a secure state of mind as an adult, even in the face of a difficult early development.

There is no denying that earlier life interpersonal experience influences later development. However, it isn't the only fate. Many therapeutic experiences can profoundly alter an individual's life course. From the therapist's experience we can learn attachment, researchers' insights into the human development which features of relational experience are the most effective at optimizing a well-integrated and developed brain. Once parents become sensitive to a child's needs—when they pay attention to and tune in to the child's signals, understanding the sense of these signals and getting a glimpse of the child's inner experience, which only then respond in a timely and effective manner. The essential features of such therapeutic relationships mirror this process in many ways. For most instances, the brain continues to remodel itself in response to experience and contribute throughout our lives.

We have explored some interpersonal relationships and neural stimulation systems. Thus, emerging studies of neuroplasticity are showing how relationships can stimulate human *neuronal activation—* even remove the synaptic legacy of early childhood social experience. Human's fast development is in persuasive neuroscience knowledge from the beginning of the universe from the birth of a star to the origin of life and hereditary of genetic.

However, the human brain which allows us to achieve this is still a mystery. The simplest experience of creating music requires creativity, emotions, objectives, and memories to provoke a connection of sensation and pleasure in are own mind and in the mind of others. How the brain makes this happen by using memory, intelligence is not easy answer?

This is the art of integration between mind and brain stimulation, and it's a place for human essence. The brain is under scientific investigations over decades with the most mysteries.

Although the base of its biological theories and the model of its function are well understood, it is still not clear enough why something is remembered and others are simply not. Aside why are such strong mechanism worries about its origins, about its mind or life, and the meaning of death. It's true that we gather all data to support our journey. However, we lack a theory to put together this integration system. We can disclose information about how the human brain and mind develop, but when I turned this information to a book, I set beside my desk, start reimagining the words, thoughts, pictures, and people I combined with this information flow. so Amazingly, to the point I don't know how I did this. We might never know how to combine the scientific information flow with the subjectivity of our own interpersonal experiences.

Decades of studies by physiologists and psychologists have been made to the mind and brain and are the same, yet the result of today's learning disabled such discipline where the *physical support of the mind* is the human brain. Some studies have supported the human brain is the result of million years of *biological evolution*. That started typically reptiles and advanced to more *Homo sapiens*. This is a gradual change within *Homo sapiens*, describing a point from an elongated endocranial shape toward a more spherical one.

The two expect of such development stand out as parietal and cerebellar bulging shapes. The parietal brain section is involved in orientation, attention, perception of stimuli, sensorimotor transformations underlying planning, visuospatial integration, imagery, self-awareness aside from working and long-term memory, and tool use.

This is an important part of learning. The *cerebellum* in this area is associated not only with motor-related functions such as the *coordination of movements* or balance, but also with spatial processing, working memory, language, social cognition, and affective processing. The brain is conceivably the most important organ for the abilities that make us who are as humans. Nonetheless, the modern human brain shape was not established at the origin of our species together with other key features of craniodental morphology alone, but the brain shape also has evolved within our own species. Also, with modern development its clear process to the characteristic globular shape of the brain develops within a few months around the time of birth.

The *evolution of endocranial* shape inside *Homo sapiens* shows the evolutionary changes of human's early brain development—a critical period for neural wiring and the cognitive development journey. If that is so, the evolutionary changes to early brain development were key factors to the evolution of the human cognition system. As a result, we can conclude the integration of attachment, interpersonal relationships, and experiences in bigger pictures of today's brain development. This gradual development point of evolution journey of modern human seems to bridge the balance to the steady emergence of behavioral modernity.

For *today's brain integration*, we look within those separated areas with their unique functions. This linkage is well organized in the skull and throughout our body, thus becoming linked to each other through the synaptic connection system. The integration of whole linkages authorizes the intricate functions to emerge to such as our insight, empathy, intuition, and morality. For this purpose of integration, human experience, relationship, kindness, resilience, and they are well-being. The brain stimulation to create this term of integration are the coherent mind, the empathic relationships.

From *enlightenment to* today's society integration has been proven at the heart of interpersonal neurobiology. *Being aware of our unique nature is still in an individual's mind. Integration involves the linkage of separate aspects of our interpersonal experiences and mental processes to each other, such as our thought with feeling and our bodily sensation with logic. While in a relationship perspective, integration shows each person's being respected for his or her autonomy and differentiated self while at the same time being integrated to others in an empathic communication way. Much of this experience-dependent control of brain development relies upon the experiences (how or what of experience).* For example, children brought up in countries that have extreme physical and social isolation might have smaller brains than children from well-developed countries who have a larger amygdala.

We have explored some of the brain activity and its responsibility. Hence, the *amygdala* is the brain area concerned with emotion and fear, and a larger amygdala would therefore suggest altered emotion and fear processing. To be aware of our experience and nurture of our brain development, new neurons are born in the brain throughout our life span. This might shed light on the enormity of early life growth that is never replicated in later life. Neurons that would typically die under normal conditions could be kept in their possession under deprivation or conditions of abuse.

With current discovery, *every time we learn a new skill, we change our brain and that is part of neuroplasticity of human nature of development.* How simple the neuroplasticity causes the brain to change- adapt is almost in three steps. Let's take a look first at the chemicals of the brain that transfer signals between brain cells, the neurons and wave of action and reactions. With this activity, change can happen at any point rapidly, thus supporting the short-term memory system or the short-term improvements of motor skills. Second, the brain supports learning by altering its structures by changing the connections between neurons. These changes, however, take longer periods, therefore becoming part of the long-term memory system and long-term improvement in motor skills, for instance, trying to learn a new motor skill such as playing the guitar. This places us in short-term memory at that point of learning experience. However, the next few days, the brain might not remember how that happened, since it has not become part of the long-term memory system.

Structure changes can also lead to an integrated network that the brain regions to function to support learning and also lead to certain regions of the brain that are essential to particular behaviors that are important to the brain to change their structure to enlarge. One good example of this will be a taxi driver has more capability to map systems because of repeated driving than normal drivers. And lastly, how the brain can change to support learning is by altering its function.

As we use a certain structure of our brain, it becomes more relevant, excited to reuse this region again. Since the brain has these areas to increase these patterns of excitability, the brain shapes how or when they become active. This is the integration of whole brain stimulation from altering to shaping to changing patterns for our brain to development and supporting learning experiences that take place throughout life.

However, knowing how functional and organized our neuroplasticity is, why would it fail us from time to time? For instance, *why would children fail their class*, or why are we learning differently when we age? What is that secret to limit and facilitate human neuroplasticity? This is not an easy solution as there is no such doze of neuroplasticity medicine to increase or solve each process, especially since each brain is depending on its own function. What might be a possible solution and the primary driving change of the brain to start from the behavior?

Neuroplasticity of the human brain can change its purpose to better function and also has a negative side. These bits of incoming information are "implicit memory" changes in synaptic connections making sense like puzzle pieces. Each one is a separate sensory memory housed primarily in the nerves reporting in from the body parts where it happened—optical nerve, olfactory nerve, auditory nerve, and so on. Each of those nerves also reports the different implicit data we have gathered through interpersonal relationships to the nonthinking instinctive brain stem, which also stores parts of these memories and—this is another key—without being able to integrate them.

Thus far, if the memory is hostile, like the memory of bee stings, then we get an additional flood of unrelated information such as our gut gets tight, our heart rate goes up, our breath quickens, our leg muscles tense to run, which happens through our instinct, instantly, and it bypasses our experiences. Integration from all those visceral nerves of the body cavity is the vagus nerve, which dumps all this lower body sensory data into the primitive brain stem.

There are twelve cranial nerves in our body that come in pairs and help to *integrate* the brain with other areas of the body, such as the head, neck, and torso. Each carrier has its own purpose. Some send sensory information, including details about smells, sights, tastes, and sounds, to the brain which these nerves are known as having sensory functions. As well, other cranial nerves control the movement of various muscles and the function of certain glands, and these are known as motor functions.

The *stimulation of learning new experiences* is therefore like learning piano or becoming addicted to the use of some painkillers. The human brain is much plastic density depending on what we do or what we don't. One thing is a fact—that our brain stimulation works well with all of us, but based on each differential levels that are between us, one size never fits all. What's essential part to study further is that, our individualized human brain is much depending on its daily dose of behavior. As much is our medicine individualized the same token is our brain cells depending on its own chemicals and role of interpersonal learning experience.

This brings us back to the other purpose of this book journey to *interpersonal neurobiology* and *how-to relationship*. Also, it solves the misunderstanding that learning experiences among children aren't necessarily the same but are based on how their brain behaves and what their capacities are. Would this be a simple but a great experience of grading students based on brain development (age and stage of development) over age alone? I definitely think so. That is how we have children who thrive in fewer hours of learning, and we have children who function just enough.

This gives neuroscientists a great experience to view learning as a point of interpersonal relationships between ourselves, our brain development, and our daily behavior. With this modern nature of human evolution, we might be in a better generation to forward such discipline as part of learning experiences for teachers, parents, and college professors and that it is an essential part to human development.

I might also add one more important aspect to this *learning curve and our overall growth which* is depending on how much can we determine the balance *experience between the older models of education and the current developmental journey of interpersonal neurobiology—and learning abilities.*

For instance, children's preschool theories of Montessori have been an essential part of evolution learning experience. However, they are not necessarily the *only continuum learning abilities* for generations hereafter. This educational system has already proven its purpose to learning experience and for children development in much deeper and well-defined ways, yet not necessarily good enough starting point for future evolution, depending on the *new-balance flow of much up dated information* for generations to come. What we know now is still in its infancy compared to what we will learn forty years from now. Likewise, how much human developed over past forty years ago is an actual fact. As a result of any point or given situation, the brain function for the typical social environment in our Western culture might be compromised.

I can conclude memory is an essential part of human development and interpersonal experience. However, how the brain remembers is the major purpose of human growth and well-being over what we remember. This knowledge has proven to be potential for human development, and contributing such discipline is necessary for education systems and development of the mind. The great news is that when we correlate our interpersonal communication and attachment findings with the independent field of brain research, we find that in fact the adult brain continues to make new connections among its neurons— and even to grow new neurons throughout the life span. As a result, adults can use their minds to actually examine their lives and examine their own memory systems to make sense of their lives and then alter the way their brains function, so they can actually free themselves up from what used to be a prison of the past. This is clearly shown by many studies.

The *role of nature and nurture (in this book, nature needs nurture)* is equally important to human development. For example, let's say adoptive parents have shown that how they made sense of their life is the best predictor of how their adopted or foster child will turn out, so it's not just genetics alone. Now when we have this understanding of self, what it does is it gives us the tool to make sense of our life, to actually parent ourselves from the inside out so that we can parent (or caregiver) our children in a way that helps them flourish. First, it is important for parents, caregivers, and educators to understand some basics about brain development. Importantly, the original view of brain development as subject to tight genetic control has been abandoned.

Brain development is a constantly changing interaction between genes and the environment (nature and nurture) with postnatal experiences altering the structure of our brain. The human brain begins as a neural tube, which allows cells to be born *(neurogenesis)*. These cells travel to the proper place in the brain and sprout branches (axons for the input and dendrites for the output) that enable proximity to other neurons and build pathways and circuits throughout our brain.

Thereafter, the neuron forms the chemical-electrical connections between cells (synapses) to relay information. Some of these processes occur prenatally, especially neurogenesis and the migration. However, the later steps continue at high levels during the first two to three years of the child's development, because the brain exponentially increases in size. Hereafter, the process continues through adolescence. The extent of this postnatal maturation is large, with tens of thousands of new synapses being developed daily during the child's early years. It's important to understand much of this growth is dependent upon predetermined events programmed by genetics, yet experience shapes this process as we explored our *experience-dependent plasticity.*

Experience has much effect and can determine the selective survival of neurons and the relative complexity of the axonal injury. It shows the effect on dendritic branching and the number of synapses that exist between the cells. Simple understanding of educational activity for educators and parents is an essential part of brain stimulation. For example, while roll-and-tumble play or watching a television show might be appropriate sensory stimulation for a four-year-old child, they are likely inappropriate for an infant.

A more suitable sensory *stimulation* for a one-year-old would be socially interacting with a nurturing, fun-loving caregiver. This implication of experience instructing shapes the brain development which is critical for custodial issues. Therefore, the role of *interpersonal communication and relationships* between children and caregivers is an essential part of development, yet what's necessary here is the caregiver's brain development education. If children at their early life experience cannot activate their attachment system, it is likely that the development of their future attachment formation will be compromised.

As a result, a more refined control of brain development is accomplished by changing the activity of specific connections between neurons. However, balance activities are necessary for development, because activity patterns between neurons can cause some neurons to grow more dendritic branches and synapses yet prune others. Therefore, particular types of information processing are enhanced.

We also explored the role of integration between brain cells and interpersonal communication and within mind and body. Also, we know that no brain area functions in isolation and that brain changes influenced by early life experiences are present throughout the brain. Therefore, information about brain development for a given brain area needs to be interpreted within the context of other neural changes. This is because brain activity is a *coordinated process of functional connectivity between areas (relation of integration)*.

While developmental transitions vary in some behaviors, fewer basic concepts hold their purpose for others. For example, *social behavior* must transition from the stage of the infant-caregiver social relationship, second to the toddler stage that expands social relationships to include other adults and children, then to the adolescent stage of development where the focus is on peers, and finally to the complexities of adult social behavior and childcare.

Based on these behavioral changes and *adaptation to the developmental* stage, the brain changes alongside. This is because the brain produces these behavioral transitions. Now if we consider child abuse, it is necessary to place the child's social behavior within the context of the stage of social behavior and the critical consideration of attachment to the caregiver.

Consequently, in the early years of a child's life, it is the social interactions with the caregiver and the caregiver's stimulation of the child's sensory receptors in the eyes, ears, tongue, nose, and skin that provide this experience-based programming of the brain.

Through the *stimulation of sensory experience*, we introduced experiences to the human brain. Teachers, educators, parents, and caregivers are the primary sources of this stimulation and are the gateways to other sensory stimulations. The continuum effects of this coding can sometimes lie dormant until the later developmental stage of life when certain behavioral brain circuits get mature.

I have studied early childhood education in one of the recognized colleges in Alberta, Canada. What I learned from its diploma program and what I practiced within daily learning activities were not necessarily the same. I could distinguish easily the education from early childhood was another door to add to my own *interpersonal* experience. When I started to explore more complex possibilities for the development of the brain, *I can conclude the modern brain education of today's century and to further follow up is the best way to define the brain based on its daily learning experience and therefore its daily development. This places us in the psychology of nature needs nurture and the psychology of education— necessary for learning experiences for educators.*

The human brain is one reason for today's overall growth, however distraction is seen, due to not being able to *define* itself further. We have a hundred billion neurons, or brain cells, with close to a quadrillion connections between them, and we have yet to fully understand a single cell. Neuroscience is the best place to explore where psychology meets biology to further our understanding of physical, psychological, and neurological health conditions, such as the brain's role in how we perceive different types of pain and the underlying cause of Parkinson's disease, yet it is not enough.

Computer simulations, imaging, and other tools give researchers and medical experts new insight into the physical anatomy of the brain and its relationship to the rest of the mind and body. We can contribute our brain knowledge to such discipline and create complex systems like computers. Just as computers are hardwired with electrical connections, so is the human brain hardwired with neural connections that link together its various lobes. This also links sensory input and motor output with the brain's message centers which allow the information to come in and be sent back out.

One role of *today's neuroscience* research is to study damage to the brain's wiring. New developments in brain scanning allow neurologists and researchers to see more detailed images and determine not only where there may be damage but also how that damage affects, for example, motor skills and cognitive behavior in conditions like multiple sclerosis, dementia, or brain tumor. The more advanced the technology, the more relevant the information for psychology and the cure for mental health. Conditions such as boredom, mood disorder, self-esteem, passion, and creativity are not factors from childhood upbringing but are possibly there from birth, from genes—just like our height and our blue eyes are. This might be obvious but is still today far from being universally accepted. Personality might be significantly more from nature than nurture. We must be open to all learning experiences that have shaped our development—no human nature. Our behaviors and motivations are formed by parents alone and the type of society we live in. And no selfish instincts, in a state of nature without rules and social organization. One way to look at it is there are millions of cells, or neurons, densely packed into various regions of the brain.

As we learned, *each region is responsible* for a particular function. Some regions interact with our outside world, interpreting vision, hearing, and other sensory inputs to help us communicate through responses—figure out what to do and what to say, while other regions interact with our internal world, our body, in order to regulate the function of our organs (heart, lungs). Integration is the main key to the various regions to do their jobs well. Thus, they must be linked *(well communication)* to one another. As a way of there are myriad pathways or neural circuits that carry the flow of information from one brain region to another.

However, brain scientists have found that deficiencies in specific neurotransmitters underlie many common disorders, including anxiety, mood disorders, anger-control problems, and obsessive-compulsive disorder. For example, ADHD might be the other disorder found to be the result of a deficiency of a specific neurotransmitter. Therefore, norepinephrine might respond to medications to correct this underlying deficiency. This might be likely to neurotransmitters; norepinephrine is synthesized within the brain.

The *basic building block* of each *norepinephrine molecule is dopa.* This small molecule is converted into dopamine, which, in turn, is converted into norepinephrine. It's important to understand how doctors treat patients with physical symptoms might not be the same with mental health concerns. For example, a pediatrician can do a throat culture and tell whether a child needs an antibiotic, so an appropriate treatment follows the diagnosis. By contrast, psychiatrists are often required to initiate a specific treatment to clarify the diagnosis later on. It's not necessarily figuring out what might have caused the fire, but it's essential to put water on to fire and blow the smoke away to see clearly first.

With mental health, more often than I admit, I have to tell that it's not clear what is wrong. It's not that we lack the expertise or diagnostic skills. It's just that psychiatry isn't quite as far along as other medical specialties are. For instance, if a child is having problems in school, he or she might have ADHD. However, it's also possible that he has a learning disability or other concerns such as mood disorder, anxiety, or family issues.

We learned the *importance of interpersonal relationships* and experiences. Thus, what also might be *ADHD* is the result of family tensions. Aside parents who understood neurotransmitters; however, that parents often feel better about ADHD meds the remarkable compounds that govern brain function. We mentioned a bit about how each neuron produces small quantities of a specific neurotransmitter. This is released into the microscopic space that exists between our neuron that is called a synapse, stimulating the next cell in the pathway and no other.

Information is transmitted along these pathways via the action of neurotransmitters. Knowing the quantity of human neurons, each neurotransmitter has a unique molecular structure. A specific one— that is able to attach only to a neuron with the corresponding receptor site. When the specific one finds the neuron bearing the right one, the neurotransmitter binds to and stimulates that neuron. It is amazing to know how a specific neurotransmitter knows precisely which neuron to attach to, when there are so many other neurons nearby. We learned the importance of an integration system between the brain and its structure. For example, these four regions of the human brain interact with one another, so a deficiency in one region may cause a problem in one or more of the other regions.

Children with ADHD may be the result of problems in one or more of these regions. Let's take a look first at the *frontal cortex*. This region arranges high-level functioning such as maintaining attention, organization, and executive function. A deficiency of norepinephrine within this brain region might cause inattention, problems with organization skills, and impaired executive functioning. Second is the limbic system. This region of the human brain is located deeper inside the brain. The responsibility of this region is to regulate our emotions. Therefore, a deficiency in this region might result in restlessness, inattention, or emotional balance. Third is the region of the *basal ganglia* in our brain.

The responsibility of these neural circuits is to regulate communication within the brain. Basically, the information from all regions of our brain enters the basal ganglia and is relayed to the correct sites in the brain. For this purpose, a deficiency in the basal ganglia can cause information to short-circuit which then results in inattention or impulsivity. Fourth and last is the region of the reticular activating system. The responsibility of this is the major relay system among the many pathways that enter and leave the brain. A deficiency in this region can cause inattention, impulsivity, or hyperactivity.

Despite being aware of such information, we still don't know which brain region is the source of *ADHD symptoms*, nor can we tell whether the problem lies with a deficiency of norepinephrine itself or of its chemical constituents, dopa and dopamine. Although medicine can be another treatment, there are many therapies for understanding ADHD and dopamine release with children and adolescents. A child's focus on the positive is in fact a neutral consequence of the increase reward driving in the adolescent brain. During this age, there is an increase in the activity of the neural circuits utilizing dopamine, a neurotransmitter central in creating our drive for reward.

Research also shows that the baseline level of dopamine is lower. However, its release in response to experience is higher, which explains why teens are feeling bored if they are not engaged in stimulating activities. Therefore, being engaged with novel activities can increase dopamine and the flow of experiences of being alive for adolescents. The brain *increase drive for reward* in adolescents display in teens' lives might be in three ways. First, it increases impulsiveness, which means behaviors occur without thoughtful reflection.

This is based on a simple understanding that pulse enables our thoughts to stop and think beyond the immediate dopamine-driven impulse pounding on our mind. This impulse places our brain in better cognitive controls and safety awareness. This impulse or hold at adolescents can set if create space on brain and create mental understanding of impulse and action which begin to grow to counteract the revved up go of the dopamine reward system. The second way in which dopamine can be increased is sensitivity to addiction. Many behaviors and substances that are addictive involve the release of dopamine.

Therefore, individual continue to engage in the behavior despite knowing its negative impact. And the third type of behavior shaped by the increase reward is hyperrationality. This means adolescents can put more into the benefit of excitement than the potential risks of such action. What is going on with this way of thinking is not necessarily lacking of reflection (impulsive), and it's not being addicted to a certain behavior, but the brain places more weight on positive outcomes than negative ones. This process unfolds once teen years come to an end.

We move from literal thinking of hyperrationality to more on the side of *considerable way* of thinking. The aim goes deeper toward bigger pictures over immediately focusing on the release of the dopamine reward. This is essential in understanding adolescents' behavior or being point as impulsive behavior or just knowing the risks they can take from time to time. Many teens can be rational and thus need to incorporate the nonrational input of their intuitive gut feelings or heart sensation to enable themselves to focus on positivity which values allows rewards to in much better experience.

Another factor of seeing teenage brain is on top of the emotional spark for driven rewards, social networking experience and peer pressure is also playing part for essence. The decision which is made in a group is the combination of rewards driven, peer process, and hyperrationality to nongist thinking as a result. This is the nature of risky behaviors which emerges often from the teenager's brain. Mostly risky behaviors emerge from hyperrationality, the unbalanced nature of pros and cons or impulsivity for adolescents. The important learning experience educators, parents, and schools might take on is the changes that occur in adolescents' brain are not merely about maturity over immaturity yet rather are essential developmental *transitions* that enable certain abilities and behavior to take place.

Throughout this age group, integration plays the development process by linking different parts to the whole region of the brain. Another aspect is the *growth of fibers of cognitive control* that brings awareness to impulsivity, making space into mind to pause and reconsider. It's essential to knowledge for honoring adolescents' development chain rather than viewing it as a process of immature brain and they can *grow out of it*. Adolescents absorb information from experiences. Thus, during their transition of development journey, the support of parents and educators contributes to the development of their brain. As we learned, our brain development is based on "experience shapes—induce neural activation" and by genetic information processing. How we decide to do things also reveals who we are and how our brain functions at that moment.

Therefore, understanding adolescents' brain might determine their actions or purpose. Just know that in this period, the brain changes in two dimensions. Such as how to reduce the amount of brain basic cells, the neurons and their linkage, the synapses which also calls pruning. This is also getting its effect from experience and how to handle stress. The growth of neurons and their synapses is much during childhood, and this overproduction of neurons and synapses can extend till age eleven for girls and age twelve for boys.

Brain transformation during adolescence is that it lays down myelin which is a sheath covering the membrane among interconnected neurons. The responsibility of this myelin sheath is enabling the passage of the electrical flow and the neuronal activation between other neurons for better synchronized information processing. As we also learn new skills, we grow new connections, even new neurons. Once we could establish a new *synapse linkage*, we can lay down myelin for making the circuits faster and more effective. These two fundamental changes of pruning and myelination support brain well-being in *adolescents*.

Just as we explored, there are *different types of neurons*. By the same token, there are also different *types of chemical neurotransmitters*. Researchers studying mental illness believe that abnormalities in how particular brain circuits function contribute to the development of many mental illnesses. For example, connections between nerve cells along certain pathways or circuits in the brain can develop to problems with how the brain processes information; and this might be the result for abnormal mood, thinking, perception, or behavior. Can it be possible one aspect of *autism spectrum disorder* is relevant or an absolute lack of ability to communicate with others at a social level? In the reason, individuals who have inability to relate themselves in the ordinary way to people and situations or lake of ability to imagine themselves in the situation of other individuals are not fully aware or might be mind-blind? As we read, awareness has stages: awareness of self and awareness of others.

Therefore, autism might include difficulty in attributing the mental state of others too. Can it be possible then that this disorder links more with *social and emotional deficit* than developmental delays? Well, any leaking of integration (nature and nurture) will result in such delay. For instance, deficit in social-emotional reciprocity and deficit in nonverbal communication behavior that we use for social interaction will lead to development delay somehow. We have come down to the point where science education, physics, and mathematics are not alone in contributing to learning, but further to what we have achieved in this century.

I met a boy who sees himself as a ADHD kid sometimes. His few friends have understanding of his ADHD and are less judgmental toward what he might be doing at some point during their activities.

He might be suffering from some neurological unbalanced chemicals to understand ADHD, but not too severe. What I gained from this child was *this simple understanding*:

I Am, and I Am Not

I am not my pills nor I have ADHD
I am a child who can't sit still, I have energy
I have suffered from not playing soccer
I have suffered from not playing hockey
I have suffered from not playing wrestling
I have suffered from not doing any activity
My teacher wants me to sit, my mom sends me to bed
My games make me play
My times make me stay
I am not my schedule; I am a child
I am not my discipline; I am a wild
I have suffered from childhood
I have suffered from wildhood
I have suffered from misunderstandings
I am not my pills nor I am ADHD
I am Jack, an active boy
That's who I am, yes, that is who I am
I give away my energy, now I am not me
I give away the pills, now I can see
I am a child who can't sit still, I am not a wild
Jack who I am, that's only who I want to be
A unique me with unique activity
Jack!

What was surprising to see was his best friends were *mimicking* his higher-energy activities. I observed the small group for a while. His friends were all acting higher-energy activities such as fidgeting in class, dancing, moving between activities, smiling, and laughing. It put me in *wonder*, has this higher-energy happiness to some point affected his close friends and classmates? I don't think that ADHD can be contagious. Consequently, it's a nature-and-nurture and mirror-neuron experience that I was getting.

I tried to *interfere* with one of the *friends* by making him realize if he was aware of his action (playful fighting) at some point. He said confidently that he is aware of his activities and fighting, but then again, *he likes it.* I asked him, "Why do you like it?" He said it's a fun way of getting him through the class routines and daily settings and keeping him alert to some point. To me it meant he is soothing himself through long hours of sitting and class routines.

Could it be that our educational experience of psychology is not there yet, despite all relevant research? The etiology of ADHD is not yet understood, though research suggests that biological and environmental factors (e.g., family and community) contribute to its development and course. Well, the etiology of ADHD is complex and multifaceted. Strong evidence implicates genetic and neurological factors, as well as their interactions with the environment, as core components of the development of ADHD. Although other contributors to the etiology of ADHD have been proposed, which might be poor parenting and food additives, these factors have limited or mixed evidence supporting the cause.

Could it be possible to *prevent ADHD without the use of drugs*? It might. Nondrug interventions for ADHD include making adjustments in the environment to promote more successful social interactions. Such adjustments include creating more structure and encouraging routines. Children with ADHD may need help in organizing their activities in daily life. Therefore, some simple interventions to try for childhood ADHD may include a simpler schedule, like making sure your child has almost the same routine every day. The schedule might include a balance between homework time and playtime. Post this schedule in a prominent place in your home where it can be viewed easily by your child. Help or cooperate with your child to organize everyday items. Work with your child to have a shelf or a relevant place for everything. This includes clothing, backpacks, and school supplies. Note that children with ADHD might need consistent rules that they can easily follow. When your child follows their rules, they should be rewarded.

Managing ADHD with many therapies—consciousness practice, such as mindfulness (meditation)—is a better solution not only for the children, but for the caregivers, teachers, and parents. However, the only important point to the all-brain health concern is understanding the concern itself prior to any treatment, therapy of some sort, or rescheduling the daily routine. It's important to understand the definition of what ADHD (or any other brain health concern) is and its symptoms according to the inaugural's age and stage of development. It's the first choice to think with an educated brain than a meditative one. Educating psychologists, nurses, teachers, professors, and health care workers about brain health education is an essential part of providing treatment and educating patients on their diagnoses. When it comes down to the definition of the brain (interpersonal brain journey), up-to-date information should be necessary.

Let's take a brief look at *attention-deficit* hyperactivity disorder (ADHD), which is a chronic condition that affects millions of children and often persists into adulthood. ADHD includes a combination of problems, such as difficulty sustaining attention, hyperactivity, and impulsive behavior. Symptoms can be difficulty paying attention; frequently daydreaming; difficulty following through on instructions and apparently not listening; frequently having problems organizing tasks or activities; frequently forgetting and losing needed items, such as books, pencils, or toys; frequently failing to finish schoolwork, chores, or other tasks; being easily distracted; frequently fidgeting or squirming; difficulty remaining seated and being seemingly in constant motion; being excessively talkative; frequently interrupting or intruding on others' conversations or games; and frequently having trouble waiting for his or her turn.

Well, it turns out one such treatment strategy—therapy—has been around for generations. Still it's a hot research topic at the UCLA Mindful Awareness Research Center (MARC) and many other educational facilities around the globe. Researchers have explored many venues about using mindfulness for ADHD children for some time, but the question was always whether children with ADHD could really do it, especially if they're hyperactive and children. Unlike many tools for ADHD, mindfulness develops the individual's inner skills. It improves the ability to control attention by helping to strengthen the ability to self-observe and self-control. In other words, it teaches to pay attention to what we are paying attention to. It also helps children to be more *aware of their emotional state* so they won't react impulsively.

If we look into *the brain development point of view*, brain development is a process that begins shortly after conception and continues into our midtwenties. The brain creates self from an embryonic structure which is called the neural tube. This process is called neurulation. Shortly after the next few months, these embryonic brain cells proliferate and differentiate into particular cell types. After they migrate to take up appropriate positions inside the growing structure of the brain, these cells then begin to create the connections that will create the brain's neural circuits. It's very clear that the first few years of life are a period of intense activity in the development of the brain. Important connections are rapidly being formed among brain cells (as interconnectedness forms) that allow them to exchange information and form circuits. Hereafter, these circuits form the architecture of our brain that allows us to interpret information from our environment and interact with the world around us.

Now we can come closer to understand that our feelings and the actions we perform originate from our *brain*. With that knowledge in *mind*, we can say the most basic circuits that rule the most basic skills of us—likely the sensory systems—form first. This basic system will provide the foundation and scaffolding for more complex circuits which will rule more complex behaviors, for instance, the language, attention, and emotional regulation to build on top from bottoms up. It is back to the understanding of nature-and-nurture development.

This book aims to explore all venues of our development as well as shed light on the whole brain-mind-consciousness as one direction of our growing-up journey, not the sum of the whole. Thus, the circuit's ruling of all of our skills is built sequentially, meaning with simpler skills to begin that provide the support for future, more complex behaviors. One of our most complex skill sets is the executive function. Unfortunately, it doesn't finish developing until our mid twenties. If ADHD or a similar disease be the disconnectedness issue from early development, wouldn't it be possible to link this connection through daily experiences? Well, we sure can, because once the connections in a given brain circuit are formed, the brain purifies these *connections* through experience.

We have explored the connection between our neurons and our experiences, our attention and the function of brain development. Would *meditation* be that linkage between them? Well, those connections that get used more become very strong and less likely to change as compared to those connections that get used the least. Aside to all other theories to practice, science to neurological studies, this is another developmental process which is called pruning.

What's important to remember is that the experiences (how experiences) we have in childhood will have an impact on how our brain's circuits get used. As much as it's essential to learning the conversation between our circuits, as much for whose teaching. Can it be important to say our childhood memories (especially emotional experiences) affect how we teach ourselves to teach children? Are we responsible for recognizing our own misconnections perhaps? Even for adults, high-quality experiences will reinforce important cognitive, social, and emotional skills that are necessary for teaching-learning, which will form *close relationships* and positive health outcomes. As adult learners, if we not create bottoms up, but still create a solid foundation that benefit for additional development.

Children who do not have better opportunities, especially those who are exposed to negative experiences, are likely have poorer outcomes in comparison. In this way, the quality of the brain's architecture can have a profound influence on our outcomes throughout life. It's best if adults recognize children with any mental health concerns earlier as it's possible to connect the discontented regions (circuits) in early stages. Children's emotion, their caregivers, attachment bond, subjective experiences, mindfulness, creativity, and the environment are brain depending in a point to how much gets its daily dose of stimulation. For instance, if HD is hyperactive disorder, what would create the linkage to put this disorder back together? We can agree that numbing the brain with any types of treatment is temporary and a Band-Aid type of solutions.

Can it be possible that *mindfulness (awareness-updated-information)* is an essential dose of daily learning experience at schools? It might be the only solution at one point that our experience changes our neurons and our brain's development. The solution might lead us again to the same path as we start our writing journey, the role of brain, mind, consciousness, and educational systems. Today more than ever, humans search for an understanding of the world inside out.

Brain architecture is the building block of understanding the story of early brain development and its result—lifelong health. Our life narrative structures itself from the early stage—either positive or negative experiences can change the development and function of our brain.

Our *emotions* such as primary emotions directly reflect the changes in states of mind (close relationship). *It's the emotional experience that allows to understand life's meaning. Emotions serve as meaning to information we attain. Where that is how range of differentiated process become integrated (become aware).* Emotion also serves as our daily drive, our motivation. Just remember the story of snake bite(if you ever get bitten by a snake) in childhood and being scared anytime coming across long rope throughout adulthood. This is due to the flow of energy throughout our system that allows us to be cautious and hypervigilant as way of responding to past experiences. The mental state activity at a given time shapes the elaboration of arousal and meaning from primary to categorical emotions. Our primary emotions act as primary colors; we mix it with other colors to build on it.

Emotions, like fear and love, are carried out by our *limbic system*. We learned a bit that this is located in the temporal lobe. While the limbic system is made up of multiple parts, the center of emotional processing is the amygdala through which we receive input from other brain functions (interconnected) like memory and our attention. Yes, the shapes look like almond. As we learned, the amygdala is responsible for multiple emotional responses, like love, fear, anger, and sexual desire. Therefore, damage to the amygdala can result in abnormal emotional responses, and overstimulation causes excessive reactions. Our hippocampus is another part of the limbic system that sends information to the amygdala region. One of the memory processing centers of the brain region, the "hippocampus" interacts with the amygdala when we have memories that involve the emotional aspect. This may be the origin of strong emotions triggered by particular memories, such as responses to traumatic memories.

As we learned about brain function and their interconnectedness with our overall development, we understood our prefrontal cortex, located near the front of the head that is involved in *decision-making in response* to our *emotions*. This region of the brain (prefrontal cortex) controls what decision a person would make when faced with an emotional reaction and also regulates anxiety. Another part of the limbic system is our *hypothalamus* that feeds the information to the *amygdala*. This region, the hypothalamus, acts as a regulator of emotion, controlling levels of sexual desire, pleasure, aggression, and anger. Interconnectedness in mind, the cingulate gyrus acts as a pathway between the thalamus and the hippocampus. This region is responsible for the role in remembering our emotionally charged events. This region of the cingulate gyrus focuses its attention on saturation and alerting the rest of the brain that a certain event is emotionally significant (pay attention).

Let's not leave the *ventral tegmental area* when we complete the regulation of emotions. This *tegmental region* is also involved in emotions, especially in how a person perceives the pleasure. Also, the dopamine pathways are located in the ventral tegmental area. We learned the dopamine is a neurotransmitter.

Thus, it is involved in mood, and increased levels elevate the person's stage of pleasure. Not leaving the *cerebrum* as the largest part of the human brain that is covered by gray deep folds and wrinkles that makes up 85 percent of the brain weight. This is the thinking part of the brain and it controls the voluntary muscles. This location is responsible for housing short-term and long-term memories. However, the *limbic system* is referred to as the *emotional brain*. This region of the brain the thalamus looks as the gatekeeper for messages passed from the spinal cord and cerebrum. The hypothalamus controls our emotions to regulate the temperature by telling the body to sweat when it's overheated and to shiver when it's cold.

This integration is wonderfully complex and educationally important for learning experience in schools for teachers dealing with children with ADHD or other mental health concerns. ADHD or related to brain health education can't be treated to a single understanding of treatment (especially medicine) as we just explored the interconnectedness function of the whole brain-to-mind-to-body system. For instance, the hippocampus sends memories to be stored in sections of the cerebrum, then recalls them when necessary. When next time we become sad, happy, thirsty, or excited, we learned good enough the important part of integration—brain, mind, experience, mindfulness, and our system of function as a whole.

Let's dive even deeper. Information about our *social surrounding* directly affects our *appraisal* process. With that said, let's look into our social integration system and the effects on the appraisal process. If we look in to emotions and empathy level of understanding. Many studies have independently argued that the *mirror neuron* system is involved in emotions and empathy. Could it be true that people who are more empathic have stronger activations both in the mirror system for hand actions and the mirror system for emotions? The function that arbitrates by mirror neurons depends on the anatomy of the physiological properties of our circuit that these neurons live.

Emotional and empathetic activations were found in regions of parieto-premotor circuits. *These are responsible for motor action control. We learned neurons become active with attention. Also, mirror neurons are activated when actions are both executed and observed.* This may explain how people understand the states of other people. It sounds like mirroring observed the action inside the brain as if it conducted the observed action. Could it be this is relevant to humans when they anticipate and make sense of the behavior of other people by activating their mental processes? When this is carried into action, would it produce similar behavior? Would this be the intentional behavior as well as the expression of emotions? This reminded me of the story of Jack and his classmates again.

Could it be that the children were *mirroring Jack's excitement*, full of energy activities, etc.? If yes, then could it be also possible for Jack to mirror his classmates' behaviors? There are high chances children at school teach themselves how to adapt to new experiences. Often children use their own emotions to predict what others will do. Therefore, we can project our own mental states onto others. *A balanced class might also contain the combination of any stage and age of development at some point over an individual's class settings.*

This will bring us back to the idea that the integration of our mind is not only within our own brain or consciousness or between ourselves, but between other people and universe. Neural processes and social relationships contribute both to our mental abilities and to our development. We learned our middle prefrontal circuits function to "integrate" the processing of social information and autobiographical consciousness, aside from the evaluation of the meaning of the information, the activation of our arousal, and the coordination of the bodily response in addition to higher cognitive processes. Let's look at mirror neurons and human awareness at this point.

Could it be possible that *mirror neurons* provide the *neurological basis* for human self-awareness? We learned mirror neurons can help simulate other people's behavior at some point. Can it be this turned *inward* to our own self-awareness? Or maybe create second-order representations of one's own earliest brain processes. This could be the result of a neural basis of self-analysis and of the trade of self-awareness and other awareness. This is essential to understand our own mental life experiences that might contribute to others' learning experiences. This might have opened up a door of metaphysical secrets in the mirror neuron brain that has shaped our development side. When we talk about awareness, it's best to shed light on consciousness and emotions.

Emotion is a nonconscious process. Emotions describe the motion of our behavior within our environment. Our brain gets information from two different sources: First, our senses tell us what's going on in the outside world, while our emotions exist inside our body to tell us what these events and circumstances mean to us. This is another reason for defining the brain as an interpersonal brain aside from its anatomy. Just as hunger motivates humans to find food, *emotions motivate* humans to take care of other needs—like safety and companionship—that ultimately promote human survival and reproduction. Second, emotions are controlled by the levels of different chemicals inside the brain, not necessarily by *love* or *hate chemical.* At any given moment, dozens of neurotransmitters are active, and some of these neurotransmitters go between individual cells, and others are broadcast to the entire brain. By layering signals on other signals, the brain can adjust how humans respond to things and can effectively alter the mood. For instance, in dangerous situations, the brain releases stress *hormones* that make humans react faster, flooding certain regions with the neurotransmitter *epinephrine* (adrenaline). When the danger subsides, the brain sends out a calming signal in the form of chemicals which dampen the response of regions that create fear.

Humans, like all mammals, produce basic emotions such as fear and anger. Humans have especially highly developed *social emotions,* like shame, guilt, or pride. This involves an awareness of what other people think and feel about us. Researchers are increasingly looking toward newer networks to understand better how the brain controls mood. These two particular networks might be the answer that stand out, which are the autobiographic *memory network and the cognitive control network.* The human autobiographic memory network processes information about our ourselves (interpersonal), including recalling personal memories and self-reflection.

The important key hubs in this network comprise brain areas inside the *prefrontal cortex,* which sits in the front of the brain; the hippocampus; the posterior cingulate cortex, which is the upper part of the limbic lobe; and parietal regions, which sit behind the frontal lobe. These regions and their functions are important for mental imagery. And our cognitive control network links up regions that coordinate our attention and concentration. Therefore, we can complete tasks. *Integration among brain circuits is important. However, "the how-to relationship of this integration" is the curving point in mind development.* It recruits a circuit of the front part of the cingulate cortex and dorsolateral prefrontal cortex. These areas are specialized for cold, unemotional, rational thought. These two networks are thought to have a drawn relationship.

The *autobiographic memory network* switches on when the brain is preoccupied by thoughts which lead the task-oriented cognitive control network to switch off. As a result, it reduces our ability to complete the given task we're supposed to be doing. This is why daydreaming is frowned on at work. On the other hand, the autobiographic memory network is suppressed when the cognitive control network is required to gather the attention needed for a given task to complete. It's best to know when the two networks don't work properly (relationship), they can result in mood disorders. There are two types of memory. The first type is autobiographical memory, such as personal experience, self-reflection, and self-focus.

The second type is ty *cognitive memory*, which includes logical, task-oriented, focus attention and beyond ourselves. Let's take a look at the connections of our memory, its type, and our mood therefore in brief. There are two important types of mood disorders. The first type is depressive disorder. This is characterized by a persistent down mood or feeling down. The second type is bipolar disorder. This is expressed as extreme high or manic moods that alternate with periods of feeling down. In the case of depressive disorders, the brain's autobiographic memory network gets stuck being on. Therefore, this results into thinking much about the self. The symptoms are unhappy thoughts, rumination, and self-loathing. Yet our thoughts on the source of emotion can be full of contradictions.

We are familiar with thinking of the mind, which we might mean emotion, imagination, reason, and other conscious and unconscious processes of the brain and still might think our body as definite and separate. We might have also associated emotions with different parts of the body. For instance, love comes from the heart and anger from the spleen, or even fear is something we feel in our spine, so to speak. Since we understood the integration system between: ourselves and our interpersonal relationships, our brain and mind and feeling the felt of something might be right which also called as a "a gut feeling" can also be a true statement.

The fact is generally agreed to lie somewhere in between these two views. As the discussion on the mind/body debate demonstrates, there is very little support for the "dualist" school of thought that holds the mind is separated from the body. There is no support from psychologists or physicians that would argue that emotions are the product of the different organs of the body, because emotion is believed to be generated from a physical source, and the part of the brain responsible for it is the *limbic system*. As we learned, the limbic system is made up of several structures located in the cerebral cortex—structures register the levels of chemicals called *neurotransmitters* that are being manufactured by our body in response to certain conditions the person is experiencing. Since we understood our emotions, the importance of *relation integration*, and the function of our brain-mind as a whole, then, let's take one direction toward what mental health might be. Can mental health be defined well if there is no definition for the mind?

Well, according to this book journey and so many other professors' research, I am sure you are agreeing to say no. We can safely say that few aspects of *mental health* include our emotional, psychological, and social well-being. It affects how we think as much as our thoughts affect our brain development. Our mental health is the integration of our overall health. Therefore, it determines *how we handle stress*, relate to others, and make daily choices. Mental health continues at every stage of life, from childhood and adolescence through adulthood. *To understand our mental health, we must learn the importance of overall integration (brain-mind-body-others-community-universe) up to today. This is an essential part of interpersonal development and our identity, not just a career for the health department.*

Any symptoms or characteristics you're about to research will convince you the system of integration is the only way to evaluate. Studies of integration are not new to scientists. Integration has been an essential part of numerous disciplines so far, for instance, from the brain to emotional and social functions or consciousness. In this book, we conclude the *relation integration* not as a sum (brain-mind or consciousness, etc.) but as a whole system of development. We learned about our *brain stimulation to bodily organs* and mindfulness connections to consciousness, as well as our social aspect of integration as our mind affects ourselves and others.

The good part of this book journey is it offers two ways in which the internal processes of the brain combine with a stimulus input from the body to give rise to a picture in the mind and consciousness. The way we will explore is that the input from the body is supplemented by the brain before it reaches the mind. And another way is the idea that the brain *generates output* to the mind that is supplemented *by input from the body*, such as when it looks to our facial expressions to determine what kind of emotions the mind should be experiencing which this interaction between the body and the brain is so subtle.

Our facial expressions play a significant role in how the brain experiences emotions. It's not surprising that the way in which the muscles in our bodies (such as in our face) are held can influence the emotional state in which we find ourselves. This might be beneficial to expand on to how input from the body is manipulated by the brain before reaching the mind. This might explain our state of mind, which is it's not as the emergent way that we feel, yet as the activity in the brain that is a result of the shift of energy stream among neuronal circuits as the neuron network receives, operates, and outputs information.

Certain systems of the brain are *activated* at the same time and can rebate *linkage* with each other to affect the processing of each other. Therefore, these patterns of activity give rise to the emotions, thoughts, or sensations that we can then consciously become aware and share with others. We well understood the importance of interpersonal relationships and experiences with brain development.

Thus, the capturing of experience inside our memory is an interesting way to learn. It shows the influence of a person's brain and mind on their perception of their surroundings, how this *networking* ability arises from the modification of neurons themselves as well as the way in which they are wired and *integrated to other neurons*. It is likely that experience can be saved as memory encoded in specific neuron-firing patterns and might activate again in the future. These firing patterns interpret into the memory of the experience.

Human *memory is a subjective process* in which experience plays a role by giving us things to remember. Just like we understood Jack's own point of view. What is essential to take on from Jack's poem was how the *brains remember* those experiences and how we understood ourselves in those memories. Our memory is also being reworked with the input of new experience and often repeats the idea that the brain communicates not just with its own, but also with other brains. It does this in the form of integration between us and others, such as through visual emotional cues or the verbal sharing of memories, thoughts, sensations, and emotions. The idea behind the saying "No one lives their life alone" serves its purpose and is another contributor to the *evolutionary mind.*

We have the ability to change ourselves, our past experiences, memories, and others by sharing our brain's journey with each other. Eventually everything is shareable and bearable because the brain is constantly changing; and consequently a human's state of mind, memory, and future experiences are not static as a result. Other ways to learn more about our memory is that memory can be about linkages in the brain over mainly understanding to being *alphabetical albums* to be accessed when needed. Human retrieved memories are by learning experiences, and somehow vulnerable to deformation than being saved details—accurate photocopies of the past, especially knowing there are different types of memory *(implicit memories and explicit memories)*.

Implicit memories require less awareness than explicit memories. Think of implicit memory as the type of memory that lets you do stuff without thinking, like brushing your hair. On the other hand, explicit memories are about the first time you tried something new, starting your first work. What to take on from this point of memory system is to understand how children's relationships are with implicit memories day by day. Going to school, playing games, eating, watching television, and playing with friends are becoming more relevant information. However, the memories and experiences children have now are what they'll remember later on in their life, which result as part of long-term memories just by repeating. The more fun experiences children will have at schools, the more they'll want to continue to the future.

In *Jack's case*, if he views himself in one instance as a child with higher energy and feelings of missing the full understanding from his educators, parents, or classmates, this daily memory is not what he wants to learn from. What a small thing a professional can do to bring up full *awareness of self* and whichever follows up after *I am* is accepted in fun-loving therapies for role modeling, *balance between medicine,* mindfulness, and development-appropriate creativities as a result of today's learning experiences of *interpersonal neurobiology* and human development.

This is how the principles of an interdisciplinary approach to psychotherapy which is called interpersonal neurobiology. Interpersonal neurobiology is a new science and new approach that examines independent fields that emerge to paint a bigger picture of human experience and development. The mind appears in the agreement of at least neurobiological and interpersonal processes. This flow of energy and information can be within us and between us. As part of the whole process, other features of our world such as the *nature and environment* can also impact how the mind emerges.

Within studies of *psychotherapy*, we can see that relationships with another person profoundly shape the flow of energy and information between two people, and within each person. The perspective of interpersonal neurobiology is also to build a fundamental purpose which the *objective domains of science and the subjective domains of human knowledge* can find a common ground. The learning process of *interpersonal neurobiology and integration system* is to offer a balanced understanding of the mind and of mental well-being that can be used by a wide range of professionals, schools, colleges, or professors as learning experiences with *human development. Human development is not just defined by brain development or mind*, but *by brain, mind, and spirit as a whole.* Any misleads are halfway through the development process.

The *mind develops not in early years, but across the life span,* because the genetically programmed maturation of the *nervous system is shaped by the continuum experience process.* And our brain has trillions of connections to one hundred billion neurons and an average of ten thousand synaptic connections that link one neuron to others. *The story of nature needs nurture is an essential part of the learning experience of this book journey. Therefore, the definition of brain continues—open-minded.* We learned how synaptic linkages are created both by genes and by experience. Interpersonal experiences shape new connections among neurons by how genes are activated.

In addition to such, this is how proteins are produced and how interconnections are established within our neural networking system. The brain has self-regulatory circuits that may directly contribute to enhancing how the mind regulates the stream of its *two important elements: the energy and the information.* Despite being aware of our mind, many different definitions exist to what mind is. However, there are better results to today's approach of the mind that can be an embodied process. The responsibility of such is to maintain this stream of energy and information.

Furthermore, information that has a close relationship with where, why, how, when, and what serves the purpose of our knowledge and defining our personal brain. This maintaining process might also be at the heart of our mental life. Earlier in our book journey, we learned through the important part of brain regions and the association with ADHD or related mental health concerns. When separated regions of the brain are allowed to specialize in their function and then to become integrated together, the system is said to be working as a whole over its sum part. An integrated brain is a whole brain, meaning it's *closely connected with its parts* to its mind and its consciousness. For example, brain communication systems with its parts are much essential to communication with the mind.

The human brain has a left side that helps with logical thinking, language, sequence, details, rules, order, and organizing thoughts into sentences. On the other half is the right side that helps humans experience their emotions, nonverbal communication, images, interpersonal relationships and memories, music, art, dance, creativities, and nonverbal cues; and it's more connected to the lower brain area which receives, understands, and processes emotional information. The two sides are connected by a bundle of fibers also in a way that humans need them to work together.

Children, however, are most likely to operate from *their right brains* as they haven't developed the abilities to use logic, understand time, and use words to express feelings fully yet. Thus, learning how to create communication via daily experiences is depending on how much today's learning experience, educators' and parents' experience, and educational systems allow us to learn through classrooms or nonclass activities. There are lessons to learn how to create relationships between ourselves and *brain stimulation*. For example, children are experiencing emotions as adults do. It's essential to understand this is the operating of their right brain. When *language or logic* tells them it isn't so bad, trying to distract them, none of these strategies might be beneficial yet as they're left-brain strategies. Therefore, activities are necessary to be integrated with mental abilities, considering brain development throughout education, especially from *preschool to grade 6*.

For *preschool children*, the emphasis of *education should also be brain stimulation* and for growing further into deeper intellect level and mindfulness *(aware of self and energy information)* for future development, over numerical, mathematics, geography lessons alone, etc. *Such and such activities perhaps need to use the right brain to connect with the left (integration) to tune in to their emotions, to resonate with children's personal experience and acknowledge their feelings. This also plays a role in increasing dopamine and energy flows into brain cells.* To redirect with the *left brain*, sometimes it only needs logic and understanding while using *language* as a way of activity or suggestion. How our neurons are shaped by experience, environment, and relationships is also part of the emotional importance of life's difficulties. Trying to talk children out of their feelings or avoiding painful experiences is not a well-defined development journey. Instead, picking a time to have a storytelling about the difficult events is a great strategy for integrating both sides of the brain, which the left tells the story of the right brain's strong emotion just by using language and logic. We explored enough of *brain anatomy* to understand the *structure and function* of each part. Thus, the lower brain develops early and is responsible for bodily functions like breathing, as well as for strong emotional reactions like fight (anger), flight (fear), or freeze (fear). A small region in the lower brain can cause us to react emotionally without being aware of it. The upper region of the brain which is the top part of the *cortex* (the area behind your forehead) *develops* later in *childhood* and through into *adulthood*.

This is the place where *mental processes happen*, meaning making better decisions, the understanding of self, the controls of the body— emotion, empathy, a sense of right and wrong, etc. As much as the left side of the brain is depending on the right side, by the same token, the strong upstairs brain balances out the downstairs brain and is essential for social-emotional intelligence. Throughout the class activities teachers adding opportunities to help children practice upstairs brain skills, such as decision to make is essential. This is also as simple as giving choices about what to eat, what to drink, etc. From grade 1 onward, it's often best to observe but not interact with choices and conflict kids' face. Don't rescue them (unless it's necessary). However, help them predict possible outcomes.

There are many *strategies for regulating emotions*, such as calming techniques like taking a deep breath (take a belly breath). Older kids can learn to slow down using counting as a metaphor or even better learn *mindfulness practices* such as meditation. The best perditions coming from mindfulness practices are a reflection on their feelings, helping them predict what they might feel in a new situation or how they might have handled it. These simple but necessary practices build relationships between self as a form of interpersonal experience and between other relationships and also create empathy and morality. This teaches not what is simply right or wrong, but understanding how our actions as part of neural networking systems *impact the society* as a whole. For instance, one who prefers to be left alone without paying attention to his lonesome will impact his friends; they will become lonely too. This is a true interpersonal love experience of my own. How much we are different is a learning experience, yet knowing how we are made of one fabrication is the important lesson to take on.

Practicing to do the right thing has already developed us into having an *evolutionary brain*; compassion, kindness, and empathy are carried out not necessarily because of rules alone, but because knowing right from wrong places us to be the only species which survived. This *evolutionary movement* also changed the *brain chemistry* and served the purpose of an integrated brain well. When children are missing information and aren't connecting well with their upstairs brain, it's the role of adults to get them moving to integrate their brain. The implications of such discipline are significant, yet one way to explore is that we don't *own* our minds—that we as individuals are interdependent on others for the functioning of our minds. This *relational* part of the integration might be uncomfortably subjective. However, if you are in a family or married relationship, it is known that our subjective, inner mental life is profoundly influenced by others regardless of gender differences.

It's best to mention mental health concerns such as depression and anxiety are soaring. The questions of whether antidepressants work or not and whether sex is more vulnerable to anxiety and depression are still learning experiences. This is a well-understood subject from the scientific side of *anthropologists*. They know from research how real this relational component of our mental lives truly is. What we need is a *linkage, our connections to the social with the brain synaptic.* To achieve the essential ability to move readily between these two levels of human reality, we will have to explore possibilities within this book journey to find the common ground that links them. Not being able to understand brain development, interpersonal communication systems, and our relationships with the memory, *children integrate their difficult memories into adulthood.* Their emotions will show up in their behavior, which can affect both them and us (we).

With simple practices, we can determine greater outcomes as what's a challenging memory for a child might seem pretty harmless to adults. The important aspect the education system plays is to introduce brain and mind development as one another's important aspect (subject) of school and college daily curriculums. What might have been more essential if we could carry such educational experiences—aside from our *evolutionary brain of today.* It means understanding our own minds is a key factor, which then we can use to understand the minds of others.

Teaching students from K to grade 12 to know: what's on their mind, what is awareness, what is consciousness, and how to focus attention on the body. Likewise, they use: the images they have from their experiences (memory), the imagination (from the right brain), the feelings they have (right brain), and the thought they are using to understand their world (left brain) which all these leads to process of our developments not a product. Interpersonal neurobiology, the brain-to-mind integration system, is necessary to help *educators* and students to develop the continuum aspect of human development to integrate self, others, and environments and to develop *relationships* based on kindness, compassion, and empathy. *Integration between the two brains is based on an understanding of the communication. What makes it effective is how we communicate to share our experiences of energy and information.*

When *teachers* speak to *students*, the voice box stimulates this movement of air molecules which manifests as kinetic energy flow. Then the eardrum responds to this energy pattern by creating electrochemical energy movement within the acoustic nerve and downstream *neural circuits* of the brain. Much of the molecules flow in and out of the *neural membranes* and then release *chemical transmitters* which activate downstream neurons. Hereafter when these patterns of neural firing match with prior learning experience, then this *energy flow carries informational value* that results in an understanding between the teachers and students. However, where are these shared elements of mental life taking place?

Many research and brain imaging studies examine the metabolic, energy-consuming processes in specific neural regions in addition to the blood flow to certain areas that are thought to be a *clustering of localized neuronal activity. Electroencephalograms (EEGs) assess the electrical* activity across the surface of the brain which is measured by electrodes. *These studies of neuroscientists are the way in which the brain functions through the energy-consuming activation of neurons.*

The best understanding of this learning process shows the degree and *localization of the arousal* and activation within the brain—this flow of energy has directly shaped *human mental* processes. Let's not forget that thoughts are processes and refer to mental operations and problem-solving skills that are suitable for the handling of *comparison, combination, transformation* of different types of information, *relations, and problems*. What do mental operations look like or peruse? They serve an identifiable special function or purpose toward the organism's adaptational needs. They are much responsible for the *action and processing* of a single type of objects and relations among *environmental entities*.

Importantly, they are responsible for enabling the organism to deal with a particular type of environmental relations. This also requires specific operations and processes which are appropriate for the representation and processing of the type of concepts concerned. In a way, these *operations and processes of thought are the mental correspondents* of the type of *relations concerned*. The mental aspect might be analyzed into three main types of components. Specifically, each component involves *core processes (speed, control, spread), mental operations, processing skills, and rules and principles integrating their functioning and use, and the knowledge and beliefs*.

First, the *core processes, meaning* speed, spread, and control, are special kinds of mental processes throughout each system. Therefore, they are very fundamental processes that ground each of the systems into its respective environmental realm. These processes are also the *outcomes of our evolution as a species*. This might also be contributor to characterizing the cognitive functioning of other species. *During brain development, the core processes (speed, spread, control) are the first manifestations of the systems. Therefore, they are mainly action and perception bound.*

As we pointed out, core relationships are integration systems. Thus, core processes are inferential traps within each of the systems that respond to informational structures with core-specific interpretations that carry "value" or meaning to the human species. This operating system, its rules, and its processing skills are systems of human mental actions too which are used to purposefully deal with "information and relations" in each level of the brain structures.

Let's *zoom into brain development* a bit more than we might explore. The operations, the skills, the rules, and the *knowledge arise via influence between each brain region—specific core processes* such as the *environment, the executive and self-monitoring,* and self-regulation processes of the *hypercognitive system.* Therefore, the initial characterized property is gradually transformed into conclusions that are increasingly self-guided and self-reflected upon, and each system involves knowledge of the reality. It is integrated therefore as a whole. Human evolution and development are also a process of such knowledge, accumulating over the years as a result of the interactions between a particular system and its respective domain of reality.

Conceptual and belief systems are too necessarily integrated to the physical, *biological, psychological,* and *social* worlds thus found at this level of the organization of the various systems. We have explored many comprehensive theories of the developing self-aware and self-regulated human mind that integrate the three traditions in psychology, since the end of the nineteenth century. These are the *traditions of cognitive,* differential, and developmental psychology. Among so many other books, we also viewed the architecture of the human mind as to propose that the mind is organized in three stages. Two of the stages are comprising general-purpose mechanisms and processes. The third stage might reflect on comprising specialized systems of thought and problem-solving.

Although integration is one bigger stage throughout the development process, each of the stages is a *complex network of processes* including systems that *involve multiple dimensions* and might be a bank of the organization system alone. However, to just understand the basic purpose of these *three stages* involves *general processes* and *functions* which define the processing potential available at any given time. So the state of the processes composed of this stage drives the condition and functioning of the systems included in the other two levels.

If we look into this *structure and its stages* in detail, we might add the other *two stages* are knowing levels. They involve systems and functions underlying understanding and problem-solving. One of these two knowing levels is the result of the environment. It necessitates systems of cognitive functions and abilities specializing in the representation and processing of the different aspects of the physical and the social environment we live in. Also, the other knowing level is directed to the self. It involves processes aiming self-monitoring, self-representation, and self-regulation.

Therefore, these three stages point for *awareness and consciousness, intentionality,* and self-control. As a result, knowing, learning, or performing any abilities at any time is a mixture of the processes involved in all these three stages of brain-to-mind development. For example, in the *core process of speed,* organisms seek to recognize a simple stimulus as quickly as possible. This can be locating or identifying someone, such as a letter or word which this conditions. Speed of processing indicates the time needed by the system to record and give meaning to the flow of information.

Typically speaking, the faster we can *recognize a stimulus,* the more structured the information processor is thought to be. This is not hard to understand as this is the nature of the human brain because the neural of the *stimuli tend to decay* faster or perhaps expend or might not be relevant any longer by the traces of information later on. Therefore, speed of processing serves its purpose for being a mechanism that would enable thinking organisms to keep control of processing and stay focused on the information—by the same token, filtering out interfering and goal-irrelevant information and shifting focus if required. This might also take our mind toward the memory system, which is the ability of the brain to store, retain, and subsequently recall information. *Traditional studies of memory in the nineteenth and twentieth centuries* began in the realms of philosophy which put memory within the paradigms of *cognitive psychology.*

Thus far, in the *twenty-first century,* it has become one of the principal pillars of a new branch of science that represents an integration system of cognitive psychology and neuroscience that our book journey also learned it as *cognitive neuroscience.*

Cognitive science often leads to the scientific study either of *mind or of intelligence.* The introduction to cognitive science stresses that it is a highly interdisciplinary academic area, in which psychology, neuroscience, linguistics, philosophy, as well as artificial intelligence, anthropology, and biology are its specializations. Cognitive science is the *interdisciplinary* study of cognition in human species, animals, and machines. Another reason of cognitive science is to understand the *principles of intelligence* that might lead to comprehension of the mind and of learning. The main principle of cognitive science is that a whole understanding of the mind and brain cannot be processed by studying a single level.

Even with today's technology to map out every single neuron in the brain and if it were known when each neuron was firing, it would still be impossible to know how a particular firing of neurons translates into the observed behavior. In such case, an understanding of how these two levels (brain and mind) relate to each other is crucial. For example, the problem of remembering a phone number. One way to explore this process would be to study behavior through direct observation. We could present a phone number and be asked to recall it after a delay, and we then measure the accuracy of the response.

A second approach would be to *measure the cognitive ability* to study the firings of individual neurons when an individual is trying to remember the phone number. Neither of these studies on its own would fully determine how the process of remembering a phone number really works. As part of the integration system between *brain cells*, our mind and our whole body are essential parts of brain development and interpersonal experience. The new sciences of today's mind need to enlarge their zone to encompass both lived human experience and the possibilities for transformation inherent in human experience.

Studying such a specific occurrence from multiple levels creates a wider understanding of the processes that occur in the brain to give rise to a particular behavior. Few of such necessary levels to analyze might be the *computational* concept, identifying the *goals of the computation*, the *representation*, and the *algorithms* (giving a representation of the inputs and outputs, also the algorithms that transform one into the other), as well as the *hardware implementation* (how algorithm and representation maybe physically becomes aware).

Despite new interpersonal experiences and recent studies, not all those who consider themselves *cognitive scientists* hold a functionalist view of the mind—the view that mental states and processes should be explained by their function to understand fully what they do. What cognitive means in cognitive science is used for any kind of mental operation or structure that can be studied in exact terms; this conceptualization is very wide. Therefore, it's important to not be confused with how "cognitive" is used in some traditions of analytic philosophy. For instance, where cognitive has to do only with formal rules and truth conditional semantics. Despite applying the findings of psychology and cognitive science, social and affective neuroscience, it's the mindset of science itself that should be on board broad to cultural and intellectual life as part of integration—whole. This is composed in growth of skepticism and examination bout accuracy conventional wisdom. How much of what we think is true really is true if we examine the fact? In addition, it would be beneficial to the intellectual life if searching for explanations is added as another aspect of the scientific mindset just to relate phenomena to more basic phenomena and to try to integrate those phenomena with still more basic phenomena as learning experiences. For example, in the scientific point of view, biological phenomena were explained in part at the level of molecules, which were explained by chemistry and afterward explained by physics. Therefore, there is no excuse for not *continuing explanations.*

Human biology offers learning experience of the brain, yet human nature is a product of the organization of the brain. As explanations of mid or *neuronal networking integration* societies unfold themselves, they consist of brains linking with other brains and negotiating positions to *coordinate their behavior* and so on. This might perhaps benefit us from an understanding of cognitive science and evolutionary psychology. It can be educational experiences for professionals that education depends on a theory of learning, what does children find more naturally from the guidance of their teachers. What is essential to learn from psychology classes are topics such as love, sexual attraction, religion, spirituality, work, jealousy, anger, guilt, morality—all of the things that give life its purpose. This can be in addition to attention, attitude formation, and short-term memory. Evolutionary psychology could address these topics to not interact with the scientific ways of things alone. Neither human nature nor the human brain always fits into distinct boxes.

Studies of recent *MRI and PET* scans and specific clinical tests of language abilities and impairments show that our ability to move our face and tongue in the sequence necessary to produce speech, for instance, saying "t" and "ta," and our ability to hear and convert the same sounds are in Broca's area of our brain. This indicates the integration system of *speech production and comprehension* which are not independent systems. This integration of science and *letters is symbolic* of what we could hope to be a wider trend, particularly in psychology and cognitive science to the traditional domains of humanities.

Despite our *modern technology,* can it be possible in the *field of neuroscience* to know far less about language than about other brain mechanisms? For instance, is understanding human emotion, memory, or sensation far more successful than language? Also, language is a human species phenomenon. Thus, researchers can't use animal species as a form of guinea pig to study and to investigate brains at the neuron levels. It could be also the reason beyond inborn difficulty of studying language is that it is so closely integrated to human thoughts. There are certainly parts of the brain in which language is concentrated. However, it is hard to distinguish these areas from those involved in *nonlanguage cognitive processes.*

There's no aspect of human communication and cultural creation that can't benefit from a greater exploration of psychology and the other sciences of the mind. The category of our autobiography would be strengthened by an understanding of the nature of human memory.

Seemingly, *language-specific areas* were the first localized areas to be discovered in the brain. Humans' capacity for speech and language provoked classic debates on nature vs. nurture by strong proponents of nativism by *Chomsky (1959)* and learning by *Skinner (1959).* Research is still breaking ground with regard to the neural mechanisms that underlie language development. This decade may represent the dawn of a golden age with regard to the developmental neuroscience of language in human species.

While we are far beyond these debates, infants their innate susceptibility, and their incredible abilities to learn once they get exposed to natural growth. Human languages are rich in words that give us understanding of what they mean. These sounds—meaning associations and symbolism—are somehow similar across languages. How does our *brain link phonetics with meaning?* Because language is so difficult to localize, scientists have focused instead on language as a means to understand the workings of the mind. For example, in sound symbolism, the sound of words can bring images to our mind—think of petite, meaning small, as opposed to grand, meaning large. Even though sound symbolism is more *implicit* and less reflexive than *synesthesia*, it still can be thought of as a process that cross-activates other—auditory and visual—areas of the brain.

To some degree, this discrepancy reflects how the human mind maps sounds to meanings. *Language* is the window into the human species' nature. This is what makes humans unlike other species (cats and horses). Thus, language is a pretty good place not only because of language itself—the fact that we make different sounds with our mouths in order to get ideas across—but also because language has the fine tune for the kinds of thoughts and social relationships that humans want to communicate with one another. It's essential to learn that language is highly *metaphorical.*

For each word we speak, we think firsthand; thus, can language be separated from our thought? Would it be possible to answer about localized language functioning? Many neuroscientists have taken a different approach in trying to find localized *language areas in the brain.* If we look at the language in a more sociological study of language and the brain, this would investigate language as a means of understanding the way the mind works. With advanced research and new methods, we might learn where individual words are stored between the *10 and 100 billion neurons* that composed our brains.

Generally speaking, the *left hemisphere of the brain is responsible for language and speech* and is called the *dominant hemisphere.* The right side of the hemisphere plays a large part in interpreting visual information and spatial processing. *Broca's area* is located in the left frontal lobe. Any damage in this region, one may have difficulty moving the tongue or facial muscles to produce the sounds of speech. The individual would be able to read and understand spoken language yet might have difficulty in speaking and writing. Wernicke's region is located in the left temporal lobe. Any damage to this area causes *Wernicke's aphasia*. The individual may speak in long sentences that have no meaning, add unnecessary words, and also might be creating new words. These individuals are capable of making speech sounds, yet they have difficulty understanding speech and are as a result unaware of their mistakes.

It still insisting that *identifying speech sounds is delivered out in the superior temporal lobe bilaterally*. The superior temporal sulcus bilaterally is involved in the phonological-level feature of this process. In addition, the frontal/motor system is not central to speech recognition, although it may regulate the auditory perception of speech. The conceptual access mechanisms are probably located in the lateral posterior temporal lobe (middle and inferior temporal gyri). Speech production involves sensory-related systems in the *posterior superior temporal lobe in the left hemisphere*.

The connecting point between perceptual and motor systems is supported by a sensory-motor circuit for vocal tract actions (not dedicated to speech). This is the same as the *sensory-motor circuits* found in the primate *parietal lobe*. This way verbal short-term memory can be understood as an emergent property of this sensory-motor circuit. Therefore, the examination is understood within the condition of a dual stream model of speech processing in which one pathway supports speech comprehension.

The feature of this process is that the frontal/motor system is not central to speech recognition, although it may *regulate auditory perception of speech comprehension* and the other supports sensory-motor integration. When it comes to learning more on language development, we might ask ourselves, *what are we trying to understand? Even though human languages are viewed informally as a family of communication,* this system developed over thousands of years ago and passed down from one generation to the next as a form of *evolutionary process*. However, it is more accurate to think of human language as a *computational system* inside the brain. These computational systems *transform* between thought, ideas, and concepts, and also as an *acoustic signal*. For example, if one views an event, say, a bee stings a child, perhaps this event can be understood; that is represented in some way in the conceptual system of the viewer.

Thus, this *conceptual representation*, in turn, can be translated into many ways of spoken expression. Such can be composed of sounds like the bee stung the child, the bumblebee bit his hand, or a bee attacked the little boy. This observation leads to learning experiences that there are many ways to express a concept through speech, which is a sign that the stuff of thought is not the same as spoken language.

In addition, *pervasive ambiguity* is another way to explore this further. For example, they went to the bank at noon, which could imply a financial transaction or a riverside meeting. This ambiguity exists in the *speech signal*, yet not in the mind of the speaker, hereafter teaching us that language is not the same as thought. However, language is the means by which *thoughts* can be *converted into an acoustic figure.*

This might also bring us to explore more relevant information *regarding mental abilities, language, and brain-to-mind integration system. The mind is rarely defined in fields that focus on mental experience.* Obviously, understanding of language to the internalized system of rules is only one of the many factors that decide how a comment will be used in a certain circumstance. The *linguist* point of view to determine what constitutes knowledge of a language—to construct a *correct grammar*—might be studying one fundamental factor that is *involved in presentation.* It's important to study the interaction of several factors involved in complex mental acts and underlying actual performance. It's beneficial to recognize that even the most familiar phenomena require explanations.

There has been substantial *progress over the past several years* in understanding aspects of the *functional neuroanatomy of language.* However, it is still a learning progress. The human species who has acquired knowledge of a language has internalized a system of regulation that relates sound and meaning in a certain way. The linguist fabricating grammar of a language is in effect offering *hypothesis* concerning this *internalized system.* The *linguist's hypothesis,* if presented with adequate *explicitness* and accuracy, will then have certain observed consequences with regard to the form of expression and their explanation by individuals.

The *grammar* put forward by the linguist is also an *explanatory theory*. This might suggest an explanation for the fact that an individual speaker of the language in question might have perceived, interpreted, formed, or used a comment in definite ways and not in other ways.

The *native speaker* has acquired a grammar on the basis of very restricted and degenerate evidence; the *grammar has empirical consequences* that extend far beyond the evidence. At one level, the phenomena with which the grammar deals are explained by the *rules* of the *grammar* itself and the interaction of these rules. At a deeper level, these same *phenomena are explained by the principles* that determine the selection of the grammar on the basis of the restricted and *degenerate evidence available* to the person who has acquired knowledge of the language, who has constructed for himself this particular grammar.

The concept which determines the form of *grammar* and that selects a grammar of the *relevant* form on the basis of *particular information* composes a subject that might, *following a traditional* usage, be called as universal grammar. This study *(universal grammar by Chomsky)* is also understood as a study of the *nature of human intellectual* magnitude. In certain ways, it figures to compose the necessary and adequate rule that a system could meet to qualify as a *potential human language*.

A such a system that is not accidentally true of the existing human languages yet that is rather rooted in the human *language capacity*. Therefore, such system composes the *innate organization* that determines what counts as *linguistic experience* and what knowledge of language which arises on the basis of this experience. It's important to understand a linguist is also involved in the study of both *universal and particular grammar*. For better understanding, a linguist is involved in the establishments of explanatory theories; and at each stage, there is *psychological interpretation and theoretical and descriptive work*.

Linguistics also explores more to discover better philosophies of particular (grammar) language and the concept of the *genetic basis for language acquisition (universal grammar by Chomsky)*. Other cognitive systems are intended to conceive along similar lines that each has its own principles. At some point, cognitive systems are understood to be, in effect, *organs of the body*, primarily the brain. For this purpose, to be investigated the manner of other subcomponents with typical properties that *communicate* in the life of the human species, for instance, the systems of vision, motor planning, circulation of the blood, etc. Continuing with their role in behavior, *the cognitive organs link into activities traditionally considered as mental such as thought, planning, interpretation, evaluation*, and so on. It's best to focus our attention on the following question: what contribution can the study of language make to our understanding of human nature? This question also threads its way through modern Western thought.

However, in that age that was less self-conscious of what we learned today, the nature of language, the respects in which *language mirrors human mental processes* and creates the flow and character of thought, such disciplines were only topics for study. Later in the nineteenth and twentieth centuries, as linguistics, philosophy, and psychology have worked to go their separate ways, the classical problems of language and mind have automatically taken place and have served to link these diverging fields and to give route and importance to their efforts. Chomsky played a bigger role in linguist and language development.

According to him, language is more like walking. Although humans learn by example, he proposed that we are all born with a fundamental understanding of such mechanisms. Chomsky's original work, the *universal grammar*, is the reason why humans can recognize *grammatically correct* from nonsensical phrases. Humans have the ability to distinguish words from nonwords even without an understanding of the language. Such knowledge comes by observing and memorizing grammatical cues due to our understanding of language is also built on human experience.

Human *brains lock onto words to understand phrases and sentences*. We go through *grammar-based construction* in the forming of language. In addition, it's essential to recognize that grammar is also a collaborative work, achieved by using acoustic cues such as intonation, and statistical cues, like word transition. Chomsky is best known for his influence on linguistics, specifically the development of *transformational grammar*. He alleged that formal grammar was straight responsible for a person's ability to recognize and interpret mere utterances. Likewise, he *did not believe that language was innate.* Therefore, he stated that *animals and humans* were both *capable* of the same comprehension when it's not hidden from specific linguistic information. However, it's only the human species who could continue to develop those abilities through a process that is called a *language acquisition device.*

At some point, the fundamental structures of language are innate and universal to human tongues. For example, *children* develop a competent use of language regardless if they are exposed to incomplete or inaccurate grammar. It's clear to many points that children do not receive much direct teaching about how to speak. As language becomes more compound and children become more skilled, it's likely that children use different parts of their brain to support this experience. *Language is a complex system* It includes the study of how language itself works, such as grammar, the assembly of words, phrases, sentences, and phonology. The study of sound, semantics, the study of meaning, pragmatics, language—conversation and so on. Interestingly, the association between asymmetry and language was generally weakest during the critical language period. Scientists interested in language also study how it is processed in our real life. This field of study is called *psycholinguistics.* The topic might be how is it acquired by children and language acquisition? Aside from all, how such experience computed in the brain which led us to the field of *neurolinguistics.*

It's an important journey for learning language development to *not confuse language with three other things that are closely related to language.* These include written language, proper grammar, and thought. Regions of the brain became more successful about the time children start school. However, children have no instinctive tendency to write as they learn it through construction and schooling. Between the ages of two and four, myelin asymmetry might not predict language very well. For this reason, if the children's brain anatomy does not predict their language skills, it suggests their environment might be more influential.

The researchers hope the study will provide a reasonable solution for future research aimed at pinpointing brain structures that might predict *developmental disorders.* Most disorders such as autism, dyslexia, and ADHD have specific deficits in language ability. It's best that studies look at abnormalities and how a typical child develops. This is essential pointer of integration system, first to investigate the relationship between brain structure and language throughout the early childhood then demonstrate how such linkage changes when children grow up.

This also brings us back to understanding *nature and nurture relationships* with human development and education transformation. We cannot deny that human nature is heavily determined by our biology; and by the same token, we cannot argue that social structures determine human values, personality, and even social problems. Furthermore, the *computational transformation* between our thoughts and acoustic waveform is a complex, multistage procedure. This process not only involves several stages of processing in the sensory and motor periphery, but also requires other linguistic stages of *integrated—central brain systems*.

The aim for neuroscience of language might involve mapping the neural circuits that support the various levels or stages of such computational transformations to understand the integration within input and output systems, aside from related nonlinguistic functions. *In the near future*, the result of this research might summarize what is currently understood regarding the *neural foundation of speech sound recognition*. The neural region is involved in accessing meaning from acoustically presented speech and the role of sensory systems in speech production. Aside to the *neural circuits* underlying sensory motor integration for speech and related functions.

And the *verbal short-term memory* and the organization of the planum *temporales the region* classically *associated* with speech functions. Therefore, we might then discuss the neural basis of higher - order feature of language processing. *Today's understudying of grammar* is indivisible to the contributions of one study of linguist by Noam Chomsky for the past sixty years.

To explain in understanding of language, *creativity or productivity* is the main key, which is the ability to produce and understand new sentences. It is amazing how to explore how people are capable of doing it. When we speak or understand a language, we haven't just memorized each sentence at the time. However, we would rather have consciously *assimilated the grammar for combining elements into creating brand-new assemblies. This also brings us to understanding of linguistics and the integration between psychology into the human mind. A second insight* is that *languages* have a *syntax* which can't be indicated with their *meaning.* Also, syntax isn't composed of a line of word-by-word alliance like stimulus response theories in psychology.

Language in general has a long colony, meaning the word in one place in a sentence can give order to the choice of the word in several positions throughout the sentence. For example, if the sentence begins with "either," there's down the line an "or." However, *speech recognition is* bilaterally arranged in the *superior temporal gyrus.* The modification from the acoustic speech signal into a conceptual representation takes many processing steps in the auditory periphery. Some pieces of evidence from a variety of sources showed that the phonological stages of spoken-word recognition are *supported by neural systems* in the superior temporal lobe, superior temporal gyrus, and superior temporal sulcus—bilaterally.

The brain must figure out at least two things when it comes to the task of learning a natural language. First is how to transform the sound patterns of speech into a representation of the *meaning* of an utterance. Second is how to *reproduce* those *sound patterns* with the *vocal track.* The neural organization of *conceptual-semantic systems* might view as conceptual information is represented in many dispensed models integrated with the *cortex.* These representations include the same sensory, motor, and supramodal cortical systems originally invoked in processing that information. Some researchers show a more focally arranged semantic hub in the anterior temporal area. Also, few believe that *semantic knowledge* is organized into functionally specialized neural systems. This is dedicated to processing information from evolutionarily relevant conceptual categories and domains of knowledge that have survival.

The superior temporal lobe (bilaterally) that processes acoustic and phonemic-level information during speech *recall,* and considering that conceptual-semantic information involves cortical regions outside of the *superior temporal lobe,* the questions might be then, how do these two types of *information come together?* Of course, there is an integrating system, but the neural mechanism remains to be specified. In many studies, evidence shows the posterior lateral and inferior temporal regions as the answer in mapping sound onto meaning. Therefore, damage to posterior temporal lobe regions, especially along the middle temporal gyrus, has long been connected with *auditory comprehension deficits*.

What's particularly notable is the evolution of our language capability. I can recall reading books about what it is that makes the human species more special. There have been suggestions such as *bipedalism* and tool use, yet I think that the one defining capability is language. Some cognitive scientists view language as a *mental organ* and some as instinct. *Language develops* in our *early life spontaneously* without a conscious attempt or any formal order. I was interested in all features of human language. I worked with children, despite teaching my own children.

I was exploring how children learn language, how adults learn new languages how we understand sentences in conversation, as well as where language is situated in the brain and how it changes over *history* (evolution). Why do adult immigrants learn lessons in long periods while their *four-year-old kids learn the language so quickly*? What language would a child speak if he was raised by different environments and so on? We can't deny that language spread by public daily conversation which can contribute more as language is a cultural artifact that was invented at a certain point in history. Such understanding passes on to children by explicit instruction via schools and caregivers' role models. I can also add that the language is human instinct. We get some of our language from famous icons, famous characters, or famous athletes, for instance. Therefore, we're all going to be expecting new vocabulary.

Another way to explore language is if we think language is a mental organ. We already learned the integration of mind and body; therefore, we gained enough understanding that it came from the same source as *physical organs*, although it is an *object of natural selection* in the evolution of the human development. With this information, language is an innate faculty of humans that comes from the same source that every other *innate* aspect of the human brain and body develops. Can this give language a recognition of *materialized by-product* of the laws of growth? It has been a while that language has been the main topic of discussions of the human mind and human nature. Many questions such as if the language is an instinct, so can't be the rest of the mind, or can it be possible if there's no such thing as intelligence, a capacity for learning or even a general ability to imitate, always make the mind wonder. We explored that the mind is an integral system of a whole. Thus, language is being one link which also shaped by natural selection. As a result, language can be an instinct that serves its purpose for universality in addition to complex grammar. We acknowledged that all languages contain nouns and verbs, subjects and objects, cases and agreement, and vocabulary as one way to understand the universality of language and its design.

The *grammar* we speak every day, in the sense of the unconscious rules, strings the words together into phrases and sentences, which is also a *mental algorithm* that causes people's ability to talk. I learned from children that they begin to babble in their first year of life. First words begin at about one year of age; and first combinations, things like *more food*, happen around age eighteen months. Much takes place in those six months of children's development, despite the lack of grammar lessons or even teaching from their parents. What's going on in the mind of the child isn't a complicated procedure. Children learn better with better communication.

However, an unconscious program that synchronizes the child's language with the language is of the community. Children are also introducing complexity into the language. Furthermore, language seems to have *neurological* and even *genetic sensitivity*. For example, if we point at a bad gene or an injured brain, then language suffers. However, the rest of the brain is all functional, which might always be that protest which language is the most mentally effort thing human species has. We can conclude that the anatomy of language is complex, like the anatomy of the eye. Nonetheless, language is quite clearly adaptive in the sense of inherently serving the goals of reproduction. The impression from anthropology that humanity is like a carnival, meaning everything might come from a tourist *mentality*: when you come back from a holiday, we remember what was different about this location; otherwise, we might as well have stayed at home. That is, many anthropologists overstated the degree to which the ethnic group they studied was different and might be strange, both to justify their profession and to raise people's *consciousness* about *human potential.* Yet the anthropologists might have spent so much time looking for differences among human species that they have not noticed the basic categories of human experience which are found in all cultures, such as humor, love, jealousy, responsibility, joy, or laughter.

This reminds me about Jack and how his playful, joyful *communication* was an effective contributor to his classmates. Language is simply the most recognizable example of human universal. The main discovery of cognitive science and synthetic intelligence is that humans apt to be blasé about abilities, like seeing things, picking up a staff, walking, talking, remembering a face, and participating in ordinary conversation. These ordinary tastes are fantastically complex which require their own special kinds of mechanisms. All the wonderful regular to complex things that people do might come out of the interactions among a smaller number of basic modules. Thus, one other amazing thing about the mind is it is *a system for intuitive mechanics.* This also is our understanding of how *physical objects behave* or how things fall apart. For instance, the intuitive of biology which the expectations are about how plants and animals work. The knowledge of number to the basis of mathematics, and the mental maps to the large territories or recognizing the kinds of environments we feel comfortable to live in. In addition, the knowledge of danger, the emotion of fear and a set of phobias, such as fear of venomous and dangerous animals. Likewise, the intuitive of disease and waste products and what is icky and unhealthy. And the *intuitiveness of self-knowledge*, well-being, our interests, desires, love, and knowledge of others.

If we recall the poem we read about Jack, no wonder he understood his behavior and motivations for what he does or who he is. Therefore, the answer to the question why should we care so much about language might be that language is a human *intellectual instinct* and one important way to communicate. We can also offer realistically that we can apply linguistics to literature, biology of groups to understand fictions, *phonology* and *psychology* to our poetry, psychology and *biology* to understand art and music as a whole, and the last one which is essential to *interpersonal relationships is to add the biology of memory to understand biography.*

Even beyond today's research and applying the findings of psychology and cognitive science as addition to, social and affective neuroscience, it's the goal of science that should be exported to our cultural and intellectual life as a whole. We understood biology gives us an explanation of the brain. Also, we learned human nature is a product of the organization of the brain. Therefore, societies spread, because they consist of the brain's integration with other brains for *negotiating arrangements* to coordinate their character. If we look into *human brain and our progress,* then we must be able to learn about facts from centuries ago to today's progress. So what does progress mean to us? We may think the question is so subjective and culturally relative with many answers.

Well, we know life is better than death, and health is better than sickness. Sustenance is better than hunger, and abundance is better than poverty. Of course, peace is better than war, and safety is better than danger. We can't deny the fact freedom is better than tyranny, and equal rights are better than bigotry and discrimination. Knowledge is better than ignorance, and intelligence is better than living in the dark. In addition, happiness is better than misery. Therefore, if all this shows increase over time, that is progress. This is the human well-being measure—from life, health, sustenance, safety, prosperity, peace, knowledge, freedom, happiness over such periods, which shows progress.

From brain development to enlightenment ideals need a positive defense and explicit commitment. The world has made progress in every single measure of human well-being. For example, life expectancy in the United States in 2015 was 78.96 years, which shows nine years longer than it was a half century ago. In addition, from the mid–eighteenth century, global life expectancy rose from 29 years to around 71.4. Looking back in the 1700s, a third of children born in the richest parts of the world died before their fifth birthday while according to much updated research, that changed to 6 percent of the children in the poorest parts.

Also, one *another progress* seen on *fertility rates* which have fallen in developed countries such as Europe and Japan. Even Muslim countries have seen a 40 percent drop in fertility over the past three decades. This includes a 70 percent drop in Iran and a 60 percent decline in Bangladesh. The world population growth rate peaked higher but declined. This trend is attributed to the growing wealth and education in the world, in which parents no longer breed larger families and women delay having children. This might be another result of the eighteenth-century Enlightenment ideal of reason over irrationality.

As addition the understanding of humanism and peace over sectarianism. Studies show the global *average IQ* score is rising about three points every decade. We can also be the witness of incline via growth of education—represented by the growth of literacy as another way of human progress. We are aware that *education plays a big role* in society. Educated people tend to be less racist, homophobic, and sexist and place higher values on imagination and are more likely to vote, volunteer, and trust their fellow citizens. The search for racist and homophobic jokes took a steep fall from 2005 to 2017. Sexist jokes show an uptick from 2010 and 2014 and continue another fall from 2014 to 2017. Before the seventeenth century, literacy was the advantage for a small group—now 83 percent of the world is literate.

Even in many Middle Eastern and North African countries, more than three-quarters of the people over sixty are illiterate. The rate for those in their early life was only a single digit. The world's income increased from 1820 to 1900, and fifty years later, it tripled again. The story of global wealth goes from nothing to less, to some, then increase. From 1995, 30 of the world's 109 countries have benefited income growth rates which doubled every 18 years. As the world has grown richer, nature and safety have started to rebound. The question for is the world really falling apart might have answered via major research, facts, charts, and the ideal of progress has been obsolete.

In many elegant assessments of the human condition in the third millennium, cognitive scientist it's better to step back from the brutal headlines which play to our psychological, instead absorb the data. The seventy-five fact graphs by researchers show that life, health, prosperity, safety, peace, knowledge, and happiness are on the rise worldwide. This *progress* is the *result* of growing enlightenment, a good-enough declaration that reason and science can increase *human development*. With intellectual depth and enlightenment, we can make the case for reason, science, and humanism: the ideals we might need to confront our problems and continue our progress. We might need an understanding, a discussion, because progress is, in my view, one of the most important concepts of our time.

If it is interpersonal neurobiology or enlightenment now, the exploration for reason, science, humanism, and progress, insists that the human race has never had it so good as a result of values we attribute to education and brain health development from the past eighteenth century. Maybe it's time to reclaim the *mantle of progress*. This *twenty-first century* is the most peaceable era in our species' history of existence. No aspect of life is untouched by the knowledge and from the education system. Daily existence is very different if we always have to worry about being sick, raped, or killed; and it's hard to develop sophisticated systems of learning or commerce if the institutions that support them are built with confusion and burned as quickly as they build.

The historical route of violence, shallow education system, and economic issues affect not only how life is lived but how it is understood. What could be more fundamental to our sense of knowledge and purpose than a conception of whether the strivings of the human race over long periods have left us better or worse off? How, in particular, are we to make conclusions of modernity—of the erosion of today's family, our tribe, tradition, culture, or religion by the strength of individualism, cosmopolitanism, reason, and science? It might be depending on how we understand the legacy of this *transition*. It can be understood whether we see our world as a nightmare of crime, war, or as a period that, by the standards of history, is blessed by unprecedented levels of peaceful coexistence. Many pieces of evidence show how our *history* has *engaged our psychology*, and so many things in human affairs are connected to everything else. Across time and space, the more peaceable societies also tend to be richer, healthier, educated, and more likely to engage in growth.

Therefore, the theory of mind also invoked here is the synthesis of cognitive science, affective and cognitive neuroscience, social and evolutionary psychology, and sciences of human nature and how brain to mind works. According to such discipline of understanding, the mind can be a complex system of cognitive and emotional faculties implemented in the brain. Thus, humans might owe their basic design to the processes of evolution. Yet it's better to view life as an "integration process of whole" over its sum. Whether it's enlightenment or being aware, evolution or mindfulness, science or physics, all inspire people to be aware of how they compose their daily lives. Another aspect of this book journey has been to make sense of who we are. Our mind is, embodied in our extended neural circuitry and is *embedded in our connections* to others, aside to the way we relate to our planet Earth. Thus, such integration indeed needs careful attention to establish and maintain a great mental health. Otherwise, poverty, hunger, and homelessness threaten the essential needs of many throughout the world.

War and natural disasters would fill many lives with fear and suffering even for individuals in more stable environments. The regular life could become filled with an overwhelming focus on the outer world and an experience of being isolated from meaningful connections with others. Therefore, the embodied and socially embedded requirements for a healthy mind are not being created in daily life throughout the world. Many would be deficient in a daily regimen necessary for psychological strength or mental well-being.

So what would be included in *the healthy lifestyle outline*? In the field of brain health, interpersonal neurobiology, science, or evolution, we might define a major aspect of all and also propose that a healthy life or mind emerges from a process of *integration*, meaning the linkage of different components (sums) of a system. Importantly the *close relationship* among links over just integration alone. That system can be, for example, the mind, brain, consciousness, enlightenment, evolution, science, interpersonal experience, genes, nature, nurture, belief system, and relationships among and between us that we connect to one another in the form of interpersonal neurobiology.

The connection between us, within us, and among us. In the form of brain science, this integration can be viewed, the separated areas with their unique functions such as in the skull and throughout the body which become linked to each other through synaptic connections. These integrated linkages enable more intricate human functions to emerge—such as insight, empathy, intuition, and morality. A result of such stimulus, integration born kindness, resilience, and health, well-being. In modern society, mindful awareness has been scientifically proven to promote social, emotional, and physical well-being and is an effective part of many psychotherapies.

The state of awareness harnesses specific social and emotional circuits in the brain; practicing such receptive state of mindfulness becomes a trait of resilience. The development of these *resonance circuits creates an integrated brain state.* Thus, it creates the benefits of improved immune and cardiac function, enhanced empathy and self-understanding, and a deeper connection to oneself and others. In addition, mindful awareness is useful in the prevention of relapse of drug addiction and chronic depression or in the treatment of anxiety, borderline personality disorder, etc.

This knowledge of being fully aware in the present moment is no longer an ancient practice and has been found in cultures throughout the world. In this book, the emphases are not in mindfulness alone, yet it's the updating energy information flow to our brain and mind through a life span. It is the driven knowledge to the mind that we can identify our world based on the interpersonal brain definition (*our identification*). Especially interpersonal neurobiology is the interdisciplinary field that invites all branches of science and other ways of knowing to come together and find the common principles from human development and understanding human experience.

Today's research and science which contribute to this exciting field are not limited yet include anthropology, biology, science, computer science, mathematics, mental health, developmental, psychopathology, psychology, sociology, linguistics, neuroscience, psychiatry, etc. Interpersonal neurobiology weaves research from these areas into a consilient framework that examines the common findings among other independent disciplines. This also provides the basis of mental health, well-being, brain development, and the developing mind, for instance, if we take a look at the *neurobiology of behaviors*: the mind, brain, and our relationship. We know our behavior carries out responsibility toward ourselves and the society.

Everything we know is part of mental experiences, our thoughts, emotions, feelings, beliefs—the intentions to carry out a behavior and the ability to carry that behavior out. Our relationships to others require the mental function to regulate our behavior and to think clear. It's critical to understand what the mind is if we are the caretaker of the mind. However, I must confess reading between the line—less than two hundred thousand health occupational facilities, education facilities, and related health professionals might not have the definition of mind.

Throughout the book, we might have *explained what the brain is*, so we can draw our conclusions of *mind to behaviors*. Let's shed light on the connection between the brain and the mind. What is brain? Simply, the collection of cells called neurons and supportive cells. The neurons are connected to each other by synapses and look like *spiderweb. There is integration between mental process and synapses. There are more than 100 billion neurons, and a regular connection with other neurons will be 10,000. Our brain works by action potential, meaning electrical energy flows down to the axon, and at the end, this energy is converted to chemical energy. That's how physics defines energy as, the capacity to do things.*

Accordingly, a simple way of saying what the brain is all about is it's a set of interconnected cells that allow electrical chemical energy to flow. This brain is embodied much as it's skulled. Okay, what is mind? The mind is consciousness, thoughts, feelings, and subjective experiences for sure, yet it is also an embodied, relational, emergent process that regulates the flow of energy and information. This energy and information flow happens throughout the nervous system.

The mind is not the output of the brain, yet it's the emergent process that arises its energy and information flow past through the body through its relationships. This relationship is between people to people, between our planet Earth and the universe. Thus, human experience is energy and information flow. This experience is shaped by relationships between the brain and the mind, aside from the fact that it's a complex and open system of self-organization. The relationship itself is the sharing of energy and information flow. Another way of saying it is the mind is the emergent process that regulates the flow. Close relationship is the sharing of the flow, and the brain is the embodied mechanism of the flow. Our interpersonal relationships and our relationships throughout the universe are integrated to this information and energy flow.

Let's not forget the *mind structures the brain, and awareness* is an essential resource. On the other hand, we learned the structures of the brain and its relationships throughout the body and outside the body relationships. Therefore, the integration system builds from *top-down experiences*, learning what we learn from outside us (include evolution) and from bottom down, learning from our interpersonal experience (include attachment)—more in a raw way.

As a result, our relationships have formed from "me" to "we." Also, this means our brain has been integrated. Therefore, the brain tissues get its stimulation to function well from the integration system. This is how the integrated brain functions as a whole.

Our brain integrated to its parts, mind, as much as to people, planet, universe, and so on. We have explored how humans flourished from poverty, health issues, economy, and a poor education system compared to early years. Therefore, health and well-being are *integration* for now century and is the continuum contributor for the future. The interpersonal neurobiology and integration process opens the door to functional activities throughout the education system while being beneficial to learning disabilities, ADHD, and other developmental concerns.

We used as an example, Jack and his classmates in a way of *mirror-neurons interpersonal relationships* or me to we connection. If we embrace interpersonal neurobiology's proposed definition of a key facet of mind as an embodied and relationally embedded process that regulates energy and information flow, how can we make a practical definition of mental habits that can help students and teachers with their teaching of daily essential mental activities? How do we use the focus of attention on intentions to strengthen integration in our bodies and in our relationships on a daily classroom setting? This practice helps Jack, his classmates, and his educators toward integrated brain development. The number one *fundamental process* that shapes energy and information flow is *attention. Attention shapes and directs the energy and information which allows us to get less distracted.*

One example for *working memory is* mindfulness. This really involves scientific practices that need to be applied over any type of facts (math, science, etc.) at educational facilities. The only assent that is shared between teachers and students daily is the energy and information flow that has symbolic values (like math and science) through relationships. We know our nervous system is all about electrical chemical energy flow. Yet energy and information can be beneficial and chaotic. *Since the human mind is open*, a small chaotic experience can influence us big time, just being part of a complex system that is emergent property, not intuitive.

Teachers might not understand that the mind is an emergent process that arises from energy flow between us and among us. In the classroom setting, this mind integration is shared between teachers and students, among students, and within the students themselves (mind-brain relationships) in the form of a self-organizing system (not intuitive experience). This energy system arises from elements of the system and come down to organize that system. This is called a *self-organizing system* which is an essential part of math (it's a mathematically correct form). This might brighten our relationships with our planet, evolution, well-being, and the philosophy *of nurturing the nature. This understanding defines the internal education which allows students to regulate the flow of energy and information patterns from kindergarten. In the classroom, teachers practice to drive this energy and information flow to the brain to train the circuits of the brain which is the essential part prior to the other educational facts.* The few minutes of stabilizing energy flow is the focusing on the breath which trains the attention circuits of the brain, laterally.

This practice brings us to be aware of awareness and paying attention to intentions. That's how the mind of a student becomes stable to accumulate energy and information flow through the education system between relationships which requires integration.

Integrated students feel emotionally stable and feel hormonal. A simple technique of mindfulness is stabilizing the observing circuits to sensing circuits that create awareness for we relationships and break the barriers to delusions of me in skin boundaries. Once again, the case of Jack and his classmate was a great example of focusing, observing, and applying the interpersonal experience to the learning system. The transition process of integration, however, requires recognition necessary to attain for educators and educational awareness.

Despite the fact majority of educational systems have grown to learn the importance of learning experience, and updates become aware itself. For instance, even philosophers have to face the facts that some of the greatest philosophers aren't the greatest philosophers. Some are recognized important to philosophical thoughts, like Isaac Newton. On the other hand, Charles Darwin's idea was considered greater according to other philosophical ideas. What might have made his idea so great was he united the world of purposeless causation with the *world of meaning*, from physics to ethics and poetry in one unified perspective. Later on, even some of his ideas and theory proved to be artificial by other philosophers. For example, in the century and a half since Charles Darwin's publication of *On the Origin of Species*, evolutionary theory has become the base of modern biology.

However, the application to the human mind remains steeped in some dispute. Darwin wrote of cognitive evolution on *The Descent of Man* suggested that any human mental faculties are the outcome of evolution by natural and sexual selection. He insisted that they should be understood in light of what he called *common descent*. This evolutionary interpretation of human cognition was taken up in the *1980s by contemporary evolutionary psychology. Hereafter*, it rapidly became dominated *by a school of thought* famous to our experience as *Stone Age mind*. Evolutionary psychology views the human mind as organized into many modules. Each has been underpinned by psychological adaptations designed to solve problems that were faced by our Pleistocene ancestors.

We argue that the key tenets of the established evolution psychology paradigm require moderation in the understanding of recent findings, for instance, from a number of disciplines such as human genetics, evolutionary biology, cognitive neuroscience, developmental psychology, and paleoecology. Human genes have been subject to recent selective sweeps, because humans play an active, constructive role in *codirecting their own development and evolution. Findings and experimental evidence often favor a general process rather than a modular account of cognition.*

There is always a continuum window of opportunity for transformation. From the beginning of life when humans were conceived, there is a certain pattern of communication throughout life by caregivers and society. From that point, the synaptic architecture of the brain and how it's *connected to the two atmospheres of the corpus callosum* and the connection downward to the body shows how attachment is from the past which has then molded the way the synaptic connection is formed. And how the humans now with these synaptic tendencies will begin to stimulate the world which gives the feedback according to what we are familiar with.

Therefore, the brain as embedded will continue to form based on these synaptic connections (close past experiences) as other ways of *evolutionary development.* With today's understanding of mind integration and brain development and continuum integration, we can contribute to learning experiences for transformation. For example, if we take a look at the plane of reality that is open to many possibilities, yet if any synaptic changes that happen above this plane of reality, will give certain ups and down patterns (trauma in early age).

On the other hand, beneath this is the mind part which is the physical aspect of reality (I don't know my feelings or my body). *From the patterns of synaptic changes to feelings of being disconnected is the plane of reality between, which brings us to the experience of openness by relaxing the subjective experiences into openness while bringing synaptic firing down into openness (receptive open synaptic state). This openness allows many possibilities such as the mind can change the firing patterns of the brain which results in new ways of being—redefinition of the interpersonal brain. The open plane of possibilities is a continuum journey to continuum integration and authenticity throughout our interpersonal relationships. From the enlightenment of philosophical thoughts or evolution perhaps, a simple healthy mind outline is an essential part of the process. Therefore, the healthy mind platter is a daily essential mental activity necessary for optimum mental health.* For example, the daily activities make up the full set of mental nutrients that the brain and relationships need to function at their best. These essential mental activities strengthen the brain's internal connections and human connections with each other and the world.

From paying attention (focusing), meaning closely focused on tasks in a goal-oriented way while taking on challenges, we make deep connections in the brain. On the other hand, playing time allows us to be creative. Connecting time with other people and to the natural world around us, we activate and reinforce the brain's relational circuitry. Downtime, when we are unfocused, helps the brain recharge. Almost like sleeping time, we give the brain the rest it needs. Physical time strengthens the brain in many ways. And time, in meaning, when we quietly reflect internally, helps to better integrate the brain.

Therefore, communication integration is at the heart of both interpersonal neurobiology and developing mind. It is defined clearly as the linkage of differentiated components of *many systems* including daily lifestyle. *The important aspect of the scientific developing mind and integrated system that ought to be exported to the rest of the intellectual life is the search for explanations. That is, not just to say that history is one damn thing after another, that stuff happens, and there's nothing we can do to explain why, yet to relate phenomena to more basic or general phenomena, and to try to explain those phenomena with still more basic phenomena.*

Therefore, we have repeatedly seen what happened in the sciences, where, for instance, biological phenomena were explained in part at the level of molecules, which were explained by chemistry, which was explained by physics, and so on. There's no reason that this process of explanation and the birth of integration can't continue.

There is *no such conflict between the sciences and humanities*, or we hope there shouldn't be. There should be no turf battle as to who gets to speak first or about what matters. What really matter are the ideas. It is our best to seek the ideas that give us the deepest, richest, best-informed understanding of the human condition and developing brain. Therefore, it's regardless of which community or what discipline comes from. That has to include the sciences, but we must know it can't come only from the sciences. It's better if we focus on ideas, disciplines, or academic traditions.

Likewise, it comes down to *freedom of exploration* and free will, which explains why people get so anxious. Freedom does evolve, and it could go extinct, if we aren't careful. We might explore the evolutionary theory, not the physics, to understand the phenomenon of freedom alone. Also, it's essential to our daily experience that the world is not determinist, nor is everything inevitable. What has been defined by the word "determinism" is at any instance exactly one physically possible future. On the other hand, inevitable means unavoidable, and determinism does not imply inevitability. It has ruefully been noted that we have lots of philosophy professors. By the same token, we have many books written on evolution and *human free will*. Even science itself presupposes that every phenomenon has a cause. We may speak of spontaneous combustion or a spontaneous abortion.

Spontaneous is simply another way of saying the cause is unknown over *uncaused*. Philosophers and neurobiologists have sought to rescue free will as a scientific prospect, not merely an emotional necessity, by enlisting quantum indeterminism, arguing that the physics of very small particles introduces room for *genuine* spontaneity. Yet when we consider brain development, free will, and human potential, the difficulty goes even deeper, for instance, penetrating the realm of personal responsibility, punishment, and praise. Let's say, for example, if to do something *of our own free will* means that it was utterly uncaused, then how can we be blamed, or praised, for it? But if it is caused by previous events, evaluation, neurochemical necessities, and ionic perturbations of voltage differentials across cell membranes, then the question remains the same.

When we think of free will, we might think free will is a free and *independent choice,* a voluntary decision, and we took on the responsibility of our own free will. Philosophy wise, the doctrine that the conduct of human beings expresses personal choice and is not simply determined by the physical or by the divine forces. If we look into the neuroscience of free will, we may come across a part of neurophilosophy. This is the study of topics related to free will, for instance, volition and sense of agency, using neuroscience, and the analysis of how findings from such studies may impact the free will debate. As it has become more possible to study the living human brain, researchers have begun to explore *decision-making processes.*

Studies have revealed unexpected things about human agency such as moral responsibility, and consciousness in general. Other studies have predicted participants' actions before they make them. Studies explore how we know we are responsible for voluntary movements as opposed to being moved by an external force, in other words, how the role of consciousness in decision-making may differ depending on the type of decision being made.

Despite much attention to the nature of human development and findings, the field remains highly controversial. The precise role of consciousness in decision-making and how that role may come across types of decisions still remains unclear. Furthermore, most studies explain that *free will* means many different things to different people if we consider some notions of free will are dualistic and not. It requires more research. Some important and common conceptions of free will are compatible with the emerging evidence from *neuroscience.*

Looking inside the head from neurotransmitters through neuron firing rates to overall activity, we can understand the brain *ramp-up* before movements. Such image or study explains the readiness potential, a ramping-up activity which is measured using EEG. Some have claimed that this causes the brain to unconsciously commit to a decision before consciousness awareness. Others subjected that this activity is a result of random fluctuations in brain activity that drive arbitrary, purposeless movements. It's necessary to add that brain health plays a daily role in decision-making, which is another aspect of free will. For example, some areas of the human brain are implicated in mental disorders that might be related to free will.

If we look back to the history and its findings, from billions of years ago, Earth was a lifeless place. Therefore, it was less struggle nor wanted too. Slowly, that has changed. Staring to the eye of science, seawater drains chemicals from rocks. Those chemicals pushed and combined, hit upon the trick of making copies of themselves in turn and more copies as rerun. Such replicating chains were caught in oily bubbles that protected them. This made replication possible, and eventually they began to journey out into the open sea. As a result of such, a new level of order had been achieved on Earth which had been understood by some studies as way that life had begun. *The tree of life has many stories*, its branches stretching toward complexity (this also explains well the evolutionary development). Human organisms developed systems, subsystems, and sub-subsystems, layered in ever-deepening regression.

Studies have used many systems to anticipate their future and to change it. Researchers looked within. Some found that they had patterns of memories, ideas, and purposes that emerged from the systems inside. Slowly, experiences, language become to live and used it to know themselves; the live organisms began to ask how they had been made. This is at least another explanation on how a soulless world could have given rise to a soulful one. *The emphasis has been on the human brain and mind which studies have crammed nearly every related discipline: evolutionary biology, neuroscience, psychology, linguistics, and artificial intelligence.*

Each research, from bottom to top and back to front, tells us there is a path leading through science, philosophy, history, and religion, that we people are physical objects. There is much to learn and understand about our biological history, brain, and conscious minds.

So many philosophers have walked that path toward life itself, brain journey consciousness. Many authors described consciousness as something like the product of multiple, layered computer programs running on the hardware of the brain while readers felt that they had shown how the brain creates the soul. Others thought that they missed the point entirely. To them, these books were less focus left untouched to the question of how a three-pound lump of neurons could come to possess a point of view, interiority, selfhood, consciousness—qualities that the rest of the material world lacks.

Therefore, today, *philosophers are divided into two groups: the physicalists who believe that science can explain consciousness* in purely material terms and *the dualists who explore that science can explain, yet only half of the picture.* Despite today's technology and research, the experts found themselves circling a familiar puzzle known as the hard problem. Suppose that you're a scientist studying animals. How would you know whether an animal is conscious? Well, we are aware enough that animals interact with humans, respond to their environment, and slowly, evidently pursue goals. However, human-made nonconscious robot could also do those things.

The theory of consciousness is an ambiguous concept. It can mean a lot of different things, depending on the context. For instance, I can say that I am conscious of something, as in "I am conscious of the fact that I am currently writing this page about consciousness." It can also mean self-consciousness or self-awareness: the notion that we know our existence and that we have a self. The problem is that there's no way to observe consciousness directly or mathematics wise measure it accurately. Let's say, looking at the outside, it's possible to draw our imagination that the whale is a "zombie"—physically alive yet mentally empty.

On the other hand, in theory, the same could be true of any apparently conscious being. The zombie problem is a conversational vortex among those who study animal minds. These definitions of consciousness vary among philosophers Some might have called it the "easy problems" of consciousness, meaning they are not easy in the sense that we could easily figure out how the brain creates these psychological phenomena. However, they're easy in the sense that it seems like neuroscience could figure out how the brain creates these phenomena. It seems they all like specific psychological functions that could in principle be explained in terms of neuroscience and psychology.

From imagining to neuroscience and to experience of our interpersonal journey, how can the brain create the redness of red, the blueness of blue, the sting of pain, or the thrill of laughter? *How do we distinguish these problems from easy problem* to what some called the *hard problem of consciousness?* How can the brain create these raw, sensory experiences? How can the brain create the redness of red or the blueness of blue, the sensation of pain, or even the excitements of laughter? These raw experiences and the hard problem of consciousness seem a principle phenomenon that needs more explanation, because science is in the business of studying things objectively. To the extent that we can, we take subjective experience out of the equation. Some researchers, anticipating the discussion's inexorable transformation into a meditation on *Westworld,* clutched their heads and sighed.

However, can we calculate consciousness in a scientific way? In mathematics, we have a system of rules which leads to answers. For example, an algorithm in mathematics is a procedure, a description of a set of steps that can be used to solve a mathematical computation. The key proof of this system is computing to check whether it's true or false. Following the steps might lead to the right answer or might not, yet result in redoing the given formula to succeed. The idea behind it is if you *believe* the system is true, then it's true. Going through the steps and realizing to how much this make more sense, it convening. If we trust enough this system or *algorithm* the way it constructed that is true, yet also we can see the way it constructed that cannot be proven by this procedure.

Consequently, *the answer lies on "believing" the rules over the rules of formula. What goes behind our understanding is not about the rules or algorithms. It is more on appreciation of our consciousness that we got them in the first place. Understanding is a conscious activity. It is the close relationship within us. Therefore, knowledge is internal with the right amount of practice. By the same token, algorithms are used in many branches of science and everyday life for that matter. The understanding behind each theory is the art of human consciousness and "convincing answer."*

We do not have to give away our mind to practice our psychic ability or explore our consciousness; we can be discerning and psychic. We learn enough from the famous *mathematicians, Albert Einstein a physicist* who developed the general theory of relativity. He is considered one of the most influential scientists of the *twentieth century*. Also, the English natural philosopher *Isaac Newton* claimed that Grimaldi's diffraction was simply a new kind of refraction. He claims that the *geometric nature* of the laws of *reflection* and *refraction* could only be understood if *light* is made of *particles*. He referred to as the corpuscles, as waves don't tend to travel in straight lines. This is a critical experiment that is devised to decide between two contradictory theories.

Therefore, the failure of one determines the certainty of the other. *As a result, almost everyone agreed that light must be composed of either particles or waves. Newton used the failure of wave theory to prove that light is made of particles. The conclusion leads to light is composed of colored particles that combine to appear white.* Furthermore, *quantum mechanics* (QM) developed over many decades, beginning as a set of disputable "mathematical explanations" of experiments that the math of classical mechanics could not explain. Quantum mechanics theory explains all sorts of things that couldn't be explained before, starting with the stability of atoms. However, when we accept the weirdness of quantum mechanics (in the macro world), we have to understand the idea of space-time as we know it back from Einstein.

Oftentimes, it's weird that it doesn't make sense, even following the rules we come up with, something that isn't there. For example, in quantum mechanics, an object can exist in many states at once, which sounds bizarre.

Correspondingly, the *quantum* description seems completely contrary to the world as we experience it. *The mathematics of quantum mechanics has two parts to it: first is the evolution of a quantum system. This has been described precisely by the Schrödinger equation, which tells us if we know what the state of the system is now, we can calculate what it will be doing ten minutes from now. On the other hand, the second part of quantum mechanics is the thing that happens when we want to "make a measurement,"* we use the equation to work out the probabilities of certain outcomes.

Looking back to understanding of that consciousness emerges from the quantum physical actions which is within the cells of the brain.

Now decades later, do we still stand by these statements? In many views, the conscious brain does not act according to classical physics. It doesn't even act according to conventional quantum mechanics. I think it acts according to a theory that we don't have yet. Researchers are still hoping to find a structure that preserves coherence, because it ought to be there.

Human consciousness is something that computation can't do. "I think, therefore I am" is the activation of consciousness. Asking ourselves, if the brain waves, derived from deeper level quantum vibrations found somewhere within the cells of the brain, wouldn't be too warm and wet . . . for quantum processes to occur? This might result in studying quantum vibrations within the microtubules of neurons. These vibrations are important to this theory because *there is a quantum process called quantum coherence occurring somewhere in the neurons of the brain or within the microtubules.* It might be difficult for other researchers, especially neuroscientists, to see microtubules as the source of something as seemingly immaterial as consciousness itself.

Despite the *controversy* surrounding the theory itself, if it were to be proven correct, it could solve one of the important questions: *how can free will exist in a universe that may be deterministic?* We have shed light on a general understanding of free will, yet there is another theory that free will is nonexistent and that every decision we make is the result of some previous situation. For instance, if we made a decision to get something to eat, it's because we were hungry. Our decision to get something to eat was determined by our hunger. The food that we went to buy was also determined by an exposure to that particular food group at our certain age.

Everything that happens from early life is determined by some preceding event. With that said, how can true free will exist if every choice we make is *determined by a preceding event?* Can the answer in *quantum vibrations* provide an indeterministic approach to consciousness? Can it be true that consciousness arises from quantum-mechanical processes? Can it be true the quantum nature of the vibrations allows free will to exist in the mind? How can we measure our understanding? Would it be easier if psychiatrists and medical specialists look at the organ they treat? Think about it, cardiologists, neurologists, orthopedic doctors, virtually every other medical specialty, look into imaging. Can it be true that psychiatrists guess? Well, after Newton, and after Einstein, the way people thought about the world transformed. Once the puzzle of quantum mechanics is solved, will there be another revolution in mind? It will not be easy to make predictions.

There are ideas like how quantum mechanics could be used in *biology*. I am sure eventually these ideas will make a huge difference in all sorts of unimaginable ways. Yet let's hope not the *philosophy as a sport, which its ball would be the human intuition*. It is proven that philosophers compete to shift our intuitions from one end of the table to the other. Despite the changes some intuitions, resist being shifted. Among these is our true story—that there are only two states of being: either awake or asleep, conscious or unconscious, alive or dead. Can it be more to human experience, yet our brain development has not processed it further? How can we define human development or evolutionary development, especially "brain to mind, consciousness development," if we have not lived long enough to explore our relationships through multidimensional space regardless of any discoveries? Would our ability limit us to only planet Earth and to human life alone? Biology is the science concerned with the study of life, yet we have many definitions behind this theory.

Life is a characteristic that distinguishes physical entities that have biological processes, for instance, self-sustaining processes, from those that do not. Other ways of saying an organism's astonishing knowledge of controlling a stream of order on itself, therefore surviving the decay into atomic chaos while producing orderly events—in the form of evolutionary process.

Many forms of life exist, such as plants, animals, fungi, protists, archaea, and bacteria. There is currently no agreement regarding the definition of life. Another definition is that organisms are open systems that maintain homeostasis, are composed of cells, have a life cycle, undergo metabolism, can grow, adapt to their environment, respond to stimuli, reproduce, and evolve. However, several other definitions have been proposed, and there are some borderline cases of life, such as viruses, etc.

The definition of life has long been a challenge for brain development, mind, consciousness to scientists and philosophers, with many varied definitions put forward. This is partially because life is a process—our development, experience, mind, time, consciousness, not a substance. This is a continuum process and versus the product definition. Also, it's complicated by a lack of knowledge of the characteristics of living entities, if any, that may have developed outside of humans' planet, Earth.

Importantly, the philosophical definitions of life have also been put forward, with identical concerns on how to differentiate living things from the nonliving. The most current definitions in biology are illustrative. Life is considered a characteristic of something that preserves and reinforces its existence in the given environment and exhibits most of the following traits:

- Homeostasis: regulation of the internal environment to maintain a constant state such as sweating
- Organization: being structurally clam of one or more cells, the basic units of life
- Metabolism: conversion of energy by converting chemicals and energy into cellular components and decomposing organic matter
- Growth: preservation of a higher rate of anabolism than catabolism
- Adaptation: the ability to change over time in response to the environment
- Response to stimuli: from the decreasing of a unicellular organism to external chemicals, from complex reactions involving all the senses of multicellular organisms, etc.
- Reproduction: the ability to produce new individual organisms

These complex procedures, called physiological functions, have underlying physical and chemical bases. If we take a look at the *physics perspective, living beings are thermodynamic systems with an organized molecular structure that can reproduce itself and evolve as survival dictates.*

Thermodynamically, life has been described as an open system which makes use of rise in its surroundings to create imperfect copies of itself. What distinguishes life in a greater level on Darwinian evolution is that life by the evolutionary process rather than its chemical composition. Another definition of life is that living things are self-organizing and self-producing, much similar to the definition of the brain.

However, viruses do not metabolize, and they need a host cell to make new products. Therefore, they have been described as organisms at the edge of life. Other studies on the origin of life include *biophysics* (it has commented that living things function on negative entropy), living systems theories (they claimed living systems are an *open self-organizing living system which is maintained by flows of information, energy, and matter, as we almost give such explanation to the interpersonal definition of the brain*), and Gaia hypothesis (they disclose the idea that the Earth is alive and found in *philosophy, religion*, but the first scientific discussion of it was by the Scottish scientist James Hutton).

Other definitions explore life as a property of ecosystems, nonfractionability, complex system biology, Darwinian dynamic, and operator theory. There is a trend to some known life-forms that share a fundamental molecular mechanism which reflects their common descent. Thus, based on these observations, hypotheses on the origin of life attempt to find a mechanism *explaining the formation of a universal common ancestor, starting from simple organic molecules via precellular life to protocols and metabolism. Models have been divided into "genes first" and "metabolism first" categories, but a recent trend is the emergence of hybrid models that combine both categories.*

On the other hand, living organisms synthesize proteins, which are polymers of amino acids using instructions encoded by deoxyribonucleic acid (DNA). Protein synthesis entails intermediary ribonucleic acid (RNA) polymers.

Another possibility for how life began is that *genes* originated first, followed by proteins or the alternative being that proteins came first and then genes, similar to the story of the egg and the chicken. *Environment* plays a bigger role in forms of life on Earth, such as cyanobacteria. This dramatically changed the composition of life-forms on Earth by leading to the near extinction of oxygen-intolerant organisms.

Generally, in biology, cell theory is the historic scientific theory. *Today it is universally accepted* that living organisms are made up of *cells* which are the basic structural units of all organisms. *Furthermore, cell is the basic unit of structure in all organisms and also the basic unit of reproduction. After years of looking into research, the modern version of cell theory includes the idea that energy flow occurs within cells. Heredity information (DNA) is passed on from cell to cell, and all cells have the same basic chemical composition. From the psychologists' point of view, they generally consider the organism the basis of the mind.* Therefore, it is a vitally related area of study.

Neuropsychologists work at the interface of the mind and body. Neuropsychology is the study of the *biological* substrates of behavior and mental processes. The major research topics in this field contain comparative psychology that studies humans in relation to other animals, as well as perception that involves the physical mechanics of sensation and neural and mental processing. To understand our relationships with ourselves, planets, ancestors, universe, plants, animals, *it's necessary to explore human potential for growth toward brain, mind, consciousness, spirituality, awareness, etc. Some of the most important information can be answered or formed easily through thoughts, mind, and openness which our history of evolution keeps its track well.*

Life-forms present on Earth today have evolved from ancient common ancestors through the generation of hereditary variation and natural selection. Although some studies state that life may have begun as early as 4.1 billion years ago, it can be traced to fossils dated to 3.5–3.7 billion years ago, which is still only slightly younger than Earth, which gravitationally accreted into a planet about 4.5 billion years ago. This is life as a whole, *not just human experience alone.* Research shows more than 99.9 percent of species that have ever lived are extinct.

The several branches of science that reveal the common historical, functional, and chemical basis of the evolution of all life include electron microscopy, genetics, paleobiology, and molecular biology. Life, living matters, that shows particular attributes that include responsiveness, growth, metabolism, energy transformation, and reproduction. *Despite the fact it is a noun, as with other defined entities, the word "life" could be better cast as a verb to reflect its essential status as a process. Life comprises living beings, assignable to groups that each individual is composed of one or more minimal living units.*

As we mentioned above, the units are called cells and are capable of the transformation of carbon-based and other compounds (metabolism), growth, and participation in reproductive acts. Well, the phenomenon of life can be processed in several ways. First, life as it is known and studied on planet Earth. Second, life imaginable in principle. Third, life by hypothesis, which might exist elsewhere in the universe. To human as far as is known, life exists only on Earth. Most life-forms reside in a thin sphere that extends about 23 km from 3 km beneath the bottom of the ocean to the top of the troposphere. An estimated 10–30 million distinguishable species currently inhabit this sphere of life, or biosphere.

On the other side of the coin, much is known about life from reflected in the various biological or the "life" sciences. It therefore includes the following:

anatomy (the study of form at the visible level)
ultrastructure (the study of form at the microscopic level)
physiology (the study of function)
molecular biology and biochemistry (the study of form and function at chemical levels)
ecology (the study of the relations of organisms with their environments)
taxonomy (the naming, identifying, and classifying of organisms)
ethology (the study of animal behavior)
and sociobiology (the study of social behavior)

Furthermore, there are particular sciences that participate in the study of life and focus more only on certain taxa or levels of observation, for instance, botany (the study of plants).

lichenology (the study of lichens, leafy or crusty individuals composed of permanent associations between algae or photosynthetic bacteria and fungi)

herpetology (the study of amphibians and reptiles)

microbiology (the study of bacteria, yeast, and other unicellular fungi, archaea, protists, and viruses)

zoology (the study of marine and land animals)

cytology (the study of cells)

However, most scientists implicitly use one or more of the metabolic, physiological, biochemical, genetic, thermodynamic, and autopoietic definitions as mentioned briefly.

Metabolic is relating to metabolism, the whole range of biochemical processes that occur within us or any other living organism. Metabolism consists of anabolism which is the buildup of substances and catabolism the breakdown of substances. The term "metabolic" is often used to refer specifically to the breakdown of food and its transformation into energy.

The definitions are well known with biochemists and some biologists. Living systems are objects with definite boundaries, continually exchanging some materials with their surroundings but without altering their general properties, at least over some period.

Physiological definitions of life are popular. Life is defined as any system capable of performing functions. For example, eating, metabolizing, excreting, breathing, moving, growing, reproducing, and responding to external stimuli. In addition, physiology tests how organs and systems within the body work, how they communicate, and how they combine their efforts to make conditions favorable for survival. Human physiology, specifically, is often separated into subcategories; these topics cover a vast amount of information.

Researchers in the field can focus on anything from microscopic organelles in cell physiology up to more wide-ranging topics, such as ecophysiology, which looks at whole organisms and how they adapt to environments. The most relevant arm of physiological research is applied human physiology; this field investigates biological systems at the level of the cell, organ, system, anatomy, organism, and everywhere in between.

Biochemical or molecular biological definition sees living organisms as systems that contain reproducible hereditary information coded in nucleic acid molecules and that metabolize by controlling the rate of chemical reactions using the proteinaceous catalysts known as enzymes. In many respects, this is more satisfying than the physiological or metabolic definitions of life. Molecular biology is a branch of biology that concerns the molecular basis of biological activity between biomolecules in the various systems of a cell. This includes the interactions between DNA, RNA, proteins, and their biosynthesis and the regulation of these interactions.

Genetic in biology means a gene is a sequence of nucleotides in DNA or RNA. That encodes the synthesis of a gene product, either RNA or protein. During gene expression, the DNA is first copied into RNA. The RNA can be directly functional or be the intermediate template for a protein that performs a function. The passing of genes to an organism's offspring is the basis of the inheritance of phenotypic trait. We are aware that all organisms on our Earth, from the tiniest cell to the loftiest trees, display extraordinary powers. They effortlessly perform complex transformations of organic molecules and exhibit elaborate behavior patterns.

In addition, they indefinitely construct from raw materials in the environment more or less identical copies of themselves. Therefore, how could such a system of staggering complexity, stunning beauty ever arise? The answer, for which today there is excellent scientific evidence, was carefully chronicled by the *English naturalist Charles Darwin.*

A modern rephrasing of his theory of natural selection. The theories that developed in the early twentieth century to integrate Mendelian genetics with Darwinian evolution are called the modern syntheses. Evolutionary biologists have subsequently altered this concept. Hereditary information is carried by large molecules known as genes, composed of nucleic acids. Different genes are responsible for the expression of different characteristics of the organism.

During the reproduction of the organism, the genes also replicate and thereby pass on the instructions for various characteristics to the next generation. Darwin's theory of natural selection mentions that complex organisms evolved through time because of replication, mutation, and replication of alteration.

A genetic definition of life, therefore, would be a system capable of evolution by natural selection. It is important to mention that life defined as a reproductive system dependent on replicating components does not rule out synthetic reproduction. Genes are adjusted so that they are expressed only when the product is needed, since expression draws on limited resources. Also, a cell regulates its gene expression depending on its external environment, meaning available nutrients, temperature, and other stresses, as well as its internal environment, such as cell division cycle, metabolism, and infection status. Human beings, like mammals in general, are ambulatory collections of some over one thousand cells. For instance, humans, chimpanzees, gorillas, orangutans, and their extinct ancestors form a family of organisms known as the *Hominidae*.

Researchers generally agree that among the living animals in this group, humans are most closely related to chimpanzees. This might be according to judging from the comparisons of anatomy and the genetics. Let's say if life is the result of *descent with modification*, as Charles Darwin put it, therefore, we can try to *represent its history* as a kind of family tree obtained from these morphological and genetic characteristics.

The top the tree would show organisms that are alive now. The fork of the tree shows the common ancestors of all the tips connected to that node. Biologists refer to such junction as the last common ancestor of a group of organisms. Also, all tips that connect to a particular node form a clade. In the diagram of the *Hominidae* at the right, the clade nominates by node 2 that includes gorillas, humans, and chimps. Looking in to the clade, the animal with which humans share the most recent common ancestor is the chimpanzee.

Human cells are in all fundamental respects the same as those that make up the other animals. Each cell typically consists of one central, spherical nucleus. Looking in to a living nucleated cell, it is well detailed and has a complex architecture. This appears frenetic with activity when explored through a microscope. *Furthermore, in the chemical level, it is known that life's large molecules, the "proteins and nucleic acids," are coherent at a very fast rate.*

Despite the fact some feel debased by the implication that people might be nothing more than a frenetic collection of interacting molecules, still it's thrilled with the power of science to reveal the inner workings of the chemistry of life. *The dramatic work of biochemistry and molecular biology in the twentieth century shows that laws of biology are obtained from the communication of atoms, thermodynamic concept, and life's chemistry.* This information has persisted with faithful continuity since its origin approximately 3.7 billion to 3.5 billion years ago. It brings us back to the same question on life itself and life on Earth. Life on Earth, the existence of diverse definitions of life, surely means that life is complex and difficult to briefly define.

A scientific understanding of living systems has existed since the second half of the nineteenth century. However, the miscellany of definitions and other factors among professionals suggest a different answer. For example, all organisms on Earth are extremely closely related, despite their superficial differences.

The elementary sequence, both in form and in matter, of all life on Earth is essentially identical. This identity suggests that all organisms on Earth are evolved from a single instance of the origin of life. To generalize from a single example is impossible, especially knowing when the answer itself is changing, growing, and evolving. In this respect, the biologist is basically invalid. This if we may compare with the chemist, physicist, geologist, or meteorologist, each of whom can now study aspects of his discipline beyond Earth. If truly only one type of life on Earth exists, perspective is lacking in a most essential way.

On the other side, the existent flow of all life-forms means that ancient life or even the origins of life may be peeked by studying modern cells. If we look briefly to the *origin of life and hypotheses,* perhaps the most fundamental and by the same token the least understood biological problem is the origin of life. Most of the hypotheses of the *origin of life that fall into one of this four categories are as follows:*

- The origin of life is a result of a *supernatural event*. This is one irretrievably beyond the illustrative powers of physics, chemistry, and science.
- Life, particularly simple forms, *spontaneously* and readily arises from nonliving matter.
- Life is coeternal with *matter* and has no beginning. In addition, life arrived on Earth at the time of Earth's origin.
- Life arose on the early Earth by a series of progressive *chemical* reactions.

Hypothesis 1 is the traditional contention of theology and some philosophy. This is in its most general form not inconsistent with modern scientific knowledge yet. Hypothesis 2 was the existing opinion for centuries, which might be a typical seventeenth-century view follows. Hypothesis 3 gained its momentum toward the end of the nineteenth century. One of the Swedish chemists named Svante A. Arrhenius stated that life on planet Earth arose from *panspermia*, microscopic spores. He mentioned that this formation wafted through space from planet to planet or solar system to solar system by radiation pressure.

However, his idea avoids rather than solves the problem of the *origin of life*. It's interesting that although the naturalist Charles Darwin did not commit himself on the origin of life, most subscribed to hypothesis 4 more admirably. The other famous biologists of 1869–1874 asserted that life could be generated from *inorganic chemicals*. Nonetheless, they had extremely unclear ideas about how this might be accomplished. *The meaning of organic molecule implied, especially then, a class of chemicals uniquely of biological origin.*

Although that urea and organic carbon-hydrogen molecules had been routinely produced from inorganic chemicals since 1828, the term "organic" meant *from life* to many scientists and still does. In the following discussion, the word "organic" suggests a not necessarily biological origin. The origin-of-life problem largely reduces to resolution of an organic, nonbiological source of certain processes. This can be as the identity maintained by metabolism, growth, and reproduction we mentioned before.

Would it make sense, if one thinks at present of the origin of the life, one might as well think of the origin of matter? The two problems are in some fact curiously connected. As expected, modern astrophysicists do think about the origin of matter. There is much evidence that is convincing to the point thermonuclear reactions, either in stellar interiors or in supernova explosions, give rise to all the chemical elements of the periodic table. This rise is more massive than hydrogen and helium. Some thermonuclear reactions are more probable than others.

In the 1920s, some *biochemists* such as the British geneticist J. B. S. Haldane and the Russian biochemist Aleksandr Oparin observed the nonbiological production of organic molecules in the present oxygen-rich atmosphere of Earth is highly. However, if Earth once had more hydrogen-rich conditions, the abiogenic production of *organic molecules* would have been much more likely.

In addition, if large quantities of this organic matter were somehow combined on early Earth, they would not necessarily have left much of a trace today. In the present atmosphere—with 21 percent of oxygen produced by cyanobacterial, algal, and plant photosynthesis—organic molecules would regularly, over geological time, to be broken down and oxidized to carbon dioxide, nitrogen, and water. As Darwin claimed, the earliest organisms would have tended to consume any organic matter spontaneously produced prior to the origin of life. Some of the facts lead to the idea that a certain cosmic distribution of the major elements occurs throughout the universe. For instance, very early in Earth's history, there was a much larger abundance of hydrogen. This has subsequently been lost to space; most likely the atoms carbon, nitrogen, and oxygen were present on the early Earth.

However, not in the forms of CO_2 (carbon dioxide), N_2, and O_2 as they are presented today but rather as their fully soaked hydrides, for example, methane, ammonia, and water. The presence of large amounts of reduced (hydrogen-rich) minerals, like uraninite and pyrite, that were exposed to the ancient atmosphere in sediments formed over two billion years ago suggests that atmospheric conditions then were considerably less oxidizing than they are now.

If we go as far back as 1958, some of us witnessed the space race. NASA's first space satellite, *Explorer 1*, launched a Geiger counter and miniature tape. This tape recorder into space registered astonishingly high radiation levels above Earth. Thus, this discovery gave humanity its first glimpse of the *Van Allen radiation belts*, named after James Van Allen. This famous scientist mentored an aspiring student named Jim Green. Therefore, today he is NASA's planetary science director. *So far, we can conclude based on past and today's information that our solar system is a wondrous place with a single star, our sun.*

Aside from everything that orbits around it, such as planets, moons, asteroids, and comets, this beautiful solar system we call home is part of an even larger cosmos with billions of other solar systems. Other pieces of evidence explore the latest experience and provide an insight into the thinking of a modern-day theoretical physicist. However, many questions still need clarification, for instance, is the universe destined to subside or to enlarge indefinitely until it homogenizes in a heat death? Research might introduce a third possibility: the cosmological conformal cyclic cosmology (CCC) scheme.

Alternatively, the *universe might evolve through generations*. Through study, it might end in the decay of mass and begin again in a new big bang. The equations governing the crossover from each term to the next, called the creation of a dominant new scalar material, are assumed to be dark matter. In order that this chemical does not build up from one generation to another, it is taken to decay away completely. Some atoms of biological interest, their relative numerical abundances in the universe are as one, on Earth, and in the living organisms.

Despite the elemental composition degree from star to star, from place to place on Earth, and from organism to organism, these comparisons are informative. *Generally, 99 percent of the mass both of the universe and of life is made of six atoms, namely, hydrogen (H), helium (He), carbon (C), nitrogen (N), oxygen (O), and neon (Ne). Let's take a look at the relative abundances of the elements. Zero percent here stands for any quantity less than 10–6 percent.*

atom	universe	life (terrestrial vegetation)	Earth (crust)
hydrogen	87	16	3
helium	12	0*	0
carbon	0.03	21	0.1
nitrogen	0.008	3	0.0001
oxygen	0.06	59	49
neon	0.02	0	0
sodium	0.0001	0.01	0.7
magnesium	0.0003	0.04	8
aluminum	0.0002	0.001	2
silicon	0.003	0.1	14
sulfur	0.002	0.02	0.7
phosphorus	0.00003	0.03	0.07
potassium	0.000007	0.1	0.1
argon	0.0004	0	0
calcium	0.0001	0.1	2
iron	0.002	0.005	18

Based on the *general* estimation above, we have noticed that the Jovian planets (Jupiter, Saturn, Uranus, and Neptune) are much closer to cosmic composition than is Earth. They are largely relating, with atmospheres composed principally of hydrogen and helium. In addition, methane, ammonia, neon, and water have been identified in smaller amounts.

Could it be possible the massive Jovian planets were formed from material of typical cosmic composition? This might be a result of being far from the sun, and their upper atmospheres are very cold. Earth and the other planets of the inner solar system, however, are much less massive. The first experimental simulation of early Earth conditions was explored during 1953.

Based on research, a mixture of methane, ammonia, water vapor, and hydrogen was circulated through a liquid solution and continuously sparked by a corona discharge mounted higher in the apparatus. The search for the first steps in the origin of life has been transformed from a religious/philosophical exercise to an experimental science based on the essential building blocks of proteins (amino acids), carbohydrates (sugars), and nucleic acids (nucleotide bases). This is, the monomers can be readily produced under conditions thought to have prevailed on Earth in the Archean Eon. In addition, the nucleotide bases and even the biological pigments called porphyrins have been produced in the laboratory under simulated early Earth conditions. However, the details of the experimental synthetic pathways and the question of stability of the small organic molecules produced are vigorously debated.

We explored interests and differences among planets, something that is coming to today's understanding of how *interconnected* all of the science is. We learn about Earth; we can apply what we're studying to planets like Jupiter and Venus and vice versa. *So it really is important that we look at all of our planets, and that looking at other places in the solar system, we can therefore learn what might be Earth's future.* For example, Venus is incredibly an active planet, for whatever reason, so it has dumped an enormous amount of CO_2 gases, and we believe it may still be active today doing that.

From brain to consciousness and from universe to atoms, the question of the meaning of life is perhaps one that we would rather not ask, for fear of the answer or lack thereof. If we look ourselves in an aware way, we are all as much an extraordinary phenomenon of nature as mountains, clouds, rain, butterflies, the patterns in flowers, etc. We are all just like that, and there is nothing wrong with us or that. It is the interconnectedness and the close relationship among all as a whole over its part. The universe implies the organism, and each single organism intimates the universe. Like nature, all phenomena are interactions of elements of the whole, and the relationship between them always implies and reinforces that wholeness.

Therefore, the question that might arise is how can we define our brain under a scanner or MRI or perhaps through philosophies? If we let big bang to define us in some way, billions of years ago, human was a big bang. Yet only now human is a complicated being. Hereafter, we cut ourselves off and no longer feel that we're still that big bang.

In the nineteenth century, scientists and philosophers couldn't figure out how nonliving things became living. They thought that living things possessed a mysterious life force. Hereafter, some did discover that life was the product of diverse physical systems that, together, created something that appeared magical. Others believe that the same story will be told about consciousness. The term is often regarded as capturing what it is to be human, or the essence of humanity. The term is controversial because it is disputed whether or not such an essence exists. In addition, if there was a big bang in the beginning and if the human is something that's a result of the big bang too, still we are not something that is a sort of product on the end of the process. *Humans are still a work in progress*

Therefore, this might be another answer or a definition to our development journey, an open-ended being. From the origin of life to human nature is a bundle of characteristics. Human development includes ways of thinking, feeling, and acting, which humans are said to have naturally. Arguments about human nature have been a mainstay of philosophy for centuries, and the concept continues to provoke lively philosophical debate. This concept also continues to play a big role in science, with neuroscientists, psychologists, and social scientists.

Debates about human nature are related to, although not the same as, debates about the comparative importance of genes and environment in development ("nature needs nurture"). When I see you, I see you not just what you define yourself as Mr. or Mrs. or by your name. I see everyone as the primordial energy of the universe and all there is. We all are continuous with the universe. That is, we do have individual existences, yet we also interconnected. We can't be separated from the whole process.

We are an "open-ended being" through which the universe is gazing at and exploring itself. In other words, humans are a vibrant of what the whole universe is doing in the same way that rain is a function of what the whole storm is doing. Humans are an inextricable portion of the reality process. This may or may not have begun or end with the big bang. We are also consisting of the same atoms as everything else. *For this point, we are the universe, and definitely each of us is distinct from everything else.*

The idea of humans coming into this world might be vague. The idea that humans came out of it, as grass from the soil, is a better explanation maybe. *The interconnected life, neurons, universe, and each human are an expression of the whole realm of nature, a unique flow of the total universe.* Aside from a sense of fulfillment, to over continue to be aware of themselves as isolated body inside bags of skin. *No considerate theory would destroy the human development by making it so rigid and unadaptable as to depend upon one book, the developing mind or brain, for all the answers.*

For the use of words, and thus of a book, is to point beyond ourselves to a world of life and experience that is not mere words or even ideas. Just as money is not real, consumable wealth, books are not much of a realty. To idolize any theory for living is like eating paper currency.

Understanding our experience on earth in order to our relationships with our development, we must explore everything there is. However, how can we understand what is everything? Human species never lived outside of the planet Earth, the same as fish cannot survive outside of the water. Also, if we held a human brain in our hand, we would find it to be a soggy clump of gray matter, which weighs about 1.3 kg. How is it possible that this gray soggy stuff can give rise to the richness and depth of our conscious experience? As we mentioned throughout this book, this is known as the hard problem of consciousness.

Many eminent philosophers and scientists have rejected the idea that consciousness is directly produced by brain processes. They have turned to the alternative view that it is actually a fundamental quality of the universe. This might sound far-fetched, but if we think about the other "fundamentals" in the universe, we take for granted, for instance, gravity and mass. Humans have seen that the universe is at root a magical illusion as addition to a fabulous game.

The idea of consciousness as a fundamental quality might offer elegant solutions to many problems which are difficult to explain using the standard scientific model. The idea at some point can explain the relationship between the brain and consciousness. The brain does not produce consciousness but acts as a kind of receiver which "picks up" the fundamental consciousness that is all around us and "transmits" it into our own being. Because the human brain is so sophisticated and complex, it is able to receive and transmit consciousness in a very intense and intricate way so that we are (probably) more intensely and expansively conscious than most other animals.

One of the arguments for assuming that the brain produces consciousness is that if the brain is damaged, consciousness is impaired or altered. However, this doesn't invalidate the idea that the brain may be a receiver and transmitter of consciousness. A television doesn't produce the program that comes through it. However, if it is damaged, its ability to transmit the shows will be impaired. On the other hand, the puzzle of altruism might also be explained. If, as many scientists believe, human beings are just genetic machines, only concerned with the survival and propagation of our genes, wouldn't then altruism be difficult to account for? The only real "human" is the one that comes and goes, manifests, and withdraws itself eternally in and as every conscious being.

For humans is the universe looking at itself from billions of points of view, points that come and go so that the vision is forever new. *A continuum of one journey that requires to nurture its nature.* If we look at this from a "spiritual" perspective (which sees consciousness as fundamental), though, altruism is easy to explain which is related to empathy. Hereafter, humans sharing fundamental consciousness means that it is possible for us to sense the suffering of others and to respond with altruistic acts. In addition, we share fundamental consciousness with other species too. It is possible for us to feel empathy with and to behave altruistically toward them as well. Does this mean the awakening experiences as encounters with fundamental consciousness, in which we sense its presence in everything around us, including our own selves is reality? Humans tend to experience a sense of oneness because oneness is the fundamental reality of things.

One of the main areas of interest in psychology is in what is called awakening experiences, when human awareness intensifies and expands, and humans experience a sense of oneness with other human beings, nature, or the universe as a whole. Conventional science also explains and struggles to the powerful effect of mental intention or belief on the body (as illustrated by the placebo effect and the pain-numbing effects of hypnosis). For instance, if the mind is just a by-product of matter, it should not be able to influence the form and functioning of the body so profoundly.

The idea of *consciousness as a fundamental quality* of the universe might have a great deal of weight. Today there are many books and research related to *spiritual science that argue that the best way to understand the world is not through science or spirituality alone—but through an approach which combines them both. Now does this mean in order to know our consciousness which plays a bigger role in our development and daily life, we make the universe another subject of human growth?* Centuries ago, Einstein spent the last part of his life trying to find a "theory of everything"—one that could tie together his theory of general relativity and quantum mechanics. These two theories are not fully compatible in our current understanding of physics anymore yet brought us to much better understanding. Many researchers and physicists have picked up where Einstein stopped.

Therefore, much other possibilities arise. One other solution they have come up with is string theory. *String theory combines the two theories by assuming there are multiple universes and dimensions beyond the ones humans know. Human development also needs a biological transformation to understand most of the underlying problem in all human affairs of the human condition. The idea behind "think with an educated brain over a meditative one" requires education prior to meditation. Einstein too agreed if a theory cannot be explained, then the theory is probably worthless, meaning that great ideas are pictorial. Great ideas can be explained in the language of pictures, things that we can see and touch, objects that we can visualize in the mind. That is what science that contributes to human development is all about.*

The world's best-known and most prolific physicist *including Einstein* was driven in his later *years to find* a single set of laws for the universe. The laws that would apply as readily to the chaotic subatomic particles as to the majestic waltz of galaxies in deep space. *Today* on the one hundredth anniversary of $E = mc^2$, a new generation of physicists is carrying the torch and offering some answer to life, the universe, and everything. Besides, in the twentieth century, *Newton's laws were replaced by quantum mechanics and relativity as the most fundamental laws of physics.* Nevertheless, Newton's laws continue to give an accurate account of nature, except for very small bodies such as electrons or for bodies moving close to the speed of light.

Quantum mechanics and relativity reduce to Newton's laws for larger bodies or for bodies moving more slowly.

Newton's laws of motion relate an object's motion to the forces acting on it. In the first law, an object will not change its motion unless a force acts on it. In the second law, the force on an object is equal to its mass times its acceleration. In the third law, when two objects interact, they apply forces to each other of equal magnitude and opposite direction. Newton's first law states that if a body is at rest or moving at a constant speed in a straight line, it will remain at rest or keep moving in a straight line at a constant speed unless it is acted upon by a force. This is known as the law of inertia. The law of inertia was first formulated by Galileo Galilei for the horizontal motion on Earth. His second law is a quantitative description of the changes that a force can produce on the motion of a body. It states that the time rate of change of the momentum of a body is equal in both magnitude and direction to the force imposed on it. The momentum of a body is equal to the product of its mass and its velocity. Newton's second law is one of the most important in all of physics.

For a body whose mass m is constant, it can be written in the form $F = ma$, where F (force) and a (acceleration) are both vector quantities. Newton's third law states that when two bodies interact, they apply forces to each other that are equal in magnitude and opposite in direction. The third law is also known as the law of action and reaction. This law is important in analyzing problems of static equilibrium, where all forces are balanced, but it also applies to bodies in uniform or accelerated motion. In principle, Newton created that new science. He developed his three laws in order to explain why the orbits of the planets are ellipses rather than circles, at which he thrived, yet it turned out that he explained even more. The series of events from Copernicus to Newton is known collectively as *the scientific revolution*.

We can also conclude that besides the science, the evidence present is enough to support the *universal explanation* of the physical world itself. We can acknowledge that nothing can be guaranteed against an unknown *wait-and-see argument* for some unlikely *fully realized physics* or *metaphysics* that may be able to *reconcile* the *evidence* with such a fully completed formulation of *universe reality*. One day, evidence and a better understanding of string theory may allow us to travel between universes and into new dimensions, potentially even making time travel possible.

Somehow the research is supposed to follow from the proposition that the *fundamental building block of matter is not the quark (atom-smashing physicists have shown that the protons and neutrons at the heart of atoms are actually composed of quarks) but something even smaller, a million billion times smaller—a vibrating string*. It is no easy matter to create a universe where matter, space, and time are stable. For it all to work, the fundamental forces must be unified. And that merger can only take place in higher dimensions. Our whole knowledge of the world is, in one sense, self-knowledge.

For knowing is a translation of external events into bodily processes and especially into states of the nervous system and the brain: we know the world in terms of the body and in accordance with its structure. One thing that might reinforce our isolated sensation of self is to —only ever be able to see one half of the whole and remaining blind to the rest. Can it be our normal sensation of self is a hoax or, at best, a temporary role that we are playing or we have been conned into playing, with our own implicit consent, just as every hypnotized person is basically willing to be hypnotized?

Our five senses are differing forms of one basic sense—something like touch. For example, seeing is highly sensitive touching. The eyes touch, or feel, light waves and so enable us to touch things out of reach of our hands. The ears touch sound waves in the air. The nose tiny particles of dust and gas. But the complex patterns and chains of neurons which constitute these senses are composed of neuron units which are capable of changing between just two states. To the central brain, the individual neuron signals either yes or no. However, as we know from computers which employs the binary arithmetic in which the only figures are zero and one of these simple elements can be formed into the most compound forms. With that said, our nervous system and zero or one computers are much like everything else, for the physical world is basically vibration, whether we think of this vibration in terms of waves or of particles, or perhaps wavicles.

Thus, we might never find the crest of a wave without a trough or a particle without an interval. Nevertheless, the very things that we believe to exist are always either on or off. Thus, "on" alone and "off" alone do not exist. *The general conditioning of consciousness might be to ignore intervals.* For instance, we register the sound but not the silence that surrounds it. We think of space as empty or nothingness in which certain somethings—objects, planetary bodies, our own bodies—hang.

Although it's clear enough, solids and spaces go together as inseparably as insides and outsides. *Space is the relationship between bodies*, and without the space, there can be neither energy nor motion. Let's pay more attention, which basically is narrowed perception, *the way of looking at life bit by bit, using memory to string the bits together—as when examining a dark room with a flashlight. Perception thus narrowed has the advantage of being sharp and bright, but it has to focus on one area of the world at a time.* And where there is no focus, only space or uniform surfaces and searches about for more features. *Attention is also something like a scanning mechanism in radar.* However, a scanning process that observes the world bit by bit soon persuades its user that the world is a great collection of bits, and these might call separate things or events.

We often say that you can only think of one thing at a time. Looking at the world bit by bit, we might have convinced ourselves that it consists of separate things, and so we give ourselves the problem of how these things are connected and how they cause and affect each other. It would have been easier if we had been aware that it was just our way of looking at the world one step at a time which had chopped it up into separate bits, events, causes, and effects.

If nature and nurture conspire in the architecture of this illusion of separateness, does it cause us to be genuinely misled, the sense of separateness from the universe and our sense of being divided within ourselves? Returning to our inability to grasp such intervals as the basic fabric of world and integrate foreground with background, content with context might be another solution. *In the twentieth century,* scientists are aware that what things *(atom)* are, and what they are doing, depends on where and when they are doing it. If that is so, the definition of a thing or event must include the definition of its environment. Therefore, we may realize that any given thing goes with a given environment. As a result, intimately, and inseparably, it is more difficult to draw a clear boundary between the thing and its surroundings.

What is atom in a general definition? Atom is the smallest unit into which matter can be divided without the release of electrically charged particles. It is the smallest unit of matter that has the characteristic properties of a chemical element that is considered as the basic building block of chemistry. In addition, mostly atom is an empty space. The rest consists of a positively charged nucleus of protons and neutrons surrounded by a cloud of negatively charged electrons. The nucleus is small and dense compared with the electrons, which are the lightest charged particles in nature. Electrons are attracted to any positive charge by their electric force; in an atom, electric forces bind the electrons to the nucleus. An atom is the smallest unit of ordinary matter that forms a chemical element. Every solid, liquid, gas, and plasma are composed of neutral or ionized atoms. Atoms are extremely small, typically around one hundred picometers across. Individual is the Latin form of the Greek atom.

We cannot dissect a live human, which implies that the only true atom is the universe—that total system of interdependent thing-events which can be separated from each other only in the form of name. For the human is not built as an object is built; therefore, the human does not come into being by assembling parts, by screwing a head onto a neck, by wiring a brain to a set of lungs, etc. Wouldn't this also mean that the human is separate from the universal environment only in name? When this is not recognized, we may get confused names with nature. We have come to believe that having a separate name makes the human a separate being.

The teleological approach of Aristotle came to be central by late classical and old-fashioned times. Human nature really causes humans to become what they become. Thus, it exists somehow independently of individuals. *This in turn has been understood as also showing a special connection between human nature and divinity.* This approach understands human nature itself has purposes and goals, similar somehow to human intents and goals, and one of those goals is humanity living naturally. Such understanding of human nature sees this nature as an idea or system of a human. Once we have learned this, we can return to the world of practical affairs with a new essence. We might consider the universe is at root a magical illusion and a fabulous game and that there is no separate human. And this brings us back to the notion of "the only real being is the one that comes and goes, manifests, and withdraws itself eternally in and as every conscious being" again.

For human is the universe looking at itself from billions of points of view; points that come and go make the vision forever new. For the earth might not remember who have come and who have gone. However, the existence of this invariable and *metaphysical human nature* is subject of much historical debate continuing into modern life. *Charles Darwin's theory of evolution has* changed the nature of the discussion, supporting the proposition that mankind's ancestors were not like mankind of the twentieth century. However, many recent scientific perspectives—such as behaviorism, determinism, and the chemical model within modern psychiatry and psychology—claim to be neutral regarding human nature. Despite the *modern science, such disciplines seek to explain* with little recourse to metaphysical causation, they can be offered to explain the origins of human nature and its underlying mechanisms and to demonstrate capacities for change and diversity.

Plato was one of the first to claim that the systematic use of our reason can show us the best way to live. Platonic thinking is part of this rise of reason in ancient Greece—often called the Greek miracle. It replaced superstitious, religious, mythological, supernatural thinking with rational, scientific, philosophical, naturalistic thinking. His idea, the lives we live today, especially the benefits of science and technology, is from the Greek miracle. *Plato claimed that if we truly understand human nature, we can find individual happiness and social stability.* Plato was born into an influential family of Athens, which is his birth location Athens was at the center of the Greek miracle—the use of reason to understand the world. What is most distinctive about Plato's philosophy is his theory of forms, although his description of forms isn't detailed, yet Plato thought that knowledge is an active process through which we organize and classify our perceptions. Plato claimed that forms are ideas which have at least four aspects: *logical, metaphysical, epistemological, and moral.*

Logical—how does a chair or flower apply to various furniture/ plants? How does a universal concept like bed or cat or green or warm apply to many individual things? Plato's second form was *metaphysical* to which he claimed, are forms ultimately real? Do they exist independently? Plato says yes. Universal, eternal, immaterial, unchanging forms are more real than individuals. *Individual material things are known by the senses, whereas forms are known by the intellect.* Thus, the forms have a real, independent existence—there is a world of forms. The third form is *epistemological.* Epistemological—knowledge is of forms, *perceptions* in this world lead only to belief or opinion. He finds the clearest example of knowledge based on forms in *mathematics.* The objects of *mathematical reasoning* are often not found in this world—and we can never see most of them—but they provide knowledge about the world.

His last form was *moral.* Moral—*ideals of human conduct.* Moral concepts like justice and fairness are forms. Therefore, there are physical, mathematical, and moral forms. Furthermore, Plato's philosophy responds to intellectual and moral relativism—there are objective truths about the nature of reality and about human behavior. *Plato* is a *dualist*; there is both immaterial mind (soul) and material body, and it is the soul that knows the forms. He alleged the soul exists before birth and after death and that the soul or mind attains knowledge of the forms, as different to the senses. In addition, he claimed the soul (mind) itself is divided into three parts: reason, appetite (physical urges), and will (emotion passion, spirit). He mentioned the *human will* is the source of love, anger, outrage, determination, hostility, etc. *When these aspects are not in agreement (in relationship), we experience mental conflict.* The will can be on the side of either reason or the appetites. We might be pulled by lustful appetite or the rational desire to find a good partner. To explain the interaction of these three parts of the self, Plato uses the image of the charioteer (reason) who tries to control horses representing will and appetites.

Plato also highlighted the *social aspect of human nature. He supposed that we are not self-sufficient, we need others, and we benefit from our social interactions, from other persons' talents, aptitudes, and friendship.* It is not a new theory, how people construct meaning in a way that is compatible with the modern scientific understanding of *how the brain functions.* It examines the structure of systems of belief and the role those systems play in the *regulation of emotion, using multiple academic fields to show that connecting myths and beliefs with science is essential to fully understand how people make meaning.*

Furthermore, according to research, the main goal was to examine why both individuals and groups participate in social conflict, exploring the reasoning and motivation individuals take to support their belief systems. The examination of the world's religious ideas might allow us to describe our essential morality and eventually develop a *universal system of morality. In line with reasoning, there might exist a struggle between chaos and characteristic of the unknown,* such as nature and order characteristic of explored, mapped territory, and culture. Humans with their capability of intellectual thinking also make intellectual territoriality—the belief systems that regulate our emotions.

A possible threat to an important belief activates emotional reactions, which are potentially followed by uncontrolled attempts to face internal confusion. *Despite that, people generally prefer war to be something external, rather than internal, than reforming our confronted principles.* It's not an easy test to attempt to explain how the mind works, while including illustrations with elaborate geometric diagrams, the constituent elements of experience as personality, territory, and process.

If we look into Plato's understanding of soul, considered the human psyche is to be the essence of a person, being that said which decides on how people would behave. He measured human essence to be an intangible, perpetual resident of our being—even after death, the soul exists. The Platonic soul consists of three parts: the logic (logical, mind, nous, or reason)—logos is located in the head, is related to reason, and regulates the other part; the thymos (emotion, spiritedness, or masculine)—the thymos is located near the chest region and is related to human anger; and the eros (appetitive, desire, or feminine)—the eros is located in the stomach and is related to human desires.

During Plato's time, he asserted that the three parts of the human psyche are also interconnected to the many classes of society.

According to Braden's divine matrix, he explained, which is the container that holds the universe, the bridge between all things, and the mirror that shows us what we have created. His definition comprises three components that frame the *divine matrix: container, bridge, and mirror.* Thus, the concept *container* indicates that people are living in a small community in which each one affects other people and is affected by other people in that global community.

Hence, *people's relationships* affect the shape and the nature of the universe. The divine matrix in this sense works as the mirror to *shape people's relationships* and *beliefs.* As for the concept *bridge* mentioned in Branden's definition above, it directs that people have the *decision to make* life on Earth peaceful and pleasant or nonpeaceful and dull. Thus, humans may use facilities in good developments or not. His idea on the concept of *mirror* refers to the replication of individuals' *behavior on others.* The relationship among communities, of course, is affected by the relationship among individuals as the main mechanisms of a community. Therefore, he claimed, each individual is a *mirror* of their community. That is, through an individual's beliefs and traditions, one can observe the whole community's beliefs and traditions.

For centuries, a leading question in human biological psychology has been whether and how mental functions might be localized in the brain. Looking back from Phineas Gage to H. M. and Clive Wearing, individuals with mental issues observable to physical damage., have stimulated new *discoveries in this area. Modern neuropsychology* could be said to originate *in the 1870s, when in France, Paul Broca* drew production of speech to the left frontal gyrus, thereby also *demonstrating the hemispheric lateralization of brain function.*

Soon after, Carl Wernicke acknowledged a related area necessary for the understanding of *speech.* The modern field of behavioral neuroscience focuses on physical causes underpinning behavior. Physiological psychologists use animal models, typically rats, to study the neural, genetic, and cellular mechanisms that underlie specific behaviors such as learning and memory and fear responses. Cognitive neuroscientists investigate the neural correlates of psychological processes in humans using neural imaging tools, and neuropsychologists conduct psychological assessments to determine.

For instance, specific aspects and extent of cognitive deficit caused by brain damage. The *biopsychosocial model is an integrated perspective* toward understanding consciousness, behavior, and social interaction. It adopts that any given behavior or mental process affects and is affected by dynamically interconnected biological, psychological, and social factors. Evolutionary psychology examines cognition and personality traits from an evolutionary perspective. This perspective recommends that psychological adaptations evolved to solve recurrent problems in human ancestral environments.

Evolutionary psychology offers balancing explanations for the mostly adjacent or developmental explanations developed by other areas of psychology. *It focuses mostly on definitive or why* questions rather than adjacent or how questions. Moreover, *how* questions are more directly tackled by behavioral genetics research, which aims to understand how genes and environment impact behavior.

Speaking of evolutionary, the Swiss psychiatrist Carl Jung (1875–1961) was interested in the way in which symbols and common myths permeate our thinking on both conscious and subconscious levels. Jung initially worked with fellow psychoanalyst Sigmund Freud, whose 1899 work *The Interpretation of Dreams* had attached significance to the recurring themes and ideas in people's dreams and sought to understand their relevance to subjects' psyches and mental well-being.

However, Jung and Freud later took different paths, with the former conflicting with Freud's stress on the influence of biological factors such as libido on behavior and personality. Therefore, Jung looked at areas of the mind that constitute human psyche, and the way in which they influenced one another. He distinguished the image of ourselves (persona) that we present to the world, from our shadow, which may be comprised of hidden anxieties and bottled-up thoughts.

Jung also distinguished the relationship between our personal unconscious that holds an individual's personal memories and ideas, and our collective unconscious, a set of memories and ideas that is shared between all of humanity. Communal thoughts, which Jung defined as archetypes, infuse the shared unconscious and appear as themes in our dreams which surface in our culture—in the way of myths, books, films, or paintings. *Jung touched up on the conflict among thoughts in the personal subconscious and the conscious that* could create internal conflicts which could lead to particular personality traits and concerns. Such inner conflicts could be resolved by allowing bottled-up ideas to appear into the conscious and being cooperative rather than destroying them.

Consequently, it creates a state of inner agreement, through a process known as *individuation. What is individuation refers to the process through* which a person accomplishes a sense of individuality separate from the identities of others and begins to consciously exist as a human in the world. *By the same token, this book journey has described such understanding with a twist toward a continuous flow of energy and information system (interpersonal brain).* When difficulty arises in the process of developing and understanding one's self-assessment, a psychologist, professor, or other mental health professional may be able to offer guidance, reassurance, and care and support.

What is interpersonal brain referring to is one's unique self-identity, which is separate from that of any other individual. It develops through the process of energy-information system, awareness, and education. This is an ever-continuing system and can be measured as both a goal and a lifelong process of human development. The interpersonal brain upheld the same ground as individuation, as an important human lifelong goal. Individuation describes a process of self-realization—the discovery of one's life purpose or what one believes to be the *meaning of life.*

According to centuries ago for understanding of psychology and interpersonal brain when the personalities lose touch with certain aspects of the selves, they may be able to *reintegrate* these aspects of their nature through individuation (aside from energy-information flow for the interpersonal brain).

Furthermore, what *self-psychology particularly stresses through this book journey is the development of a stable and integrated sense of self through empathic contacts with others, especially significant others.* Thus, such assessment meets the developing self's needs for *mirroring* and idealization and thereby strengthens the developing self (developing mind). The process of behavior proceeds through *transforming internalizations* in which the individuals steadily adopt the self-aware (self-identity) functions provided by professionals. From centuries ago, to modern development, developmental psychologists would engage a child with a book and then make observations based on how the children interacts with the object.

Mainly focusing on the development of the human mind throughout the life span, *developmental psychology pursues to understand* how people come to observe, understand, and perform within the world and how these processes change as they age. This may bring our *focus on cognitive development and emotional, moral, social, or neural development.* One example, those researchers who study children's development use a number of unique research approaches to make observations in *natural settings* and to engage them in trial tasks, such as activities like designed games that are both enjoyable for the child and logically useful.

The researchers have even developed clever approaches to study the mental processes of infants. In addition to studying children, developmental psychologists also learn aging and processes throughout the life span, particularly at other times of rapid change on adolescents, etc. For instance, at the early stage of personalization (early stage of development) according to research, an infant begins life in a state of fusion. In this state, the infant and the mother or a caregiver essentially exist as one.

The process of separation—self-identity—begins around the fourth or fifth month of life with the phase of differentiation. From hereafter, the infant starts to recognize the mother is a separate being. During the eight-month period, the baby will naturally gain movement and start spending time away from the mother. Reconciliation, which typically starts around fifteen months, includes the baby becoming aware of increasing amounts of separateness from the mother. The final stage of this process, according to much research, model, begins around the age of two years old. At this stage, the baby will naturally identify a sense of *personal identity* and grasp a stable mental image of the mother or caregiver, even on their absence.

Hereafter, when the process of separation—self-identity—is directed successfully, a child is typically able to have a sense of healthy independence and a firm sense of being self-aware. (delete this sentence.)

On the other hand, if parents or caregivers are overly protective, the child may experience feelings of insufficiency and self-doubt. In addition, adolescents continue to self-identity from their parents as they move into young adulthood. This age group tends to choose their schools, friends, hobbies, or even careers and make a number of other life choices that may be at probabilities with the choices of their families. Those who have successfully become self-aware will likely be able to make these choices with less anxiety. However, the process of self-identity may be challenging to some. For that reason, making choices that bend from family principles and values may be difficult. An incapability to be self-aware, or the denial of the true self, can both cause suffering and harmfully impact the development of a defined sense of identity.

The process of self-identity (interpersonal brain) is measured crucial to the development of a healthy identity and the formation of healthy relationships with others. An individual who does not sufficiently become self-aware may lack a clear sense of self and feel uncomfortable following life goals when those goals differ from the requirements of family or significant others. Difficulty of self-identity may also lead to amplified dependence on others, challenges in family or professional relationships, unfortunate decision-making skills, and just a general sense of not knowing who one is and what one wants from life. Concerned or harmful family dynamics often is the reason at least partially, to a stalled or unsuccessful self-identity process.

Relationships with both parents and siblings may have an impact on self-recognition, and the seed of advanced challenges may be planted at any stage of the developmental process. Children whose parents and siblings offer support and encouragement throughout this process are likely to have a developed identity and sense of self and may be better able to make choices and follow goals with little concern and self-doubt. *Integration of such education to family dynamic, brain health awareness, and schools is therefore an essential part of the whole development journey at any age and stage of development.*

As far as in 1960–1980, the *psychology* of the self-preference was less toward the definition of the self and more on explanation of reasoning. This way the self is like all reality, not knowable in its essence. We can describe the various consistent forms in which the self appears can demonstrate the several constituents that make up the self and explain their origin and purposes. We can do all that, but we will still not know the essence of the self as differentiated from its manifestations. An interesting application of "self-psychology" has been in the *interpretation* of the friendship, relationship, nature, and nurture.

In addition, in self-psychology, the effort is made to understand individuals from within their subjective experience via indirect self-examination, building interpretations on the understanding of the self as the central agency of the human psyche. What are essential to understanding self-psychology are the perceptions of empathy, mirroring, idealizing, and ego. Self-psychology was seen as a major break from traditional psychoanalysis and is considered the beginning of the relational approach to psychoanalysis.

Arguments about self-psychology or human nature have been a central focus of philosophy for centuries, and the concept continues to provoke lively philosophical debate. While both concepts are distinct from each other, discussions regarding human nature are typically related to those regarding the comparative importance of genes and environment in human development (the story of "nature versus nurture").

Accordingly, the concept also continues to play a role in fields of science, such as neuroscience, psychology, and social science in which numerous theorists claim to have generated insight into human nature. Human nature is traditionally compared with human qualities that vary among societies, such as those associated with definite cultures. Human nature is a concept that means the fundamental characters and characteristics—including ways of thinking, feeling, and acting—that humans are said to have naturally.

Human nature includes the core characteristics, psychology, behaviors, shared by all people. We all have different experiences of the humans in our life, and this is where the self-understanding begins. The term is often used to mean the essence of humankind, or what it "means" to be human. Philosophers and scholars tend to talk human nature based on major schools of thought from human history. In Western cultures, the discussions usually begin with Plato and Aristotle in classical Greece. Platonian thought that humans were rational, social animals, and he connected our nature with our souls and ability to reason rather than our bodies.

Aristotle differed primarily in his belief that both body and soul contributed to our human identity. These theories are not mutually exclusive but have been built upon each other and adapted over time. From the twentieth century, many ideas about human nature have been discussed by historical records such as Rene Descartes, Charles Darwin, Karl Marx, and Sigmund Freud.

Neuroscientists examine minds compromised by brain injury; others' approach has been to look back into evolutionary history. In the minds of other animals, even insects, some believe we can see the functional components upon which our *selfhood depends*. We can also see the qualities we value most in *human selfhood*. Even free will evolves over evolutionary time. The amygdala, the part of the brain that registers fear, may not be free in any meaningful sense—it's effectively a computer—but it awards the mind to which it belongs with the ability to avoid danger. In this way, the curving path leads from determinism to freedom too; a whole can be freer than its parts.

Despite much contribution to human mind, there has to be a hard boundary between third-person explanations and first-person experience Why couldn't one see *oneself* as taking two different stances toward a single phenomenon Is it possible to be "impartial about brain, mind," which from the outside looks like neurons but from the inside feels like consciousness? Scientists still can't understand how neurons—even billions of neurons—could generate the experience of *being me*. Despite growing technology, images, medicine, and research, we are still in infancy levels of development due to *numerous mental health concerns around the globe*.

An interpersonal neurobiology and integration system of brain developments—point of well-being—might be another way to explore. The complex, nonlinear system of our mind achieves states of *self-organization by balancing the two opposing processes of differentiation and linkage*. The coherent flow of this process is bounded on one side by misunderstanding and on the other by not moving forward. In this manner, we can envision a flow of well-being, with the two banks being not knowing the one side, not practicing on the other. This also can be another way of viewing the symptoms of the diagnostic and statistical manual for psychiatric diagnoses is as manifestations of less clear or of less motivated to change. Therefore, this flow of well-being can be seen to reveal the correlations among an empathic relationship, a coherent mind, and an integrated brain as the important points on the journey of well-being.

To achieve the goal of brain, mind development through the eyes of nature, it needs nurture relationships. It's necessary to explore all venues of human development from the Enlightenment experience through today's century as one direction of learning experiences to the growing-up journey of the human species. This places our attention on education of the brain, mind, consciousness, evolution process again and again. Looking back at decades of time, we move from our earliest years, and our prefrontal cortices begin to develop our capacity for reflection on the nature of time. Aside this might be a form of mental time travel that enables an early form of *self-knowing awareness*, which the reflective capacity of much might has linked past, present, and future relationships.

Hereafter, it reveals itself in an awareness of the finite nature of our time. This belief can also teach history that people's lives were often limited to a century or so and that the experience of death is an inevitable part of each life. Can it be possible temporal integration confronts this organizational role of time, and our transient lives, helping the education to consider the deep questions of purpose in life? I don't know, yet it's just better to explore, for we might be able to explain what is not necessary to define which is life and the *human mind-brain development*.

What we can tell for now is that the mind flows as energy and information which are channeled through the process of *attention*. The nomenclature of science refers to the presence of three *general mechanisms of attention: exogenous, endogenous, and executive*. Exogenous attention is a form of attentional focus driven by the immediacy of an often-external stimulus, such as a loud sound. A more sustained, self-generated form is called endogenous attention in which the individual chooses to focus attention on a particular stimulus. With executive attention, one can create a flexible response not governed by the external world or by a singular focus of attention.

The integration of consciousness involves the development of executive forms of attention that are associated with the larger capacities for *self-regulation*, such as the balancing of emotion, improved stress response, and enhanced social skills. Self-awareness has its roots within the central regulatory systems of the brain and thus may play an important role in various forms of psychotherapy and in various psychiatric disorders. In many ways, how we have developed the capacity to have a *receptive, flexible form of awareness* enables us to have freedom to focus our attention in ways that are most helpful to us and to those around us.

Enhancing this receptive awareness in the present moment is sometimes called mindful awareness. Mindfulness is defined as paying attention, in the present moment, on purpose, without grasping on to judgments. Mindful awareness has the quality of receptivity to whatever arises within the mind's vision, moment to moment. Many studies of mindful awareness practices reveal that it can result in profound improvements in a range of physiological, mental, and interpersonal domains of our lives.

However, keep in mind to think and meditate with an educated brain. In addition, cardiac, endocrine, and immune functions are improved with mindful practices. Empathy, compassion, and interpersonal sensitivity seem to be improved. People who come to develop the capacity to pay attention in the present moment without grasping on to their inevitable judgments also develop a deeper sense of well-being (sense of belonging and self-identity) and what can be considered a form of mental coherence.

Let's dive in to forms of therapies here. An ancient spiritual practice is finding new uses in the *treatment of mental illness. The systematic method of regulating attention known as meditation is now being incorporated into psychotherapeutic practice and linked in surprising ways to other healing traditions, including cognitive behavioral therapy.* The most highly developed forms of meditation are associated with Buddhism, but there are parallels in other spiritual and religious traditions, as well as modern secular versions under the names of relaxation response training or mindfulness meditation.

One distinctive practice is to choose a word, sound, or short phrase (sometimes practices call it a mantra) and repeat it with each breath while sitting in a relaxed position with eyes closed, while calmly discharging distracting thoughts and feelings. Practitioners sit and remain aware of their breathing while observing thoughts and feelings as they come and go in a quiet and detached way. If they notice that their attention is wandering, they are supposed to observe the process without trying to disengage from it and simply return to awareness of their breathing. The intention is to suspend habits of selecting, judging, and interpreting, and attend to the *present moment without allowing oneself to be distracted by fantasies, memories, and anxieties.* The similarity to the aims of psychotherapy is no fortune, as practitioners of both traditions increasingly recognize. But the psychotherapeutic tradition now taking meditation most extremely, to the surprise of some, *is cognitive behavioral therapy.* There is much evidence that these practices have distinct effects on the brain. Based on a study, brain scans indicated that Buddhist monks who were longtime meditators, compared with controls who had just a week of training, showed a high proportion of a type of brain wave that reflects a large-scale coordination of neural circuits.

Furthermore, another recent research measured brain electrical activity before, immediately after, and four months after a two-month course in mindfulness meditation. They found persistent increased activity on the left side of the prefrontal cortex, which is associated with joyful and serene emotions. As a result, researchers are now looking at the effects of meditation on the amygdala, the brain's fear center, and the caudate nucleus, which is associated with obsessional thoughts and compulsive behavior.

What is *psychotherapy*? It is a general term for treating mental health problems by talking with a psychiatrist, psychologist, or other mental health provider. During psychotherapy, individuals learning about conditions, moods, feelings, thoughts, and behaviors. There are many types of psychotherapy, each with its own approach. The type of psychotherapy that's right depends on the individual situation.

Psychotherapy is also known as talk therapy, counseling, psychosocial therapy, or, simply, therapy. Within psychotherapy, the focus of attention on various domains of mental, somatic, and interpersonal life *can create the neural firing patterns in the brain that enables new synaptic connections to be established. Neural plasticity, the change in neural connectivity induced by experience, may be the fundamental way in which psychotherapy alters the brain. Based on the modification and growth of synapses and the potential differentiation of neural stem cells into fully integrated neurons, neural plasticity reveals how the brain's interconnectedness can change throughout the life span. Consciousness may play a direct role in harnessing neural plasticity by altering previously automatic modes of neural firing and enabling new patterns of neural activation to occur.*

Meditation is another way of self-improvement. In meditative traditions, the purpose of drawing attention away from the outside world and deserting habitual patterns of observing and thinking is to enable personal change. The focused attention, self-forgetfulness, and heightened awareness of body states are hypothetical to open the mind to declined concern with one's own suffering, a move from *self-deception to self-understanding*, and resulting changes in attitudes and behavior. There are a number of effective types of psychotherapy. Some work better than others in treating certain disorders and conditions.

In many cases, therapists use a combination of techniques. The therapist will consider your particular situation and preferences to determine which approach may be best. Although many types of therapies exist, some psychotherapy techniques proven to be effective include the following:

- Cognitive behavioral therapy (CBT). This helps identifying unhealthy, negative beliefs and behaviors and replacing them with healthy, positive ones.
- Dialectical behavior therapy. This is a type of CBT that teaches behavioral skills to handle stress, manage emotions, and improve relationships with others.
- Acceptance and commitment therapy. This helps you become aware of and accept thoughts and feelings and commit to making changes, increasing the ability to cope with and adjust to situations.
- Psychodynamic and psychoanalysis therapies. These focus on increasing awareness of unconscious thoughts and behaviors, developing new insights into motivations, and resolving conflicts.
- Interpersonal psychotherapy. This focuses on addressing problems on current relationships with other people to improve your interpersonal skills—how to relate to others, such as family, friends, and colleagues.
- Supportive psychotherapy. This therapy reinforces your ability to cope with stress and difficult situations.

Now some therapists have gone the extra mile, anticipating a blend between cognitive techniques and meditation that they call the "third wave" of cognitive behavioral therapy. Some names given to the new approaches are dialectical behavior therapy, acceptance and commitment therapy, and mindfulness-based cognitive therapy.

Meditation is another way of concentrating—linking the brain to mind and consciousness. The basic steps linking consciousness with neural plasticity are as such: Where attention goes, neural firing arises. And where neurons fire, new connections can be made. In this manner, learning a new way to pay attention within the integration of consciousness enables an open receptive mind within therapy to catalyze the integration of new combinations of formerly remote sections of our mental reality.

Cognitive psychology also looks for the relationships between observable aspects of the environment and individuals' behaviors, to learn about the nature of mental processes. Neuropsychology studies the relationship between structures of the brain and psychological functioning. Cognitive neuroscience combines aspects of cognitive psychology, neuropsychology, and biopsychology. Education in this stream will be a major help to better understand and appreciate the great scientific puzzle of the mind and brain. This puzzle examines how neural activity in the brain gives rise to *mental experiences* that create the human mind.

As the brain becomes activated in the moment, it merges its firing patterns into bunches of activation we can which is a state of mind. These frequent and continuing states of activation of the brain can help describe what we see as our character, our patterns of awareness, and our emotional and behavioral responses that help us symbolize who we are (interpersonal brain, self-identity). We can embrace the distinguished states of mind and their determination to satisfy different needs for familiarity and well-being, challenge, love, mastery, and study.

State integration refers to the way we *embrace and nurture* these different positions and their major needs across time. Furthermore, we explored the complex system of our brain development and its own embodied regions, relationships, self-regulation systems of development. To remind us about the self-complex system that regulates its own emerging, we therefore should be aware of open systems.

As we mentioned, our brain to mind is changing, depending on overall integration throughout daily activities. We are remaining an open system of development. This self-open system is depending on self-regulatory systems that are not determined by a fixed programmer. This self-organizing system is emerging from the basic structures that comprise the system.

This brings us to understanding of the importance of interconnectedness of the embodied brain. It's best to learn about the physical aspect of our brain development and leave this self-organizing, self-regulatory system to complete its integration.

Researchers are concerned with the *functional and structural connectivity* of the brain and strongly suggest that the function of a brain region serves is dynamic and changes over time. In order to determine the function of a specific brain area, neuroscientists zoom out and look at the larger organism-environment system. Therefore, looking to cognitive psychology for an examination of psychological functions, cognitive neuroscience might look to an ecological dynamical psychology.

Furthermore, states of action readiness involve the whole living body of the organism and are provoked by possibilities for action in the environment that matter to the organism. Since emotion and cognition are inseparable processes in the brain, it follows that what is true of emotion is also true of cognition.

Cognitive processes are similarly processes taking place in the whole living body of an organism as it engages with relevant possibilities for action. Taking the viewpoint of the vertical plane of our somatic architecture, we can envision the anatomically and functionally differentiated elements of our bodies to extend from our head to our toes. Vertical integration directly links these elements within awareness so that new connections can be established. We just mentioned that the mind is embodied, built in part from its origins in bodily reality, however, often seduced to live in the land of the purely nonphysical world we can separate as mental. Connecting the basic somatic regulatory functions of the brain stem with the limbic circuits' generation of affective states, motivational drives, attachment, and assessment of meaning and laying down of memory is a first layer of vertical integration.

The *review* of brain anatomy reveals that it has a major integrative function, linking body, its structure, and each other. For instance, overhead the limbic circuitry emerged the neocortex of our evolving brains. The cortex, unlike the brain stem, is quite immature at birth and is shaped by both genetics and especially by experiences out in the world. In general, the posterior regions of the cortex are specialized for perception of the physical world (our first five senses), and the body itself is registered in the more forward aspects of this posterior region.

In the frontal lobe of the cortex, we have our motor and premotor planning areas that enable us to carry out behaviors. The forwardmost part of this frontal lobe is the prefrontal cortex. The side part of this area, known as the dorsolateral prefrontal region, is considered an essential circuit for working memory that enables us to pay attention. Near the middle of the prefrontal cortex, behind the forehead area, are several regions that are the limbic circuitry and an essential aspect of the social circuits of the brain. These include orbital frontal area behind the eyes, the medial prefrontal cortex behind the forehead, and the anterior cingulate behind it. In addition, such more midline structures, along with a region in the insular cortex, serve important *functions in linking body*, affective state, and thought.

Furthermore, the review of the anatomy of the middle prefrontal cortex reveals that it has a major integrative function, linking the body proper, brain stem, limbic circuits, and cortex to each other.

In addition, visual functions occupy the occipital lobe, the bulge at the back end of the brain. The primary area for visual perception is almost surrounded by the much larger visual association area. Close, extending into the lower part of the temporal lobe, is the association area for *visual memory—a specialized area in the cortex*. Evidently, this function has been significant for an omnivorous foraging primate that possibly spent a long evolutionary period extending among distributed food sources.

A less specific kind of function has been qualified to the prefrontal cortex, located on the forward-facing part of the frontal lobes. This area is associated with connotation fibers with all other regions of the cortex and also with the amygdala and the thalamus, which means that it too makes up part of the *emotional brain*, the limbic system. Among its other functions, the prefrontal cortex is responsible for constraining unsuitable behavior, for keeping the mind attentive on goals, and for providing steadiness in the *thought process. Long-term memory* has not yet been found to reside in any select part of the brain, but new findings indicate that the temporal lobes contribute to this function. That the association areas for vision and hearing and the language areas are all nearby may suggest pathways for the storage and retrieval of memories that include several types of stimuli.

Even though the *cerebral cortex* is quite thin, reaching from 1.5 to 4 millimeters deep, it comprises no fewer than six layers. From the outer surface inward, these are the molecular layer, made up for the most part of junctures between neurons for the exchange of signals, and the external granular layer, largely interneurons that serve as collaborating nerve bodies within a region. This is an external pyramidal layer, with large-bodied major cells whose axons extend into other regions such as an internal granular layer, the main termination points for fibers from the thalamus a second; internal pyramidal layer, whose cells project their axons mostly to structures below the cortex; and a multiform layer, again containing principal cells, which in this case project to the thalamus. Outside the dedicated world of *neuroanatomy* and for most of the uses of daily life, the brain is more or less an abstract entity. We do not experience our brain as an assembly of physical structures if we envision it at all; we are likely to see it as large, rounded, grayish in color.

The majority of the cerebral cortex is actually a current development in the course of *evolution*. The cortex contains the physical structures accountable for most of what we call brainwork, from cognition, mental imagery, the highly sophisticated processing of visual information, and the ability to produce and understand language. But underneath this layer resides many other specialized structures that are essential for movement, consciousness, sexuality, the action of our five senses, and more—all important factors to human existence.

Certainly, in firmly biological terms, such structures can claim importance over the cerebral cortex. In the growth of the human embryo, as well as in evolutionary history, the brain develops roughly from the base of the skull up and outward.

The *hindbrain* contains several structures that *regulate autonomic functions*, which are essential to survival and *not under our conscious control*. For example, the brain stem, at the top of the spinal cord, controls breathing, the beating of the heart, and the diameter of blood vessels. This region is also an important junction for the control of deliberate movement. Through the medulla, at the lower end of the brain stem, pass all the nerves running between the spinal cord and the brain; in the pyramids of the medulla, many of these nerve tracts for motor signals cross over from one side of the body to the other. Consequently, the left-brain controls the movement of the right side of the body, and the right brain controls the movement of the left side.

It is essential to learn from the simplest to the more complex structures of the brain and its function to understand our well-being. The *middle prefrontal circuits* transmit out what we are classifying as vertical integration. Study in basic brain research reveals that these middle prefrontal areas are crucial for producing nine facets of life as follows:

- Body regulation: Balance of the sympathetic and parasympathetic branches of the autonomic nervous system.
- Attuned communication: Allow us to tune into others' states and link minds.
- Emotional balance: Permits the lower limbic regions to become stimulated enough so life has meaning.
- Response flexibility: The conflicting of a knee-jerk reaction. This measurement enables us to think before acting and constrain, impulses giving us enough time to reflect on our several options for response.
- Empathy: Seeing the mental perspective of another person.
- Insight: Self-knowing consciousness, the opening to our autobiographical narratives and self-understanding.
- Fear extinction: Fibers project down to the amygdala and enable fearful responses to be calmed.
- Intuition: Being aware of the input of our body, especially information from the neural networks surrounding intestines, as we call it the gut feeling. Or the heartfelt feelings enable us to be open to wisdom.
- Morality: The knowledge to think of the larger good.

Human development refers to the physical, cognitive, and psychosocial development of humans throughout the life span. The steps recognize the "interconnectedness" of human development systems as one. The types of development involved in each of these three domains, or areas, of life are interpersonal self. Physical development involves growth and changes in the body and brain, the senses, motor skills, and health wellness. Cognitive development involves learning, attention, memory, language, thinking, reasoning, and creativity. Psychosocial development involves emotions, personality, and social relationships. This is simply an understanding of the human growing-up journey that doesn't require division between its integration.

As we continue to grow throughout the first five years of life, explicit autobiographical recollection becomes even further integrated into *narrative memory* which involves the detection and creation of thematic elements of our lives. *The brain appears to be able to have a narrative function that can detect themes of our life story and to draw heavily on prefrontal functions as they continue to integrate neural maps that form the underlying architecture of our episodic and autobiographical memory systems. With narrative reflection, one can choose, with consciousness, to detect and then possibly change old maladaptive patterns.* Developmental psychology has been around for decades. Developmental psychologists study human growth and development over the life span, including physical, cognitive, social, intellectual, perceptual, personality, and emotional growth.

Developmental psychologists working in colleges and universities tend to focus primarily on research. If we observe an infant or a toddler, we can't help but wonder how they learn so much so fast, particularly when it comes to language development. Then as we observe young children to those in middle childhood, there appear to be huge differences in their ability to think rationally about the existing world around them. Cognitive development includes mental processes, thinking, learning, and understanding; and it doesn't stop in the childhood stage of development. Adolescents develop the ability to think logically about the abstract world. Moral reasoning develops further, as does practical intelligence—wisdom may develop with experience over time.

Memory plays a bigger role in individual development and interpersonal brain definition hereafter. Memory abilities and different forms of intelligence tend to change with age. Brain development and the brain's ability to change and compensate for losses are significant to cognitive functions across the life span. Experience plays an essential role in building brain construction after birth. The question we address in this book is what happens to the brain and behavior when a young child is deprived of key experiences during critical periods of brain development. We focus in particular on the consequences of recognized education, with inference for the tens of millions of children around the world who from an early age experience profound psychosocial deprivation. Indication is clear that deprivation can lead to a host of both short- and long-term consequences, including perturbations in brain structure and function. In addition, there are changes at the cellular and molecular levels and a plethora of psychological and behavioral impairments.

There are many different academic approaches regarding human development. As we evaluate them through life, recall *that human development focuses on how people change, and the approaches address the nature of change in diverse ways.* For example, is the change smooth or uneven or continuous? Is this pattern of change the same for everyone? How do genetics and environment interact to influence development, the story of nature and nurture? *Some theories hold that the arrangement of development is universal. For instance, in cross-cultural studies of language development, children from around the world reach language milestones in a similar arrangement. Children begin babbling at about the same age and complete their first word around age twelve months old.*

However, we live in diverse backgrounds that have a unique effect on each of us. The idea of one size doesn't fit all means equally the same, for the universal developmental education approach isn't unique for everyone. Despite earth is one planet and we are one organism, yet many minds that starches our education to mars and back. Researchers once believed that motor development followed one course for all children regardless of culture. Yet childcare practices vary by culture, and different practices have been found to quicken or constrain the accomplishment of developmental milestones, like sitting, crawling, and walking.

As we may have already perceived, physical, cognitive, and psychosocial developments are often *interrelated*, as with the example of brain development. We will be examining human development in these three spheres in detail throughout the modules in this book, as we learn about early childhood to middle adulthood, and late adulthood development, as well as death and dying.

The psychosocial field is a big part of developmental education. Development in this domain involves what's going on both psychologically and socially. Early on, the focus is on infants and caregivers, as temperament and attachment are significant. As the social world expands and the child grows psychologically, different types of play and interactions with other children (like the story of the little boy Jack in this book) and teachers become important. Psychosocial development involves emotions, personality, self-esteem, and relationships. Peers become more important for adolescents, who are exploring new roles and forming their own identities.

The *importance of brain health education* is crucial throughout our developmental journey. Hereafter, dating, romance, marriage, having children, and finding work or a career are all parts of the evolution into adulthood. *Psychosocial development is one other side of the developmental education domain that lingers across adulthood with similar understanding of developmental issues of family, friends, parenting, romance, divorce, remarriage, blended families, caregiving for elders, becoming grandparents and great-grandparents, retirement, new careers, and coping with losses or death and dying.* Individuals may not be fully aware of the relationship between their mental and emotional well-being and the environment. The study of the psychosocial domain is enhanced over the years, yet it has been around since 1941. It was first commonly used by the psychologist Erik Erikson in his description of the stages of psychosocial development.

Other pioneers of social work regarded there to be a linear relationship between *cause and effect* in a diagnostic process. In 1917, the concept of *social diagnosis* was renamed as psychosocial study. Psychosocial study was even further developed with emphasis on the treatment model. It is contrasted with diverse social psychology, which attempts to explain social patterns within the individual. Problems that occur in one's psychosocial functioning can be referred to as *psychosocial dysfunction*. This refers to the lack of development or diverse atrophy of the *psychosocial self*, often occurring alongside other dysfunctions that may be physical, emotional, or cognitive in nature.

Human development is a continuous developmental journey, one block at a time. This education views development as a cumulative process, gradually improving on existing skills. With this type of development, there is a gradual change, for example, a child's physical growth, adding inches or so to their height year by year. By contrast researchers who view development as *discontinuous* believe that development takes place in unique stages and that it occurs at definite times or ages. With this type of development, the change is more rapid, such as an infant's ability to demonstrate awareness of object permanence which is a cognitive skill that develops toward the end of infancy, conferring to Piaget's cognitive theory.

We have much explored human development and understood the integration of brain-mind and the physical and social aspects of all. The growth patterns are not a sudden journey. Let's break this down to stages. Developmentalists often break the life span into eight stages:

1. Prenatal Development
2. Infancy and Toddlerhood
3. Early Childhood
4. Middle Childhood
5. Adolescence
6. Early Adulthood
7. Middle Adulthood
8. Late Adulthood

Furthermore, the topic of "death" is usually spoken after late adulthood, since overall, the likelihood of dying increases in later life. Death and dying will be the topic of our last module, though it is not *necessarily a stage of development* (9. Death) that occurs at a particular age.

The list of the periods of development reflects unique aspects of the various stages of childhood and adulthood that will be explored in the developmental education system, including physical, cognitive, and psychosocial changes.

Hereafter, even though both an eight-month-old child and an eight-year-old are considered children, they have very different motor capabilities, cognitive skills, and social relationships. Their nutritional needs are different, and their key psychological concerns are also distinguishing. By the same token, an eighteen-year-old and an eighty-year-old are both considered adults. In addition, discover the distinctions between being twenty-eight or forty-eight in the life span is well noticeable

From centuries ago to now, human evolution changed the stages and cycle of development. Many questions cover from which stage of life is the most important? Some might claim that infancy is the key stage, when a baby's brain is wide open to new experiences that will influence the rest of its later life. Others might argue that it's adolescence or young adulthood, when physical health is at its peak.

On the other hand, cultures around the world value late adulthood more than any other, in conflict that it is at this stage that the human being has finally acquired the wisdom necessary to guide others. The reality of the matter is that every stage of life is equally significant and necessary for the well-being of humankind. *We can add the prebirth, the potential*—the child who has not yet been born could become anything to our stages of development.

Typical *human development* is a pretty predictable process—most humans develop at similar rates, if we consider the other explanation prior. This pattern of development allows us to make generalizations about different stages, such as infancy, childhood, adolescence, and adulthood. Let's take a closer look at each stage with an open mind.

Infancy

Characteristically, infancy is the first year of life and the first important stage of human development. Many physical milestones arise throughout this stage as an infant increases control over its body. Nevertheless, infants rely on others (parents, caregivers, etc.) to meet most of their needs. They learn to trust other people as needs are met. They need to feel this security in order to properly develop both physically and emotionally.

The first year and a half to two years of life are ones of theatrical growth and change. The newborn, with many spontaneous reflexes and an intense sense of hearing, is transformed into a walking, talking toddler within a moderately short period. Parents/caregivers likewise convert their roles from those who manage feeding and sleeping schedules to continually moving guides and safety examiners for mobile, energetic children.

Brain development happens at a remarkable rate, as do physical growth and language development. Infants have their own characters and methods to play. Communications with primary caregivers undergo changes prejudiced by possible separation anxiety and the development of attachment styles.

Social and cultural issues center mostly around breastfeeding or formula-feeding, sleeping in cribs or in the bed with parents, and whether or not to get vaccinations. The infant is a vibrant and apparently boundless source of energy. Babies thus represent the inner generator of humanity. Playfulness moments are from three months to six months of age. When young children play, they recreate the world anew. They take what is and mix it with the what is imaginable to way events that have never been seen before in the history of the development. As such, they embody the principle of revolution and alteration that underlies every single creative act that has happened in the course of progress.

In the first stage of human development, infants learn to trust (trust vs. mistrust) based on how well their caregivers meet their basic needs and respond when they cry. If an infant cries out to be fed, the parent can either meet this need by feeding and comforting the infant or not meet this need by ignoring the infant. When their needs are met, *infants learn that relying on others is safe; when their needs go unmet, infants grow up to be less trusting.*

Early childhood is also referred to as the preschool years, involving the years that follow toddlerhood and precede formal schooling, roughly from around ages two to five or six. As a preschooler, the child is busy learning language, is gaining a sense of self and greater individuality, and has the foundation to learn the workings of the physical world. Such knowledge does not come rapidly yet; and preschoolers may originally have stimulating beginnings of size, time, space, and distance. A toddler's ferocious determination to do something may give way to a four-year-old's sense of guilt for doing something that brings the condemnation of others. In addition to autonomy versus shame and doubt, another way to think of the toddler stage is independence versus dependence.

Throughout the *preschool* years, children learn to declare themselves and speak up when they need something. Some children may state that they're unhappy because a friend broke their art. If this insistence is greeted with a positive reaction, they learn that taking initiative is a helpful behavior. However, if they're made to feel shamefaced for their assertiveness, they may grow up to be nervous and less likely to take the lead. Middle childhood is between the ages of six and eleven years. Considerable of what children experience at this age is associated with their involvement in the early grades of school. The world becomes one of learning and challenging new academic skills and evaluating one's capabilities and accomplishments by making assessments between self and others.

Schools contribute in this process by associating students and making these differences public through group sports, examination scores, and other methods of recognition. When children begin school, they start to compare themselves with peers. If children feel they're accomplished in relation to peers, they develop strong self-esteem. If, though, they notice that other children have met milestones that they haven't, they may struggle with self-esteem. For example, a first grader may notice a constantly worse performance on tests when compared with peers.

If this becomes often, it can lead to feelings of inferiority. Based on research, the brain reaches its adult size around age seven. Nevertheless, it continues to develop. Growth rates slow down, and children are able to improve their motor skills at this stage of development.

Furthermore, development has a wider approach from many angles. Many researchers have contributed their inputs that create a *stepping-stone for today's study*. History well remembers Jean Piaget's theory. The theory of cognitive development is widely used in education programs to prepare teachers to instruct students in developmentally appropriate ways. From birth to age two, children learn object permanence. This is the understanding that people and objects still exist even when they're out of sight. The process is called sensorimotor.

From age two to seven years old, children develop symbolic thought, which is when they begin to develop from concrete to abstract thinking. This stage is referred to as the preoperational stage. From age seven to eleven years of age, children solidify their abstract thinking and begin to understand cause and effect and logical implications of actions. This is referred to as concrete operational. Will study the next stage of development which is about the adolescence to adulthood that individual plan at this stage for the future, think hypothetically, and assumes adult responsibilities. This is referred to as formal operational.

If we look further into *Piaget's stage*, children begin to learn to speak at age two and last up until the age of seven. During the preoperational domain of cognitive development, children do not yet understand concrete judgment and cannot mentally operate information. Children's increase in playing and simulation takes place in this age. However, the child still has trouble seeing things from different facts of view.

The children's play is mainly characterized by representative play and manipulating symbols, like play is demonstrated by the idea of pieces of cloth being a towel and a box being a television. Their observations of symbols exemplify the idea of play with the nonappearance of the definite objects involved. By detecting sequences of play, a study was able to establish that toward the end of the second year, a qualitatively new kind of psychological operative occurs, known as the preoperational stage.

This preoperational stage is sparse and reasonably inadequate in regard to mental processes. The child is able to form steady perceptions as well as enchanted principles. The child, however, is still not able to achieve operations, which are responsibilities that the child can do mentally rather than physically. In addition, thinking in this stage is still egocentric. The child has difficulty seeing the viewpoint of others; therefore, this stage is split into two substages: the symbolic function substage and the intuitive thought substage. The representative function substage is when children are able to understand, represent, remember, and picture objects in their mind without having the object visible.

The *intuitive* thought substage is when children are inclined to suggest the questions of why and how. This stage is when children want to understand everything. Generally speaking, at about two to four years of age, children cannot yet operate and alter information in a reasonable way. However, they now can think in images and symbols. Other examples of mental capabilities are language and make-believe play. Representative play is when children mature make-believe friends or role-play with groups. Children's play becomes more social, and they give characters to each other. Examples of representative play include playing dress-up or having a birthday party for a doll. Remarkably, the type of representative play in which children are involved is associated with their level of imagination and capacity to connect with friends. Therefore, the superiority of their representative play can have significances on their advanced growth.

Egocentric

Egocentrism is the incapability to distinguish between self and other. More precisely, it is the incapability to exactly accept or understand any viewpoint other than one's own. While self-centered behaviors are less prominent in adulthood, the reality of some forms of self-interest in adulthood designates that overpowering egocentrism may be a lifelong development that might not attain completion. Adults appear to be less egocentric than children because they are faster to correct from an initially egocentric perspective than children, not because they are less likely to originally adopt an egocentric perspective. Egocentrism happens when a child is incapable to differentiate between their own perspective and that of another person. Children tend to stick to their own viewpoint rather than consider the view of others.

Definitely they are not even aware that such a perception as different viewpoints happens. The study of egocentrism can be seen in a trial accomplished by Piaget, a Swiss developmental psychologist. Egocentrism would also cause a child to trust: "I like cartoons, so Daddy must like too." Furthermore, parallel to preoperational, children's egocentric thinking is their constructing of cause-and-effect relationships.

The study of Piaget invented the term "precausal thinking" to designate the way in which preoperational children use their own present thoughts or opinions, like in egocentrism, to clarify cause-and-effect relationships. Three main concepts of causality as exhibited by children in the preoperational phase embrace animism, artificialism, and transductive reasoning. Animism is the trust that nonliving substances are proficient in activities and have lifelike potentials. Artificialism raises to the certainty that environmental features can be qualified to human activities or involvements. For example, the clouds are red or black because someone painted them that color. Lastly, precausal thinking is considered by transductive reasoning. Transductive reasoning is when a child fails to understand the correct relationships between cause and effect.

From the ages of four and seven, children are inclined to become very inquisitive and ask many questions. There is an appearance in the interest of reasoning and wanting to know why things are the way they are, which is why this stage is called the intuitive substage. Centration, conservation, irreversibility, class inclusion, and transitive implication are all faces of preoperative thought. Centration is the performance of concentrating all courtesy on one distinctive of a condition at the same time, as discounting others. Conservation is the awareness that varying a matter's appearance does not change its elementary possessions. Children at this period are unaware of maintenance and display centration.

The other stage of development is concrete operational. This stage, which follows the preoperational stage, arises between the ages of seven and eleven years and is categorized by the suitable use of reason. Throughout this phase, a child's thought developments become more established. Children experience an evolution where the child learns rules. Studies determined that children are able to integrate inductive reasoning. Inductive reasoning involves sketch inferences from explanations in order to make a simplification.

Adolescents are also changing cognitively by the way that they reason about social matters. Adolescent egocentrism oversees the way that adolescents think about social matters. This is the sensitive self-consciousness in them as they are, which is reproduced in their sense of personal individuality and strength. Adolescent egocentrism can be dismembered into two types of social thinking. The first type is imaginary audience that contains attention-receiving behavior.

The other type is individual tale, which contains an adolescent's wisdom of particular individuality and insuperability. Such two types of social thinking commence to touch a child's egocentrism in the concrete phase. However, it transmits over to the official operational phase when they are then faced with intellectual thought and are fully reasonably intelligent.

From adolescence and into adulthood, roughly ages eleven to roughly fifteen to twenty, is the period of formal operational. Intellect is established through the rational use of symbols connected to abstract thoughts. Such form of thought embraces expectations that have no essential relative to realism. At such opinion, the individual is has developed theoretical and logical reasoning.

While children in *primary school years typically* used inductive reasoning and picture general assumptions from personal experiences and exact facts, adolescents develop deductive reasoning, in which they draw exact conclusions from abstract ideas using reason. This ability consequences from their volume to think theoretically. Through many studies of the field of education, researchers, including Piaget, focused on two procedures: assimilation and accommodation.

To study assimilation meant integrating exterior fundamentals into constructions of lives or environments. Assimilation is how persons observe and adjust to new information. It is the procedure of fitting new information into preexisting cognitive diagrams. *Assimilation* is when new knowledge is re-explained to fit into, or integrate with, previous ideas. It occurs when persons are challenged with new or unacquainted material and refer to learned information in instruction to make logic of it. Development surges the equilibrium, or equilibration, among these two purposes. When in balance with each other, assimilation and accommodation produce mental diagrams of the functioning intellect. When one function controls the other, they produce images which belong to symbolic intelligence.

Adolescence

The second stage of development is adolescence. Adolescence is a period of theatrical physical change noticeable by an overall physical growth spurt and sexual maturation, known as puberty. However, timing may vary by gender, cohort, culture, and so on. Furthermore, it is time of cognitive change as the adolescent begins to think of new potentials and to reflect abstract notions such as love, fear, and freedom. Unluckily, adolescents have a sense of invincibility that puts them at greater risk of dying from accidents or contracting, infections that can have lifelong consequences. Studies on brain development help us understand teen risk-taking and impulsive behavior. A major developmental task during adolescence involves creating one's own identity. Teens typically struggle to become more self-governing from their parents. At this stage, peers become more important, as teens attempt for a sense of belonging and acceptance.

New characters and tasks are discovered, which may comprise dating, driving, taking on a part-time job, or planning for future academics. During childhood, children begin to develop a sense of self and independence, and this process continues in the next stage of human development. During adolescence, young men and women are primarily concerned with finding their identity and expressing who they are in society. Furthermore, puberty causes many physical changes to take place, and adolescents must adapt to their changing bodies. All of such changes can make adolescence unclear and a stressful period of development.

As adolescents try to find their place, they might experiment with different roles and make efforts to separate from authority facts, such as trying out different hairstyles and hobbies in an attempt to create an image of themselves they're comfortable with. From age twelve years old to twenty is also known as a desirable period of development. The biological event of puberty releases a powerful set of changes in the adolescent body that reflect themselves in a teenager's *sexual, emotional, cultural, and/or spiritual thirst.*

Therefore, such passion represents a significant touchstone for anyone who is looking to rewire with their deepest inner enthusiasm for life. Identity vs. role confusion is commonly observed at this stage, where the term "identity crisis" originated. Adolescents who can clearly recognize who they are grow up with more solid goals and self-knowledge than teenagers who fight to break free of their parents' or friends' inspirations.

Adolescents who still deeply depend on their parents for social interaction and guidance may experience more role confusion. In the attachment research, it is intelligible narratives, stories that deeply make sense of our lives, which are the most robust predictor of how children will attach to us. Many findings suggest that parents who have made sense of their lives, as exposed in their comprehensible life narratives, will be those that somehow offer their children patterns of communication that endorse well-being. As a result, we can recap the exploration of this finding by signifying that it is the parents'/caregivers' neural integration that helps them create a clear narrative and helps them be approachable to their child's own mind and outgoing indications. Such a pattern may reflect the central role of inter- and intrapersonal mental attunement in the development of well-being.

Early Adulthood

Late teens, twenties, and thirties are often thought of as early adulthood. It is a time when individuals are at their physiological peak yet are mostly at jeopardy for involvement in ferocious crimes or substance abuse. It is a time of focusing on the future and putting a lot of energy into making adoptions that will help one earn the status of a full adult in the eyes of society. It takes initiative for young adults to accomplish their many responsibilities, including finding a home and mate, establishing a family or circle of friends, and/or getting a good job. This principle of innovativeness thus aids individuals at any stage of life. Love and work are the key concerns at this stage of development. In recent decades, it has been well-known that young adults are taking longer to grow up. A study has proposed that there is a new stage of development after adolescence and before early adulthood, called emerging adulthood. This is likely from age eighteen to twenty-five (or even twenty-nine) when individuals are still discovering their individualities and don't quite feel like adults yet.

In young adulthood, some begin to solidify their lifelong bonds; some enter committed relationships or marriages, while others form lifelong friendships. People who can create and uphold these relationships earn the emotional benefits, while those who struggle to maintain relationships may suffer from remoteness. A young adult who develops strong friendships in academia may feel more confidence than one who struggles to form and preserve close friendships.

Research on the early adulthood stage of life is still in its early years, so we don't know everything yet that there is to know about how this stage is different from adolescence or later adulthood. Various studies, though, have shown the time that there are developmental routes that continue past puberty and into legal adulthood. In terms of the brain and continuum growth, it's clear that white matter does not stop developing until the twenties. What this means is that even after leaving behind the life stage of adolescence, early adults' brains are still working to enhance connectivity between its regions. When white matter tract in specific that continues to develop post adolescence is the uncinate fasciculus. This tract connects the limbic system, which is associated with functions such as feeling/emotion and episodic memory to the frontal lobe. This is one of the evolutionarily newest parts of the brain and is associated with higher-order operational like cognitive, choices, and goals. The uncinate fasciculus is one of the later tracts to develop, although its particular purpose and its connotation with clinical disorders aren't completely known.

Studying the brain structure and which part is contributing from birth to adulthood is important. The ventrolateral prefrontal cortex continues to show changes in how it responds to social exclusion after the end of adolescence. With so many illnesses revealing an increased occurrence during this stage, and many changes in the brain and behavior occurring even in normal development after adolescence, learning about this stage offers the knowledge that will aid in understanding both what is trendy in the internal life of early adults and what it looks like when something irregular is happening.

Deeper to the stages of development theories and practices, we might come to the understanding of *moral development*. Likewise, to other researchers and philosophers, Lawrence Kohlberg created a theory of human development based on moral development perceptions. The stage of preconventional means that individuals follow guidelines because they're frightened of the consequences and make choices only with their best welfares in mind. Aside from this, in the conventional stage, individuals act to avoid society's judgment and follow guidelines to sustain the systems and constructions that are already in place. Meanwhile, during the stage of postconventional, there is a genuine concern for the welfare of others, and the greater good of society guides the individual.

The social stages have many studies and learning theories of their own. For instance, this knowledge builds upon behavioral theory and postulates that individuals learn best by perceiving the behavior of others. They watch how others act, assess the significances, and then make conclusions regarding their own behavior consequently. The few stages in such study are attention, retention, production, and motivation. If we draw our courtesy to the attention stage, individuals first notice the behavior of others while in the retention stage and remember the behavior and the resulting values.

Likewise, in the reproduction stage, persons develop the capability to duplicate the behaviors they want to replicate. Obviously, such results in the motivation stage which ends up performing these behaviors. Humans are an essentially social species; no constituent of our civilization would be possible without large-scale collective behavior. The basic fact is therefore that human beings are able to pool their cognitive resources in ways that other species are not. This is made possible by a single very special form of social cognition, namely, the ability of individual organisms to understand conspecifics as beings, meaning *like themselves* who have intentional and mental lives like their own.

Humans are continuously reading each other's actions, gestures, and faces in relation to underlying mental positions and emotions, in an effort to character out what other people are thinking and feeling and what they are about to do following. This is also known as other theory of mind or mentalizing. Developmental psychology research on theory of mind has established that the capability to understand others' mental states develops over the first four or five years of life.

While convinced aspects of theory of mind are present in infancy, this it is not until around the age of four years that children begin obviously to understand that someone else can hold a belief that differs from their own and which can be untruthful. Furthermore, an understanding of others' mental states plays a serious character in social communication since it permits individuals to work out what other persons want and what they are about to do next and to adopt our own behavior consequently. With growing studies, we can identify remarkable consistency in recognizing the brain regions that are involved in the concept of mentalizing. Some studies in the mentalizing task resulted in the stimulation of a network of regions including the posterior at the temporoparietal junction, the temporal poles, and the dorsal medial.

The *arrangement between neuroimaging studies* in this area is extraordinary, and the also the reliable localization of activity within a network of regions. Brain lesion studies have consistently demonstrated that the superior temporal lobes and prefrontal cortex (PFC) are involved in mentalizing as damage to these brain areas might impairs the mentalizing abilities. Interestingly, one study reported a patient with large PFC damage whose mentalizing abilities were intact. Thus, it signifies that this region is not necessary for mentalizing. However, there are other clarifications for this surprising and intriguing finding. It is possible that due to plasticity, this patient used a different neural strategy in mentalizing tasks. Otherwise, it is possible that damage to this area at different ages has different significances for mentalizing capabilities. Outlining the brain structures that contribute in social cognition raises the question of whether these structures are in any sense focused for the dispensation of social information or whether social cognition is just like cognition in general that is only practical to the field of social behavior. There are some a priori reasons for thinking that we might have evolved particular systems, because social behavior makes stresses that are so exclusive.

It necessitates the rapid documentation of social stimuli and signals, massive integration of memory, expectation of others' behavior in a mutual and often inexpensive setting, and cohort of prescriptive evaluations. Each of these four examples has been feature as an exclusive aspect of human cognition, and one might imagine that each is subserved by a particular evolved ability. The behavioral theory focuses merely on a person's behaviors rather than the feelings that go alongside those behaviors. It suggests that behaviors are accustomed in an environment due to certain stimuli.

Behavioral philosophers believe that behavior determines feelings, so changing behaviors is important because this will in turn change feelings. This might take us further into the stages of attachment theory. Attachment focuses on the deep relationships between people across their lifetime. An important attachment theory finding is that children must develop at least one strong bond in childhood to trust and develop relationships as adults. Through the entire book, we have learned the significance of human development integration within and with others.

Therefore, social cultural studies tie human development to the society or culture in which people live. It focuses on the contributions that society as a whole makes to individual human development. An important part of such theory is the zone of proximal development, which is an area of knowledge and skills somewhat more advanced than a child's current level. The zone of proximal development helps educators think about and plan instruction, so sociocultural theory plays a large role in preservice instructor exercise. Moreover, studies of attachment reveal that the parent's openness to a child's indications and the coherence of the parent's own narrative are important analysts of a child's development of secure attachment. These features seem to encourage a form of resiliency in the child which helps self-regulation disclose as the child develops.

Our brain itself is the social organ of the body. If we look into the structure of our neural architecture, it discloses how we need connections to other people in order to feel in balance and to develop well. As we've learned in the function of the middle prefrontal regions, the brain integrates contribution from other people with the procedure of regulating the body, balancing emotional positions, and the formation of self-awareness. This visceral, social, and self-integration advocates that our minds are intertwined from the integration of facets of authenticity that on the surface seem to be quite disparate.

Middle Adulthood or Middle Age

Studies refer to this period of adulthood as the generativity-versus-stagnation stage. Persons in middle adulthood or middle age may have some cognitive loss. This loss usually remains invisible because life experiences and strategies are developed to reimburse for any reduction in mental abilities. The late thirties or age forties through the midsixties are referred to as middle adulthood.

This is a period in which the physiological aging that began earlier becomes more obvious and a period in which many people are at their peak of efficiency in love and work. It may be a stage of gaining knowledge in certain fields and being able to understand difficulties and find explanations with superior competence than before. It can also be a time of becoming more faithful about potentials in life. This stage is also referred to as the sandwich stage. Middle-aged adults may be in the middle of taking care of their children and taking care of their elderly parents.

While caring about family and the future, middle-aged adults may also be interrogative of their own mortality and commitments, but not essentially experiencing a midlife crisis. After years in young adulthood of following society's scripts for creating a life, people in midlife often take a break from worldly responsibilities to replicate upon the deeper meaning of their lives. In the middle adulthood stage, individuals are inclined to struggle with their contributions to civilization. Those who feel that they're contributing experience generativity, which is the wisdom of leaving a legacy behind. On the other hand, those who don't feel that their lives matter might experience feelings of stagnation.

There is a clear indication that with increasing age, adults display a slow, very steady propensity toward declining speed of response in the performance of intellectual (and physical) responsibilities. Slowing rates of electrical activity in the older adult brain have been associated with the slowing of behavior itself. This decline in the rate of central nervous system processing does not essentially imply similar changes in learning, memory, or other intellectual functions. The learning capacity of young adults is greater than that of older adults, as is their capability to establish new information in terms of its content or meaning.

Carl Jung trusted that our personality actually matures as we get older. A healthy personality is one that is balanced. People suffer tension and anxiety when they fail to express all of their inherent qualities. Jung believed that each of us possesses a shadow side. For example, those who are typically introverted also have an extroverted side that rarely finds expression. Each individual has both masculine and feminine sides.

Late Adulthood

As adults reach the end of life, they look back on their lives and reflect. Adults who feel fulfilled by their lives, either through a successful family or through a meaningful career, reach ego integrity, in which they can face aging and dying with peace. If older adults don't feel that they've lived a good life, they risk falling into hopelessness. Late adulthood is the stage of life from the sixties onward. Also, it establishes the last stage of physical change. During late adulthood, the skin continues to lose elasticity, reaction time slows further, and muscle strength diminishes. Hearing and vision—so sharp in our twenties—decline significantly; cataracts or cloudy areas of the eyes that result in vision loss are frequent. The other senses, such as taste, touch, and smell, are also less sensitive than they were in earlier years. The immune system is weakened; and many older people are more vulnerable to illness, diabetes, and other disorders.

Cardiovascular and respiratory problems become more common in older age. Seniors also experience a decline in physical flexibility and a loss of balance, which can result in falls. While a great deal of research has absorbed on diseases of aging, there are only a few educational studies on the molecular biology of the aging brain. Many molecular changes are due in part to a decrease in the size of the brain, as well as loss of brain plasticity. *Brain plasticity* is the brain's ability to change structure and function. The brain's main function is to decide what information is worth keeping and what is not.

Therefore, if there is an action or a thought that a person is not using, the brain will remove space for it. The aging process generally results in changes and lower functioning in the brain, leading to problems like memory loss and decreased intellectual function. Age is a major risk factor for most common neurodegenerative diseases, including mild cognitive impairment, Alzheimer's disease, cerebrovascular disease, or Parkinson's disease. Therefore, as an individual ages into late adulthood, psychological and cognitive changes can sometimes occur.

A general deterioration in memory is very common. This is due to the decrease in speed of encoding, storage, and retrieval of information. As a result, this can cause problems with short-term memory retention and with the capacity to learn new information. In most conditions, this absentmindedness should be measured as a natural part of growing older rather than a psychological or neurological illness. Noticeably, separate from a usual deterioration in memory is dementia. This is a comprehensive class of brain ailments that cause a steady long-term decrease in the capability to think and remember to the degree that a person's daily functioning is affected. Even though the term "dementia" is still often used in lay circumstances, it has been renamed as "neurocognitive disorder," with numerous degrees of harshness. On the other hand, Alzheimer's is the most common type of neurocognitive disorder. Accountancy covers 50 percent to 70 percent of cases.

Neurocognitive ailments most frequently disturb memory, visual-spatial ability, language, attention, and executive function. Most of these disorders are slow and progressive. Thus, by the time a person shows signs of the illness, the changes in their brain have already been happening for a long time. A study shows about 10 percent of people with dementia have what is recognized as *mixed dementia*, which is typically a grouping of Alzheimer's disease and another type of dementia. It is clear that memory also degenerates with age. The older adults tend to have a harder time remembering and attending to information. In general, an older person's procedural memory stays the same, while working memory deteriorates.

Procedural memory is memory for the performance of specific types of achievement. This guides the processes we perform and most commonly exists below the level of conscious awareness. By contrast *working memory* is the organization that aggressively holds numerous pieces of fleeting information in the mind where they can be manipulated.

The reduced volume of the working memory becomes evident when tasks are particularly compound. Furthermore, *semantic memory* is the memory of understanding things, of the meaning of things and other concept-based information. This type of memory motivates the conscious remembrance of factual information and overall knowledge about the world which remains relatively steady during life. Late adulthood or age eighty years old and up are those with long lives who have acquired a rich repository of experiences that they can use to help guide society. Elders therefore represent the source of *wisdom* that exists in each individual, serving to avoid the mistakes of the past while reaping the benefits of life's lessons.

Death and Dying

Each stage of life has its own exceptional ability to give to humanity. It's essential to sustain the stages and to defend each stage from challenges to overwhelm its individual influence to the human life cycle. The education of death and dying is infrequently given the amount of attention it deserves. Unfortunately, there is a convinced discomfort in thinking about death. Nonetheless, there is also a certain self-assurance and acceptance that can come from studying death and dying. Influences such as age, religion, or culture play significant characters in defiance and methods to this topic. In addition, there are different types of death: physiological, psychological, and social.

The most communal origins of death vary with age, gender, race, culture, and time in history. Dying and grieving are processes and share certain phases of responses to loss. There are fascinating examples of cultural differences in death ceremonies and grief. The perception of a *good death* is designated as including individual selections and the participation of loved ones throughout the procedure. Those in our lives who are dying, or who have died, teach us about the value of living. They prompt us not to take our lives for granted yet to live each moment of life to its completest, and to recollect that our own minor lives form a part of a superior whole.

Understanding time is not a unique stage to brain anatomy. As we move from our earliest years and our prefrontal cortices begin to develop our capacity for replication on the nature of time begins to develop. The first stage is a form of mental time travel that permits an early form of self-knowing awareness. This thoughtful capacity to link past, present, and future soon discloses itself in an awareness of the limited nature of our time on this planet. Individuals learn that people's lives are often partial to a period and that the experience of death is a predictable part of each of our lives. Temporal integration directly confronts this structural role of time, and our brief lives, in serving that consider the deep questions of purpose in life.

Genetic Factors of Development

Diving deeper into human development, we must study what are the genetic factors that affect human growth and development. One other key element of human growth and development left to discover is genetics. Genetics influences the speed and way in which people develop, though other influences, such as parenting, education, experiences, and socioeconomic features, are also at play. The multiple genetic factors that affect human growth and development include genetic connections and sex chromosome abnormalities.

Genes can perform in an additive way or occasionally battle with one another. For instance, a child with one tall parent and one short parent might end up, between the two of them, at normal height. However, sometimes genes follow a dominant-recessive pattern. If one parent has brown hair and the other has red hair, the red hair gene is the dominant gene, and their child will have red hair. Human genetics is the study of inheritance as it occurs in human beings. Human genetics incorporates a variability of overlapping grounds including classical genetics, cytogenetics, molecular genetics, biochemical genetics, genomics, population genetics, developmental genetics, clinical genetics, and genetic counseling.

Genes are the joint aspect of the potentials of most human-inherited characters. The *study of human genetics* can respond to questions about human nature and can help understand illnesses and the development of actual treatment and help us to understand the genetics of human life. The inheritance of characters for humans is based upon Gregor Mendel's model of inheritance.

Mendel deduced that inheritance is contingent upon disconnected units of inheritance, called factors or genes. Autosomal traits are allied with a single gene on an autosome (nonsex chromosome). They are called dominant since a single copy—inherited from either parent—is sufficient to root this attribute to appear. This often means that one of the parents must also have the same mannerism, except it has ascended due to an unlikely new transformation. Examples of autosomal dominant characters and conditions are Huntington's disease and achondroplasia.

Further into the study, the autosomal receding character is one pattern of inheritance for a trait or disorder to be passed on through families. For a recessive trait or disease to be exhibited, two copies of the trait or disorder requirements needs to be existing. The trait or gene will be positioned on a non sex chromosome. Because it takes two reproductions of a trait to exhibit a trait, numerous individuals can mistakenly be transporters of a disease. From an evolutionary standpoint, a recessive disease can persist concealed for numerous generations before exhibiting the phenotype.

Cases of autosomal recessive disorders are albinism and cystic fibrosis. In addition, X-linked genes are originated on the sex X chromosome. X-linked genes just like autosomal genes have both leading and recessive types. Recessive X-linked conditions are infrequently understood in females and usually only disturb males. This is because males inherit their X chromosome, and all X-linked genes will be inherited from the mother side. Fathers only permit on their Y chromosome to their sons, so no X-linked traits will be inherited from father to son.

Males cannot be transporters for recessive X-linked traits, as they only have one X chromosome. Consequently, any X-linked trait congenital from the mother will show up. Females direct X-linked disorders when they are homozygous for the condition and develop transporters when they are heterozygous. X-linked dominant inheritance will demonstrate the same phenotype as a heterozygote and homozygote. Just like X-linked inheritance, there will be a deficiency of male-to-male inheritance that brands it different from autosomal traits.

One case of an X-linked trait is Coffin-Lowry syndrome, which is produced by a transformation in the ribosomal protein gene. This transformationresults in undernourished, craniofacial abnormalities, mental obstruction, or short physique. X chromosomes in females endure a procedure recognized as X-inactivation. X-inactivation is after one of the two X chromosomes in females is nearly entirely incapacitated. It is significant that when this procedure happens, a woman would produce double the quantity of regular X chromosome proteins. The apparatus for X-inactivation will arise throughout the embryonic phase.

For individuals with syndromes like trisomy X where the genotype has three X chromosomes, X-inactivation will incapacitate all X chromosomes until there is only one X chromosome active. Males with Klinefelter syndrome who have an extra X chromosome will likewise endure X-inactivation to have only one entirely vigorous X chromosome. Y-linked inheritance transpires once a gene, trait, or disorder is shifted through the Y chromosome.

Meanwhile, Y chromosomes can only be originating in males. Y-linked traits are only passed on from father to son. The testis influential factor, which is located on the Y chromosome, regulates the masculinity of persons. As well the masculinity inherited in the Y chromosome there are no additional found Y-linked features. A pedigree is an illustration that displays the ancestral associations and broadcast of hereditary traits over numerous generations in a family. Square cyphers are practically continuously cast off to characterize males, at the same time as circles are used for females.

Pedigrees are used to help distinguish numerous unalike genetic sicknesses. A pedigree can likewise be used to help regulate the probabilities for a parent to harvest a progeny with a precise trait. Four dissimilar traits can be recognized by pedigree chart analysis: the autosomal dominant, autosomal recessive, X-linked, and Y-linked. Incomplete penetrance can be revealed and intended from pedigrees. Penetrance is the fraction articulated regularity with which individuals of a specified genotype patent at least some grade of a precise mutant phenotype connected with a trait. Inbreeding or mating among closely linked organisms can evidently be seen on pedigree charts. Pedigree charts of royal families often have a high grade of inbreeding. This is because it was habitual and desirable for royalty to marry another associate of royalty.

Genetic counselors frequently habit pedigrees to support pairs regulate if the parents will be able to produce healthy children. A karyotype is an actual beneficial tool in cytogenetics. A karyotype is an image of all the chromosomes in the metaphase phase organized conferring to length and centromere location. A karyotype can also be valuable in scientific genetics due to its capability to identify genetic disorders. On an ordinary karyotype, aneuploidy can be perceived by evidently being able to perceive any absent or additional chromosomes. Giemsa banding, G-banding of the karyotype, can be used to observe deletions, insertions, duplications, inversions, and translocations. G-banding will stain the chromosomes with light and dark bands exclusive to separately chromosome. Genomics is the ground of genetics concerned with organizational and practical education of the genome. A genome is all the *DNA* controlled inside an organism or a cell plus nuclear and mitochondrial DNA.

The human genome is the whole assembly of genes in a human being controlled in the human chromosome, collected from over three billion nucleotides. *Medical genetics* is the subdivision of medicine that encompasses the analysis and organization of hereditary disorders. Medical genetics is the submission of heredities to medical care. It joins human genetics, for instance, to investigate the reasons, and inheritance of genetic disorders would be measured inside both human genetics and medical genetics, although the diagnosis, administration, and counseling of persons with genetic illnesses would be a measured part of medical genetics. Population genetics is the subdivision of evolutionary biology accountable for examining procedures that source variations in allele and genotype regularities in inhabitants founded upon Mendelian inheritance. Four unlike forces can impact the regularities: natural selection, mutation, gene flow, and genetic drift. A population can be distinct as a group of interbreeding entities and their progeny.

For human genetics, the populations will entail only of the human species. The Hardy-Weinberg principle is a commonly used model to administer allelic and genotype regularities. In count to nuclear DNA, *humans have mitochondrial DNA*. Mitochondria, the authority families of a cell, have their private DNA. Mitochondria are inherited from one's mother, and their DNA is commonly used to suggest maternal appearances of descent. Mitochondrial DNA is only 16 kb in length and encodes for sixty-two genes.

To conclude, the XY sex-determination system is the sex-determination organization that originates in humans, most other mammals, some insects, and some plants. In this system, the sex of an individual is determined by a couple of sex chromosomes. Females have two of the same kind of sex chromosome (XX) and are named the homogametic sex. Males have two different sex chromosomes (XY) and are called the heterogametic sex. Sex linkage is the phenotypic countenance of an allele connected to the chromosomal sex of the individual.

This method of inheritance is in distinction to the inheritance of traits on autosomal chromosomes, where mutual sexes have similar likelihood of inheritance.

Subsequently humans have several more genes on the X than the Y. There are numerous more X-linked traits than Y-linked traits. Nevertheless, females transmit two or extra reproductions of the X chromosome, subsequent in a possibly toxic dose of X-linked genes. To accurate this disproportion, mammalian ladies have progressed an exclusive instrument of dosage recompense. In specific, by way of the procedure called X-chromosome inactivation (XCI), female mammals transcriptionally silence one of their two Xs in a compound and extremely corresponding method. Humans' genetic evidence is continuously networking with the environment, and sometimes this can influence development and growth. For instance, if a child in utero is bare to drugs, the child's cognitive capabilities may be obstructed. Consequently, it can alter the developmental procedure.

In addition, even if a child's genes would specify a tall height, if that child was deprived of nutrition, it may influence their height. Sex-chromosome irregularities impact as many as one in five hundred births. The following syndromes are examples of sex-chromosome abnormalities that can influence development: Klinefelter syndrome is the presence of an extra X chromosome in males, which can source physical structures such as reduced muscle physique and reduced body hair and may result in learning disabilities.

Fragile X syndrome is caused by a transformation in the FMR1 gene that brands the X chromosome as fragile. It can cause academic disability, developmental delays, or characteristic physical structures such as a long face. Turner syndrome happens when one of the X chromosomes is absent or incompletely missing. It only distresses females and consequences in physical characteristics like short stature and webbed neck. Genetics is the scientific study of inherited distinction. Human genetics, then, is the scientific study of inherited human difference.

The question of why study human genetics comes to mind. One purpose is basically a concentration in improved understanding ourselves. As a subdivision of heredities, human genetics fears itself with what most of us reflect to be the most motivating species on earth: *Homo sapiens.* But our awareness in human genetics does not halt at the margins of the species, for what we learn approximately human genetic difference and its foundations and broadcast certainly subsidizes to our considerate of genetics in overall, just as the study of variation in other species enlightens our understanding of our own. Another purpose of studying human genetics is its applied value for human well-being. In this wisdom, human genetics is additionally a practical science than a fundamental science.

One advantage of studying human genetic variation is the encounter and explanation of the genetic influence to many human illnesses. This is a gradually commanding drive-in light of our growing understanding of the involvement that genes make to the development of diseases such as cancer, heart disease, and diabetes. In detail, society has been keen in the past and remains to be enthusiastic to pay substantial amounts of money for research in this range, mainly because of its insight that such study has massive probability to progress human health. This perspicacity, and realization in the findings of the past twenty years, has directed to a noticeable increase in the number of people and establishments elaborate in human genetics. This subsequent purpose for reviewing human genetics is related to the first. The longing to advance medical performance that can improve the anguish accompanied with human disease has provided solid provision to elementary research.

Many basic biological miracles have been revealed and defined throughout the course of surveys into specific disease circumstances. A typical case is the knowledge about human sex chromosomes that was expanded through the study of patients with sex-chromosome irregularities. A more existing specimen is our rapidly increasing consideration of the mechanisms that regulate cell development and imitation, understanding that we have expanded mainly through a study of genes that, when transformed, upsurge the risk of cancer.

Similarly, the consequences of basic research notify and inspire research into human disease. For instance, the development of *recombinant DNA methods rapidly transformed the study of human genetics,* eventually permitting scientists to study the comprehensive assembly and functions of individual human genes, as well as to operate these genes in a diversity of formerly inconceivable ways. The third reason for the perusal of human genetics is that it stretches an authoritative tool for understanding and recitation human evolution.

At one time, statistics from physical *anthropology* were the solitary foundation of information accessible to scholars involved in outlining human evolutionary history. Nowadays, though, investigators have a prosperity of genetic data, plus molecular data, to demand upon in their effort. Two research methods were factually significant in serving detectives comprehend the biological foundation of genetics. The first of these methods, transmission genetics, elaborates passage organisms and perusal the offspring's traits to progress hypotheses about the mechanisms of inheritance. This work established that in some organisms at minimum, heredity appears to track a few definite and relatively simple guidelines. The second method elaborates using cytologic procedures to study the machinery and progressions of cellular reproduction. This tactic laid a compact basis for the more theoretical understanding of inheritance that established as a result of transmission genetics.

By the early 1900s, cytologists had confirmed that heredity is the significance of the genetic permanency of cells by cell separation, had recognized the gametes as the vehicles that communicate genetic information from one cohort to another, and had composed solid indication for the dominant role of the nucleus and the chromosomes in heredity. As significant as they were, the methods of program genetics and cytology were not sufficient to assist scientists in understanding human genetic variation at the equal of aspect that is now possible. The dominant benefit that today's molecular procedures suggest is that they consent to researchers to study DNA straight. Previously in the development of these systems, scientists studying human genetic variation were required to make interpretations about molecular modifications from the phenotypes shaped by transformed genes.

Additionally, *since the genes accompanying most single-gene syndromes* are comparatively rare, they could be studied in only a minor quantity of relations. Countless of the traits connected with these genes similarly are recessive and consequently could not be perceived in individuals with heterozygous genotypes. Unlike academics working with other species, human geneticists are constrained by principled deliberations from accomplishment investigational, at-will symbols on human focuses. Human cohorts are on the instruction of twenty to forty years, much too slow to be valuable in definitive education experimentations. All of these boundaries complete recognizing and perusal genes in humans mutually tedious and slow.

In the previous fifty years, nevertheless, foundation with the detection of the construction of DNA and hastening meaningfully with the progress of recombinant DNA systems in the mid-1970s, an increasing battery of molecular systems has made through education of human DNA an authenticity. Significant among such practices are constraint examination and molecular recombination that tolerate researchers to cut and recombine DNA molecules in exceedingly precise and foreseeable conducts; amplification practices, such as the polymerase chain response (PCR), which make it conceivable to make infinite reproductions of any fragment of DNA; and hybridization practices, like fluorescence in situ hybridization. These practices permit scientists to compare DNA trials from unlike foundations and to discover precise base arrangements inside trials, and the automated sequencing practices that currently are permitting workers to classify the human genome at an extraordinary degree. *Homo sapiens* is a moderately undeveloped species and has not had as much period to accumulate genetic variation as have the enormous common species on earth, the greatest of which precede humans by vast spans of time.

Nevertheless, there is a significant *hereditary variation* in our species. The human genome encompasses about 3×10^9 base pairs of DNAs; and the degree of human genetic variation is such that no two humans, save identical twins, ever have been or will be hereditarily equal. Among any two humans, the quantity of genetic variation—biochemical personality—is about .1 percent. This resources that about one corrupt pair out of every one thousand will be dissimilar among any two persons. Any two (diploid) persons have around 6×10^6 base couples that are diverse, a significant aim for the progress of automated measures to analyze hereditary distinction. The maximum shared polymorphisms in the human genome are solitary base-pair alterations. Scientists demand these alterations, for solitary-base polymorphisms.

Nevertheless, the genetic modifications among people, all humans have a great deal of their genetic information in mutual. These resemblances assistance describe people as a species. Furthermore, genetic variation around the globe is circulated in a rather continuous method; there are no sharp, irregular borders among human inhabitants' collections. In detail, research consequences reliably establish that about 85 percent of all human genetic variation occurs within human inhabitants, while about only 15 percent of variation happens between populations.

That is, research reveals that *Homo sapiens* is one incessantly adjustable, crossbreeding species. Constant examination of human genetic variation has even directed biologists and physical anthropologists to reconsider outdated philosophies of human racial collections. The quantity of genetic variation among these traditional organizations essentially falls beneath the level that taxonomists use to elect subspecies, the taxonomic group for other species that resembles the description of race in *Homo sapiens*. This conclusion has caused some biologists to call the rationality of race as a biological theory into thoughtful inquiry.

Hereafter, we explored that *genes do more than just determine the color of our eyes* or whether we are tall or short. Genes are at the center of everything that makes us human. Genetic factor is accountable for constructing the proteins that track everything in our bodies. Partial of such proteins are visible, like the ones that constitute our hair and skin, while others work as of sight, coordinating our basic biological purposes. For the most part, every cell in our body contains exactly the same genes, but inside individual cells, some genes are active while others are not. Once genes are active, they are accomplishing manufacturing proteins. This process is called gene expression. Once genes are inactive, they are silent or inaccessible for protein construction.

Modern genetic studies designate that human brain evolution is obsessed principally by changes in gene guideline, which necessitates understanding the biological purpose of mainly noncoding gene regulatory fundamentals, many of which act in matter detailed method. Human influence chromatin communication outlines in individual fetal and adult cortex to assign three classes of human-evolved fundamentals to putative mark genes. Studies have discovered that human-evolved elements involving DNA arrangement change, and those connecting epigenetic changes are connected with human-specific gene regulation via effects on different programs of genes representing diverse biological traits.

Nevertheless, both types of human-evolved elements join on precise cell categories and laminae elaborate in cerebral cortical development. Besides, human evolved fundamentals collaborate with neurodevelopmental illness risk genes, and genes with a high level of evolutionary restriction, importance a relationship between brain evolution and defenselessness to disorders distressing cognition and behavior.

These consequences deliver a novel understanding into gene regulatory mechanisms driving the evolution of human cognition and mechanisms of openness to neuropsychiatric circumstances. Human evolution is hypothesized to be determined principally by changes in gene regulation relatively than divergence in protein-coding sequences. Current qualified genomic and epigenomic education has acknowledged sections on the human ancestry having either an enhanced classification, referred to as human-accelerated regions (HARs), or epigenetic changes, referred to as human-gained enhancers (HGEs).

One session of human-progressed genomic fundamentals, HARs, is developed in developmental accompaniments, signifying that they may drive evolution of human-specific traits through developmental gene regulation. Current targeted sequencing of HARs in consanguineous autism spectrum disorder (ASD) relations acknowledged substantial enhancement of rare biallelic variants, importance a possible character of HARs in defenselessness to neurodevelopmental disorders. Even though an introductory efficient classification has been directed, precisely mapping the target genes regulated by these accompaniments necessitates tissue specificity. Meanwhile, the widely held study of chromatin relations are forecast to be highly tissue specific. We sought to bridge the gap between genetic changes on the human lineage and the molecular basis of human evolution by mapping these genomic foundations to their alleged target genes using chromatin configuration in human brain.

We have discovered that while HARs and HGEs goal diverse genes and molecular pathways and display different developmental routes, they meet in relations of their cell-type enhancement outlines. These patterns highlight that these elements regulate exact genes elaborate in primate cortical expansion developed in the neural ancestors of the outer subventricular zone (oSVZ), and their progeny, supragranular neurons, providing a regulatory chart for understanding the molecular mechanisms fundamental in human cortical development. Together forms of regulatory fundamentals also join on genes that are highly preserved at the protein level, consistent with the model that noncoding regulatory elements drive evolutionary divergence by regulation of important, highly constrained records.

Constrained genes targeted by these human progressed elements are improved between those in which protein-disrupting mutations source numerous neurodevelopmental conditions, plus ASD. The putative target genes of HARs are enhanced for genes that adjust traits elaborate in human brain development, regionalization, dorsal-ventral imitating, cortical lamination, and proliferation of neuronal progenitors signifying that various facet of human brain development is theme to human-specific regulation.

Despite the fact the mainstream of genes is intricate in forebrain development, an uncommon putative target gene adjusts mid- or hindbrain development. As a reminder, we cultured on the function of genes that is to pass on the information necessary to build proteins— and bodies—from one generation to the next. A newly fertilized egg cell has an assembly of genes that comprehends all information needed to transform it from a single cell into an embryo and then an adult. The process that changes a single cell into a new person or a new fish or a new tree is called *development*.

Throughout the progression of development, complex assemblies develop from simple ones. A single cell transmutes itself into an adult organism. How does something complicated come from something simple? And how do genes regulate this procedure? Producing an organism from a single cell encompasses three significant processes:

- Cell division: Cells split to produce more cells.
- Cell differentiation: Cells modify into different categories of cell to do explicit jobs in the body, from nerve cells to muscle cells.
- Morphogenesis: Assemblies of cells transfer and change their form to produce the construction of the organism.

Genes perform a vital role in controlling all of these progressions. Genes comprise the information a cell needs to make proteins—a bit like a formula for a living thing. Different genes encompass the information needed to make different proteins, and different proteins do dissimilar jobs in the cell. The proteins a cell makes decide what kind of cell it develops, and there are approximately 350 different categories of cell in a mature human being. Cells change into different types of cell because of changes in the way their genes work.

Some genes are triggered, and some genes are inactivated. As a result, the cell produces a specific set of proteins. Consequently, for instance, a nerve cell produces only the proteins needed to make a nerve cell, and a muscle cell produces only the proteins needed to make a muscle cell. Nonetheless, how do cells switch their genes on and off? And, more notably, how do they "know" which genes to adjust on and which genes to switch off? The reaction lies in distinct control genes that produce proteins that regulate the action of other genes. For example, homeotic or homeobox genes regulate entire groups of other genes to set out the elementary body plan of the embryo, separating the front from the back, and manufacturing the right body assembly in the right place.

One way in which genes can impact the action of other genes is over the manufacture of proteins called transcript features, which stick to special control sites in the DNA at the start of a gene to switch them on and off. Human brain development is shaped through *continuing complex interactions of genetic* and environmental inspirations. The trial of involving explicit genetic or environmental risk features to distinctive or atypical behaviors has directed to interest in using brain organizational structures as an intermediate phenotype. Twin studies in adults have found that many features of brain anatomy are highly heritable, demonstrating that genetic reasons deliver an important influence to variation in brain constructions. Fewer is known about the related influence of genes and environment while the brain is vigorously developing.

We review the consequences from the ongoing National Institute of Mental Health child-and-adolescent twin study that suggest that heritability of different brain areas changes over the sequence of development in a locally precise fashion. Zones accompanied with more compound reasoning capabilities convert progressively heritable with development. The possible mechanisms by which gene–environment interactions may disturb heritability values during development are discussed. Human organizational, functional, and behavioral brain development progresses as an ongoing dialogue between a child's genetic heritage and his or her environment. Understanding how these features network at different points throughout development may help to classify how and when to arbitrate to help children grow to their completest potential. However, establishing the relations between explicit risk aspects and developmental consequences has confirmed to be extremely challenging.

Research of complex neurodevelopmental disorders such as schizophrenia, autism, and attention-deficit hyperactivity disorder (ADHD) has revealed that a certain scientific syndrome may be connected with an extensive diversity of genetic risk aspects, signifying that there may be numerous directions from nucleotide to behavior. One approach to unscrambling the complex communications is to use stepping-stones such as brain structure to help bridge the gap among genetic and environmental risk factors and behavior. Genes do not code for behaviors but for the structured blocks of the cells whose communications ultimately give increase to those behaviors; contrariwise, the transformation of environmental input into determined behavioral changes happens through alterations in brain systems and even structures.

The advent of *brain imaging* revolutionized the neuroscience of behavior by making it likely to noninvasively study the brain in vivo. For instance, cortical thickness can be measured at a level of determination high enough to perceive alterations in regions across the cortex that are also recognized to be functionally and cytoarchitecturally heterogeneous. The connotation of a certain behavioral feature with thickness in an exact cortical area may be an evidence that the mechanisms elaborate in the development of that cortical area are also applicable to that behavior. In addition, the discovery that explicit genetic polymorphisms touch a cortical region guides us to the purposes of connected gene products. The amplified heritability of later growing areas such as the prefrontal cortex, superior temporal gyri, and superior parietal lobes parallels the increase of heritability in cognitive structures such as IQ and language capabilities connected with these areas.

One suggestion is that studies using brain morphometry as an endophenotype to connect genes and behavior will need to reflect age in the investigation, as brain organizational elements may be appropriate at one developmental stage but not another. Our results are also congruent with indication from other grounds that different brain regions may be mainly sensitive to environmental influences at explicit stages during childhood and adolescence. Regardless of genetic factor of development, the environment is a critical classification of brain development. Environmental enrichment (EE) is known to deeply affect the central nervous system (CNS) at the functional, anatomical, and molecular level, both through the critical period and during adulthood.

Current studies concentrating on the visual classification have revealed that these possessions are related to the *recruitment of previously unsuspected neural plasticity procedures*. At *early stages of brain development*, EE activates a marked acceleration in the development of the visual system, with maternal behavior substitute as a fundamental mediator of the enriched experience in both the fetus and the newborn. In adult brain, EE enhances plasticity in the cerebral cortex, consenting the retrieval of visual functions in amblyopic animals. The molecular substrate of the possessions of EE on brain plasticity is multifactorial, with reduced intracerebral inhibition, enhanced neurotrophin expression, and epigenetic changes at the level of chromatin construction. These results shed new light on the possibility of EE as a noninvasive approach to perfect deficits in the development of the CNS and to treat neurological disorders.

Adult brain construction is the consequence of a multifaceted collaboration between genetic developmental programs and *experience-driven plasticity processes*. A large number of studies *confirmed the presence of time windows in early postnatal life, named critical periods (CPs), throughout which neural circuits exhibit a heightened sensitivity to obtain informative and adaptive gestures from the exterior environment*. This might lead us to discover the memory system of development and its categories to understand more "brain plasticity experience-driven CPs" in depth. Several brain regions subserving main behavioral functions (sensory perception, motor control, language) have CPs that happen at different times and are triggered and measured by distinct mechanisms.

The primary visual cortex (V1) is a typical model for studying *experience-dependent plasticity*. Although the development of the visual system begins before eye opening and the original aiming of neural networks is subjected to either genetic programs or spontaneous activity, an appropriate development of the visual *system requires sensory experience*. The brain is remarkably approachable to its relations with the environment, and its morphology is transformed by experience in computable ways. Histological examination of the brains of animals uncovered to either a compound environment or a learning paradigm, associated with suitable controls, has illuminated the nature of *experience-induced morphological plasticity in the brain*. For instance, a study reveals that changes in synapse number and morphology are accompanied with learning and are firm, in that they preserve well beyond the history of exposure to the learning experience.

Furthermore, other mechanisms of the nervous system also respond to experience: oligodendrocytes and axonal myelination might also be eternally transformed, while changes in astrocytes and cerebrovasculature are more transient and seem to be *activity-driven rather than learning-driven*. Consequently, experience induces numerous arrangements of plasticity in the brain that are seemingly regulated, at minimum in fragment, by self-governing mechanisms. As we learn through the brain structural and its functions, we understood neuronal plasticity is the knowledge that neural traits can be reinforced via repetitive use. On the other hand, experience-dependent plasticity is an active collaboration among one's environment (nurture) and the biological makeup of one's brain (nature). Such experience-dependent plasticity is pretentious by how individuals adjust to the difficulties of their environment leading to reform of the brain at the cellular level.

Cognitive tasks for awareness, voluntary movement, recall, and many other occupations can be reallocated, or preexisting circuits can be reinforced through experience and learning by means of neuroplastic changes. Neuroplasticity was once thought by neuroscientists to be evident only during childhood. Nonetheless, research in the latter half of the twentieth century exhibited that many characteristics of the brain can be transformed (or are "plastic") even through adulthood. Yet the developing brain displays a higher grade of plasticity than the adult brain. *Activity-dependent plasticity can have substantial inferences for healthy development, learning, and memory/recovery from brain damage.* Epigenetic mechanisms have long been connected with the guideline of gene-expression changes associated ordinary neuronal development and cellular variation, though until recently, such mechanisms were thought to be statically quiet in the mature brain. *Behavioral neuroscientists have nowadays initiated to examine these epigenetic mechanisms as possible regulators of gene-transcription changes in the CNS subserving synaptic plasticity and long-term memory (LTM) development.*

New indication from education and memory animal models has confirmed that active chromatin remodeling transpires in terminally distinguished postmitotic neurons, signifying that these molecular procedures are definitely confidentially elaborate in numerous phases of

LTM development, plus merging, reconsolidation, and extermination. Such chromatin adjustments include the phosphorylation, acetylation, and methylation of histone proteins and the methylation of associated DNA to afterward affect transcriptional gene readout activated by learning. The present study observes how such learning-induced epigenetic changes subsidize to LTM development and inspiration behavior. In specific, the specific epigenetic mechanisms that have been demonstrated to regulate gene expression for both transcription aspects and development features in the CNS, which are serious for LTM construction and storage, as well as how aberrant epigenetic processing can subsidize to psychological conditions such as schizophrenia and drug addiction.

Together, the results support a novel role *for epigenetic mechanisms* in the adult CNS serving as potential key molecular regulators of gene-transcription changes essential for LTM construction and adult behavior. Memory is the foundation of the complete human psyche. It encompasses the countless progressions by which an organism takes in information obtainable as environmental stimuli and adapts that information to kept knowledge, proficient of being evoked at any time to make executive conclusions, form a description or generate an inclusive portrait of the world. The overall arrangements for memory embrace sensory memory (SM), short-term memory (STM), and long-term memory (LTM).

Information from the *adjacent environment* is endlessly obtainable primary to the senses, and what each modality catalogues is distinct as SM. The original sensory port into the conscious mind performs as a defending system for our concentration, as only the fraction of SM which is appeared to will be further interpreted into STM. Transient in nature, STM rapidly declines if it is not combined and transformed into LTM. After LTM is shaped, these memories can be remembered from long-term storing to perform as a perspective on further environmental stimuli, contribute in decision-making based on developed knowledge, and afterward impact behavioral responses. Remembrance of LTM to supply existing thought progressions is so fluid a phenomenon that, as humans, we experience this as an even stream of consciousness.

Behavioral neuroscientists are interested in the biological basis of these procedures, and one main goal in the learning and memory field has been to elucidate the molecular events that are activated by learning to permit for the adaptation of memory from the working short term into stored long term for advanced recall. Deeper into memory defense, memory can be distinct as the way in which a past experience alters the probability of how the mind functions in the future. Memory shapes how we experience the present and how we anticipate the future, arranging thoughts in the present moment for what arises next constructed on what we've experienced in the past. This comprehensive interpretation permits the mind to inspect the findings of two characteristics of memory and reconnoiter how their integration can endorse well-being.

Separation of these memory functions, in difference, may be understood as one characteristic of the foundation of mental suffering. Consequently, experience generates the stimulation or firing of neurons. This neuronal activation can in turn lead to modifications in the influences between neurons, the source of neural plasticity. Through humans live the implant experience into memory via an initial coating of processing called implicit or nondeclarative memory. From one and a half years of age, this early implicit layer of memory is the solitary procedure obtainable to the increasing infant. Nonetheless, even beyond that early age, individuals continue to generate implicit memories, yet they are then often selectively combined into the following layer of dispensation termed declarative forms of memory.

The effects of *histone and DNA* adjustments are self-motivated and adjustable, suggesting that the epigenome can be rapidly transformed in response to experiential stimuli to adjust the expression of memory-permissive genes, plus immediate–early genes (IEGs) that are required for the synaptic plasticity associating active learning. Significantly, certain regulatory changes to the operating epigenome can steadily endure during the life span, a feature that might describe how patterns of deposited memories can continue unchanged and dormant for stretched stages of time till the conscious brain stresses their recollection. It tracks, then, that convinced behavioral patterns, emotional responses, and even psychiatric disorders can be accredited to the philosophical inspiration that experiential stimuli have on the operating epigenome. Later on in our book voyage, we will emphasize the character of epigenetic mechanisms in the procedure of converting STM to LTM that necessitates gene-transcription activity in adult neurons during memory consolidation.

In addition, we will highlight studies investigating how aberrant epigenetic processing can pay to psychological conditions such as schizophrenia and drug addiction, and alter adult behavior. If studies dive into learning memory, the role of epigenetic mechanism appears convincing. Epigenetic alterations are activated in the developments of memory formation. Moreover, short-term memory (STM) is merged into long-term memory (LTM), and epigenetic upregulation of transcription aspects and immediate–early genes escort this adaptation. The brief outline of epigenetic mechanisms in LTM formation shows the epigenetic guideline of the working genome is accomplished through variations made to the chromatin structure that do not disturb the DNA classification. The activity of epigenetic enzymes as well as DNA methyltransferases, histone acetyltransferases / histone deacetylases, and histone methyltransferases / histone demethylases inside a promoter section regulates how obtainable the DNA of a precise gene is to dictation influences; and these epigenetic marks have been detected to change with learning and experience.

The epigenetic regulation of immediate–early genes in memory formation is the merging and recall of LTM which requires plasticity and inclined by epigenetic mechanisms. Histone adjustments and DNA methylation changes are experiential in the hippocampus, amygdala, and cortex in reply to learning, conforming with the countenance of vital memory-related immediate–early genes and transcription aspects. Significantly, epigenetic patterns established by *early-life experiences create behavioral phenotypes*. Early-life misfortune is firmly accompanied with regulation of the hypothalamic–pituitary–adrenal axis, the overriding mechanism of the stress response. It continues stress performances through epigenetic mechanisms to reprogram the expression patterns of the glucocorticoid receptor, encouraging the sensitivity of an individual's response to environmental stressors.: In relation to this learning, the transduction of experiential stimuli into LTM imposes the molecular mechanisms of epigenetics to adjust gene expression.

Experience alters the epigenome, and epigenetic modifications have been perceived at numerous memory-related gene promoters, regulating their expression, which is serious for the plasticity that transpires in response to learning. In the future r, molecular memory scientists will endure to work on mapping the comprehensive and timely expression patterns of genes acknowledged to be indispensable to the development of LTM foundation. These upcoming studies will associate *gene-expression* changes with the fundamental epigenetic alterations. Furthermore, in learning memory, we have explored the types of memory within the human brain. Most scientists believe there are at least four general types of memory: working memory, sensory memory, short-term memory, and long-term memory. Working memory is parallel to short-term memory.

Nevertheless, unlike the latter, *working memory is where a person employs information*. This helps *remembering details of current tasks*. Some behavior that uses working memory include resolving a compound math problem where an individual must remember several numbers; baking something, which requires an individual to recall the ingredients they previously added; and contributing in an argument, during which a person must remember the main arguments and the indication each side practices. We might understand by now the limbic system is the communal name for assemblies in the human brain elaborate in emotion, motivation, and emotional connotation with memory. It affects motivation and is more active in extroverts and risk-takers than in introverts and thoughtful individuals. The limbic system plays its role in the development of memory by integrating emotional states with stored memories of physical vibrations.

Working memory is a system that provides an interface between the environment and various aspects of the mind. It is a type of memory that tolerates individuals to hold information in mind whereas the person is working on it. Working memory also agrees information to be collective from awareness and long-term memory and short-term memory. The initial model of working memory has three components. The first component was an attentional regulator system, which is also named the central executive, and this was helped by two temporary storage systems: one, a verbal and acoustic system, which eventually came to be called the phonological loop, and the other, its visuospatial equivalent, the visuospatial sketchpad. Afterward, a fourth component brings together the three components and associates them to perception and to long-term memory and also performs as the basis of conscious awareness.

The central executive is definitely the most significant and the most complex component of the original three. It is an attentional system that has a restricted dispensation volume. It is also used in other areas, and it is dominant to our understanding of intelligence as a perception and complex cognition in general. The executive is fed by two temporary storage systems. It can hold information in a speech-based or sound-based form and can uphold it by subvocal practice.

Working memory is positioned in several parts of the brain. In the case of the phonological loop, primarily on an area between the temporal and parietal lobes of the left hemisphere, though the procedure of reviewing them encompasses a more frontal area, sometimes known as Broca's area. Damage to this area can also consequence in the disturbance of fluent speech. The visuospatial system principally contains the right hemisphere. Nonetheless, it also spreads to parts in the occipital lobes, near the rear of the brain. This zone is involved in visual imagery while more medial parietal parts are accountable for spatial processing. Nevertheless, the detail that these are triggered does not essentially mean that this is where the information is stowed. One of the complications in trying to use practical imaging to understand working memory is that it is mainly *correlational.*

The classification is used to be called *short-term memory*, which highlighted its *temporal* feature, signifying that the critical question was how long it lasts before the deposited information is accepted to long-term memory. Short-term memory is being upheld for a long time if an individual is not thinking about anything else. Moreover, long-term memory can start as rapidly as short-term with the two running in equivalent, somewhat than the long-term functioning only as a later processing phase. Long-term memory also embraces a series of distinguishable systems that vary while all are elaborate in storing information for longer areas than working memory. Within long-term memory, there is a key difference among what is called explicit or declarative memory and implicit or nondeclarative memory.

Declarative memory is what we generally reflect of as *remembering*, remembering that person saw someone yesterday or remembering the capital of Italy. In distinction, nondeclarative memory contains using stored information to complete responsibilities implicitly slightly than by vigorously remembering. It is naturally designated by changing the way in which persons accomplish some motion. Individuals would frequently define this as education relatively than memory, as in learning an ability such as how to ride a car.

Additional implicit memory possessions can function over a much shorter period. For instance, if I read out a sequence of words and then inquire a person to classify them verbally in a loud environment, that person will show a better presentation of the words that he or she has just heard without comprehending why. Certainly, such consequence is revealed in patients who are closely amnesiac and are completely incapable to remember that they have just heard these or definitely any such words.

Psychologist Alan Baddeley in his own model of working memory add its capacity and location in the brain. The explicit or declarative system can be separated into two broad classes. One is termed episodic memory, and it is the capacity to straightly recall or identify exact events that have occurred in the past, therefore remembering where a person went on a holiday. Now the way in which episodic memory works is by connecting the memory to the situation in which it happened, efficiently joining it to the environment, the time, and the place where it was experienced. If a person provides the part of, for instance, where I experienced it, then it can carry back memories of the occasion that happened there. Correspondingly, if a person remembers somebody's name, it will bring back that person. Since such type of memory is contingent on the capacity to paste experiences together, it is delicate. Unfortunately, it declines as the individual gets older.

Consequently, the *frontal lobes* are significant for producing and for examining *memories*. The trickiness of retrieval can be revealed through the simple mission of trying to recall the names of as numerous animals as imaginable in ninety seconds. For instance, when you say "bird," there must be thousands of them. The frontal lobes are significant for many other responsibilities concerning executive control including performance on intelligence exams. There are surely privileges that working memory can be trained, and some training curricula do recover the performance level on the responsibilities qualified and on different tasks that are broadly in the same category.

There are serval questions related to working memory. The most recent area is in visual short-term and working memory where a growing number of people have moved into the study of *visual working memory* from studying visual perception and visual attention. Some studies so far have tended to explore themselves with the earlier stages of visual short-term memory, whereas others have focused more on the role of attentional control often using methods that were developed to study verbal *working memory*. Aside from the memory stage of development, let's shed light on the function of *mirror neurons* in the *learning process*.

In the *previous years, neurosciences* have established significantly having expounded numerous significant theories of scientific research in the field. The key aim of neuroscience is to comprehend how collections of neurons network to produce the behavior. Neuroscientists perused the action of molecules, genes, and cells as we explored at some point. They similarly discovered the multifaceted communications elaborate in motion perception, thoughts, emotions, and learning. The brick fundamental nervous system is the nerve cell, neuron.

Neurons exchange information by distributing electrical indications and chemical through networks termed synapses. Exposed by researchers, *mirror neurons* are a special class of nerve cells playing a significant character in the direct knowledge, automatic, and unconscious environment. These cortical neurons are stimulated not only when an action is satisfied; but when a person sees how the same act is achieved by someone else, they signify a neural mechanism by which the actions, purposes, and emotions of others can be understood automatically. In childhood, mirror neurons are very significant.

Consequently, research learned a lot in the *early years of development*: smile, to ask for help . . . and in statistic, all the behaviors and family and group standards. Individuals absorb what they see and sense from others. Mirror neurons are significant in understanding the actions and purposes of other persons and learning new skills through mirror image. They are involved in preparation and regulatory actions, intellectual thinking, and memory. If a child observes an action, mirror neurons are stimulated and create new neural pathways. Competent activity of mirror neurons principals to good development in all extents at a higher emotional intelligence and the capability to empathize with others.

The term "neurostiinte" comes from the English "neurosciences," a neoligism created in 1962. Studies comprehended that in order to fully understand the complexity of the brain purposes, one must remove any existent complication among disciplines by means of integration of available resources and attempts. The mirror neurons were discovered at the beginning of the '90s by neurophysicists while learning about primates, and they tolerate this precise name because they activate in order to imitate other persons' actions and gestures.

The neurologists have observed that the mirror neurons actuated electrical signals at the very moment when the monkeys achieved movement in command to feed themselves. It was only when they perceived that the same neurons were activated when the monkeys watched other peers feeding themselves that the scientists comprehended the importance of such discovery. Hereafter, the term "mirror" was chosen. There are mirror neurons that activate electrical signals in our brain when a person sees someone being touched, when a person watches other people's movements or only as a sign of empathy. By observing the expressions of another individual, the brain is able to generate within its own body an internal state that is thought to resonate with that of the other person.

Resonance contains a change in physiologic, sentimental, and intentional states within the observer that are determined by the insight of the respective states of activation within the individual being observed. Such discovery in the mid-1990s reveal the mirror neuron system and how the brain is capable of integrating perceptual learning with motor action to create internal representations of intentional states in others. Original studies in monkeys revealed that if a monkey sees someone pick up an object, his own motor system will become primed to imitate that same action. In humans, the mirror neuron system is much more multifaceted.

Developing studies disclose that many ways in which our *internal*, one-to-one, and greater social experiences may be formed by the *integrative nature* of this *organization*. In addition, the behavior of greater assemblies, such as families and social meetings, may reveal this communal state of internal functioning. The scientific inferences of this work are reflective and help study to comprehend not only the inherently social nature of the brain but that their own bodily moves may aid as the gateway toward empathic intuitions into the state of another person. Mediated through the insula, insights of another's affective expressions may modify our own somatic and limbic positions and then be examined through a prefrontal process of interception, interpretation, and attribution to another's statuses. Mirror neurons disclose the essential incorporation within the brain of the perceptual and motor organizations with limbic and somatic regulatory purposes.

The mirror neuron system likewise *illuminates the overpoweringly social nature* of our brains. This social foundation of neural purpose may proposal new traits for a person to comprehend how psychotherapy followers to the process of change. When two minds feel associated and convert integrated, the state of firing of each individual an become more coherent in the future. Accurately such might mean that the corresponding activations between the body proper, limbic areas, and even cortical depictions of intentional states between two individuals arrive at a state of resonance in which one matches the profiles of the other.

Recent studies in individuals with autism spectrum condition disclose weakening in the capacity to observe emotional expressions in others that is accompanied with evidently diminished mirror-neuron initiation. With a weakened mirror-neuron system functioning, the social brain is incapable to share in the fast social communications that relies on a communal set of neural outlines that generate an embedded atmosphere of both social behavior and nonverbal understanding of the meaning of social interactions. The *story of nature needs nurture continues* throughout our book journey.

The understanding of *self-identity*, the *interpersonal brain*, the *open-ended definition of the brain*, and the *how-to relationship* with brain structures is slowly making its way to comprehend and to tolerate these updated information for our own development and to pass on to future generations. We disclosed that human development refers to the physical, cognitive, and psychosocial development of humans throughout the *life span*. The steps recognize the "interconnectedness" of human development systems as one. The types of development involved in each of these three domains, or areas, of life are *interpersonal self*. Such as: physical development involves growth and changes in the body and brain, senses, motor skills, and health wellness.

Cognitive development involves learning, attention, memory, language, thinking, reasoning, and creativity. Psychosocial development involves emotions, personality, and social relationships. This is a simply understanding of the human growing-up journey that *doesn't require division* between its integration. As we continue to grow throughout the first five years of life, explicit autobiographical recollection becomes even further integrated into narrative memory which involves the detection and creation of thematic elements of our lives. The brain appears to be able to have a narrative function that can detect themes of our life story and to draw heavily on prefrontal functions as they continue to integrate neural maps that form the underlying architecture of our episodic and autobiographical *memory systems*.

With *narrative reflection*, one can choose, with consciousness, to detect and then possibly change old maladaptive patterns. Such understanding provides tools for scientists, professors, therapists, teachers, and parents to classify mental disorders, especially knowing that diagnosing mental illness isn't like analyzing other enduring diseases. Heart disease is recognized with the assistance of blood tests and electrocardiograms. Diabetes is detected by measuring blood glucose levels. Nonetheless, classifying *mental illness* is a more subjective endeavor. Consequently, no blood test is for depression, and no X-ray can classify a child at jeopardy of developing bipolar disorder, or at least not yet.

On the other side, it's good to know the new tools in *genetics* and *neuroimaging*, likewise, scientists are construction evolution toward deciphering particulars of the underlying biology of mental disorders. Are mental illnesses merely physical illnesses that occur to strike the brain? Some studies and professors of brain science believe it's all about biology. All mental procedures are brain processes, and consequently altogether conditions of mental functioning are biological diseases. After knowing the brain is the organ of the mind, where else could mental disease be if not in the brain? For this motive, mental illnesses are no diverse from heart disease, diabetes, or any other enduring illness. All lingering illnesses have *behavioral mechanisms* as well as biological apparatuses. The only difference here is that the organ of interest is the brain instead of the heart or pancreas. But the same basic principles apply.

Mental disorder and mental illness are terms used to refer to a *psychological pattern* that occurs in an individual and is usually associated with *distress* or *disability* that is not expected as part of normal development or culture. The recognition and understanding of mental disorders have changed over time. Categories of *diagnoses* may include mood disorders, anxiety disorders, psychotic disorders, eating disorders, developmental disorders, personality disorders, and many other categories. In many cases, there is no solitary recognized or consistent cause of mental disorders, although they are widely understood in terms of a diathesis-stress model and biopsychosocial model. Mental disorders have been found to be common, with over a third of people in most countries reporting sufficient criteria at some point in their life. There are many different categories of mental disorder and many different facets of human behavior and personality that can become disordered.

The state of *anxiety* or fear can become disordered, so that it is unusually intense or generalized over a prolonged period. Commonly recognized categories of anxiety disorders include specific phobia, generalized anxiety disorder, social anxiety disorder, panic disorder, agoraphobia, obsessive-compulsive disorder, and PTSD. Relatively long-lasting affective states can also become disordered. Mood disorder involving unusually intense and sustained sadness, melancholia, or despair is known as clinical depression (or major depression) and may more generally be described as emotional dysregulation. Milder but prolonged depression can be diagnosed as dysthymia.

Bipolar disorder involves abnormally "high" or pressured mood states, known as mania or hypomania, alternating with normal or depressed mood. Whether unipolar and bipolar mood phenomena represent distinct categories of disorder, or whether they usually mix and merge together along a dimension or spectrum of mood, is under debate in the scientific works. Patterns of belief, language use, and perception can become disordered. Psychotic disorders centrally involving this domain include schizophrenia and delusional disorder.

Schizoaffective disorder is a category used for individuals showing aspects of both schizophrenia and affective disorders. Schizotypy is a category used for individuals showing some of the traits accompanied with schizophrenia but without meeting the cut-off criteria. The fundamental characteristics of a person that affect his or her cognitions, motivations, and behaviors across situations and time can be seen as disordered due to being abnormally firm and maladaptive. Categorical schemes list a number of different personality disorders, such as those classed as eccentric (e.g., paranoid personality disorder, schizoid personality disorder, or schizotypal personality disorder), those described as dramatic or emotional (antisocial personality disorder, *borderline personality* disorder, histrionic personality disorder, or narcissistic personality disorder), or those seen as fear-related (avoidant personality disorder, dependent personality disorder, or obsessive-compulsive personality disorder).

One application about *trauma's effects on memory* is that it may briefly block the integrative function of the hippocampus in memory incorporation. *With enormous stress hormone secretion or amygdala discharge in response to an irresistible occasion, the hippocampus may be momentarily shut down.* In addition to this direct consequence of trauma of hippocampal function, some people may exert effort to adjust to trauma by isolating their conscious attention, engaging it only on nontraumatic elements of the environment at that time. The resultant neural configuration of impassable hippocampal processing, when reenergized, can present itself as free-floating, unassembled elements of insight, bodily impression, emotion, and behavioral response without the interior sense that something is approaching from the past.

Beliefs and *transformed states* of mind may also arrive the consciousness as the implicit mental models and priming convert activated in reply to environmental or internal initiations resembling mechanisms of the unique experience. This implicit-only form or memory can be one enlightenment for the remembrances and symptomatic profile of PTSD. The key to memory integration is the neural authenticity that principal devotion tolerates the puzzle fragments of implicit memory to arrive at the spotlight of attention and then be assembled into the framed pictures of semantic and self-memories. With such thoughtful focus, what was once a memory configuration capable of intrusion on a person's life can move into a form of knowing that involves both deep thoughts and deep sensations of the reality of the past.

In most extents of *medicine*, we now have a complete toolkit to assist individuals in distinguishing what's going on, from the behavioral level to the molecular level. This has really led to enormous changes in most areas of today's medicine. Certainly, in recent years scientists have made many stimulating discoveries about the function—and dysfunction— of the human brain. They've acknowledged *genes* accompanying to schizophrenia and revealed that convinced brain abnormalities upsurge a person's jeopardy of developing PTSD after a stressful occasion. Others have zeroed in on anomalies connected with autism, including irregular brain development and underconnectivity between brain districts. Researchers have also begun to flesh out a physiological description for depression.

Many studies and professors of psychiatry and neurology have been actively elaborate in investigating that singled-out section of the brain— Brodmann area 25—that is intense in people with depression. Such consideration designates area 25 as a junction box that networks with other areas of the brain elaborate in mood, emotion, and thinking. This confirmed that deep-brain encouragement of the area can alleviate symptoms in people with treatment-resistant depression. Maps of depression's neural circuits, conforms, may ultimately assist as a tool both for analysis and for treatment.

Considering the underlying *biology* could assist psychoanalysts and psychopharmacologists in resolving which patients would benefit from more concentrated therapy and which aren't likely to recover deprived of medication. Yet despite the development and potential of research, it's not ready to acknowledge that all mental illnesses will one day be labeled in virtuously biological relations. One of the major complications might be that mental illness analyses are frequently general classes that embrace numerous different underlying malfunctions. Mental diseases have always been defined by their apparent symptoms, both out of requirement and out of suitability. Nonetheless, just as cancer patients are an enthusiastically varied group marked by many different disease traits, a depression analysis is probable to incorporate people with many exclusive underlying difficulties.

That offerings challenges for *defining the disease in biological* footings. Depression does have patterns; the caution is dissimilar associates of patients obviously have different outlines—and likely the need for different precise interferences. Unfraternally, when it comes to mental illness, a one-size-fits-all approach does not smear. Some diseases may be extra purely physiological in nature. Convinced illnesses such as schizophrenia, bipolar condition, and autism appropriate the biological classical in a very clear-cut logic. In these illnesses, organizational and functional irregularities are apparent in imagery scans or through postmortem segmentation. However, for other circumstances, such as depression or anxiety, the biological groundwork is more unclear.

Frequently, *mental* diseases are likely to have manifold sources, plus genetic, biological, and environmental influences. Noticeably, that's true for many long-lasting diseases, heart disease and diabetes involved. Nonetheless, for mental diseases, we're a mainly long way from understanding the relationship among those influences. If studies can think of the brain as a computer, the brain circuitry is corresponding to the hardware.

We also have the human equivalent of software. Specifically, research has mental processing of mental pictures, meanings, conditioning, a whole level of processing that has to do with such psychological volumes. Just as software viruses are frequently the reason of computer difficulties, the mental motherboards can be complete by our psychological dispensation, even when the fundamental motherboard is working as designed. Thus, if we put emphasize solitary at the brain level, analyses are probable to error a lot of what's going on in mental disorders.

The risk in employing too considerable devotion on the biological is that significant environmental, behavioral, and social influences that subsidize to mental disease may be discounted. The developing zone of epigenetics, meanwhile, could aid in delivering a relation among the biological and other grounds of mental disease. Epigenetics study examines the traditions in which environmental influences transform the way genes direct themselves. Convinced genes are turned on or turned off, stated or not stated, reliant on environmental contributions. The alterations could be drawing to epigenetic indicators, chemical labels that confer to elements of DNA and, in the procedure, turn numerous genes on and off. Such labels don't just disturb persons through their lifetime, though; like DNA, epigenetic indicators can be conceded from generation to generation.

More lately, the study of the brains of people who dedicated suicide and found that those who had been harmed in childhood had sole outlines of epigenetic labels in their brains. In the meantime, patients themselves are clamoring for improved biological descriptions of mental illnesses. Unfolding mental illnesses as brain errors aids in diminishing the embarrassment often linked with them. Schizophrenia is a disease like pneumonia. Considering it as a brain illness destigmatizes it directly. Definitely, social and environmental influences are unquestionably significant to consider mental well-being. Nonetheless, they perform in the brain. It's too soon to say whether we'll someday have a blood test for schizophrenia or a brain scanning technique that classifies depression deprived of any uncertainty. Nonetheless, scientists and patients agree: the more we comprehend around the brain and behavior, the better.

According to the researchers who compared the findings from different *psychiatric disorders*, all results showed loss of gray matte tissue that encompasses the bodies of nerve cells—in three regions deep in the brain. This includes the dorsal anterior cingulate cortex, the right insula, and the left insula. Such network of areas is associated with executive functioning, which studies have clarified as the things that allow a person to function in life. Other studies presented the notion of the brain being collected of three different assemblies, fundamentally different in their chemistry and structure and in evolutionary footings eternities apart, the alleged triune brain.

Conferring to this explanation, the brain can be alienated into the prefrontal neocortex (involved in higher cognitive procedures aside from regulation of emotions by their networks to the limbic region), the limbic or mammalian brain (involved in emotions which direct self-defense and procreation of type), and the reptilian compound collected of the basal ganglia and brain stem assemblies (elaborate in routine motor purpose/reflexes as well as social communication such as regional and courtship exhibitions). Regional brain imaging studies have examined irregularities in a piece of these brain sectors to examine the position of depression in the brain. Cortical brain zones occupied in depression are the dorsal and medial prefrontal cortex, the dorsal and ventral anterior cingulate cortex, the orbital frontal cortex, and the insula.

A reduced metabolism in the prefrontal cortex, particularly dorsolateral and dorsoventral brain regions, is a regularly replicated conclusion in major depressive disorder. Additionally, underprovided prefrontal perfusion in these districts, coupled with a decrease in problem-solving capabilities and higher tendency to perform on undesirable emotions, has been occupied in suicidal behavior. Whether this discovery is a key irregularity or a subordinate one is not vibrant. Nevertheless, such conclusion has been efficaciously cast off to articulate a therapeutic approach to inspire the dorsolateral prefrontal cortex (DLPFC) using transcranial magnetic stimulus. The reduction in DLPFC metabolism/ blood flow in depression has also been found to be contrary to antidepressant treatment. Structural brain MR imaging research proposes that a reduced frontal lobe capacity may also be current in depression. A declined capacity of the orbitofrontal cortex has likewise been occupied in depression, even though practical changes have been less regularly labeled.

Moreover, the *anterior cingulate cortex* has been a focus of much education in the pathophysiology of depression. Studies that labeled abnormalities of the subgenual and dorsal ACC (anterior cingulate cortex) in depression. The ACC has been revealed to have a practical dissection among its dorsal and ventral fragments. The dorsal ACC has been concerned with cognitive features of emotion plus battle determination of emotional stimuli with adverse valence, though the ventral (subgenual). ACC has widespread bilateral assembly with limbic districts such as the amygdala and dorsomedial thalamus aside from cortical mood regulating zones such as the lateral and medial orbitofrontal cortex and the medial prefrontal cortex. The manufacturers of the vACC to the hypothalamus, which panels the endocrinological organizations, and the autonomic organizations, which are normally intricate in the stress response, make the vACC of particular attention in depression.

The *insula*, mainly its anterior subdivision, has been concerned in involvement of emotions like disgust, self-reflection, and control of inner instinctive statuses, and response to the stimuli of taste and smell. In depression, insular initiation has been described to be amplified in reply to disgust-encouraging stimuli and undesirable pictures, and insular bulk has been noted to associate with depression scores. One study, on the other hand, stated amplified insular initiation in reply to undesirable stimuli after antidepressant treatment. On the complete, such outcomes propose enlarged sensitivity of the insula to inner visceral and cognitive procedures throughout depression.

The *core subcortical limbic brain* districts occupied in depression are the amygdala, the hippocampus, and the dorsomedial thalamus. Mutually operational and functional irregularities in these extents have originated in depression. Reduced hippocampal capacities have been celebrated in focus with depression. Themes that concern with treatment have even been revealed to have higher pretreatment hippocampal capacities, though individuals with smaller hippocampal capacities were reported to be extra prone to relapse. Decreased amygdala core volume has been reported in depression. The precise implication of these volumetric abnormalities is not recognized. In the circumstance of damage of hippocampal capacity, a certain pathophysiology associated with hypercortisolemia-connected neurotoxicity has been postulated.

Nonetheless, such result has also been initiated in *anxiety disorders* such as PTSD and might be additionally associated with the effects of disturbance in early life. Other research has exposed that a diversity of antidepressants has neurotrophic possessions. It is conceivable that antidepressants may perform by their capability to converse neurodegeneration in serious parts of the mood-regulating circuit. In the circumstance of the amygdala, amplified capacity stated in some studies might be associated with medication effects. Practical education has typically revealed an amplified metabolism or activation of limbic districts in depression. Enlarged initiation of the amygdala in the resting state as well as in response to stimuli has been informed in a number of PET and fMRI studies.

Contrariwise, in *children*, the *amygdala* response to the experimental task was stated to be dull. This was understood to be due to conceivable advanced baseline metabolic action. Nevertheless, in an additional study, hypometabolism of the amygdala and paralimbic districts was stated in more severe treatment-resilient depression. Amplified period of amygdala reply to undesirable stimuli has been stated in many studies. The dorsomedial thalamus has been theorized as an integral part of the subcortical mood route with reciprocal networks to the dorsal and ventral prefrontal cortex aside from the striatum and the amygdala. A few studies have stated an increased activation of the thalamus in depression. Nonetheless, astonishingly maximum studies have distinguished no alteration.

The striatum has been an emphasis of brain imaging education in depression from the original time primarily because of its character in motor reply, in response to prize, and in inspiration. One of the initial tales was of a reduced caudate capacity in depression, even though this finding has not been reliably simulated. The precise character of the striatum in depression still remains to be completely elucidated. Recent studies with recompense-linked stimuli or positive stimuli have reported either no change or increased or decreased initiation in the striatum. The nuclei of main neurotransmitters which are supposed to be irregular in depression or the changes which are shaped by antidepressants are initiated in the brain stem.

The *raphe nucleus contains* the brain serotonergic neurons, the locus coeruleus, the norepinephrine neurons, and the substantia nigra and ventral tegmentum, the dopaminergic neurons. The reduced serotonin transporter, which can also be cast off as a secondary quantity of serotonergic neuron mass, was conveyed in a study of depression. Another study informed reduction in the serotonin transporter and upsurge in the dopamine transporter after lingering antidepressant conduct. In rapid, numerous cortical, subcortical, and brain stem districts have been revealed to have irregular initiation or metabolism in brain imaging education. However, few conclusions have been constantly and consistently informed. Numerous methodological details have been noted for the discrepant results plus demographic heterogeneity of inhabitants' examples, heterogeneity in the harshness and the superiority of depression, medication effects, and the effect of substance abuse.

An additional *essential interrogation* concerning the incompatible results may lie in whether advanced brain functions and their abnormalities can be abstracted exclusively in footings of activity in discrete brain regions. The dissimilar results of limited movement modification in brain regions across education and focus groups have commanded some agents to recommend that the irregularity in depression and other psychiatric disorders might lie in inequities of connectivity among brain districts relatively than enlarged or reduced action of one specific part. Subsequently, researcher have started to debate and discover imagery results in depression in relation to integration among brain regions.

Studies showed a *mutual affiliation between the reduced metabolism of the prefrontal cortex* and an increased metabolism in the limbic areas such as the striatum and the thalamus in depression leading to the hypothesis that corticolimbic connectivity irregularity may be existing in depression. Such finding of lessened metabolism of the subgenual cingulate cortex in depression, a section which on one hand has connectivity to the cortical mood regulating regions such as the dorsal ACC and the medial and lateral OFC and on the other has networks to the amygdala and dorsomedial thalamus as well as has outputs to the brain stem zones elaborate in vegetative purposes, directed to the hypothesis of irregularity of the amygdala-striatal-pallidal-thalamic-cingulate cortex circuit in depression.

We can all be unhappy or gloomy at periods in our lives. We have all had some experience of mental illness. Nonetheless, do we actually comprehend it—what is it? Many of our preconceptions are improper. A mental illness can be distinct as a health condition that changes an individual's thoughts, *feelings*, and *behaviors* and that sources the person suffering and effort in functioning. As with countless diseases, mental illness is severe in some cases and minor in others. Persons who have a mental illness don't necessarily look like they are sick, particularly if their illness is insignificant. Other people may show more obvious symptoms such as confusion, agitation, or withdrawal. Moreover, we have learned there are many different mental illnesses, including depression, schizophrenia, attention-deficit hyperactivity disorder (ADHD), autism, and obsessive-compulsive disorder.

Each *illness modifies a person's thoughts*, feelings, or behaviors in separate ways. To distinguish each disease, we may figure out not all brain diseases are characterized as mental illnesses. Conditions such as epilepsy, Parkinson's disease, and multiple sclerosis are brain disorders; but they are measured neurological diseases rather than mental illnesses. Remarkably, the lines between mental illnesses and these other brain or neurological disorders are blurring slightly. As scientists endure to examine the brains of individuals who have mental illnesses, they are learning that mental illness is allied with changes in the *brain's structure*, *chemistry*, and *function* and that mental illness does certainly have a *biological foundation*.

This ongoing research is, in some ways, instigating scientists to minimize the divisions between *mental illnesses* and these other *brain illnesses*. The period mental illness evidently designates that there is a problem with the mind. Nonetheless, is it just the mind in an intellectual wisdom, or is there a physical foundation to mental illness? As scientists linger to examine mental illnesses and their grounds, they acquire more and more about how the biological procedures that make the brain work are changed when a person has a mental illness. However, through our exploration, we have understood the integration part of mind, brain, body, and daily aspects of our lives.

Consequently, before thinking about the difficulties that happen in the brain when someone has a mental illness, it is helpful to think about how the *brain functions typically*. It is a well-known fact by now that the brain is an extremely complex organ. It makes up only 2 percent of our body mass, but it consumes 20 percent of the oxygen we breathe and 20 percent of the energy we take in. It panels nearly everything we as humans experience, including making movement, sensing our environment, regulating our involuntary body processes such as breathing, and controlling our emotions.

Limitless *chemical responses* arise every second in the brain; those responses motivate the thoughts, actions, and behaviors with which we respond to environmental stimuli. In short, the brain commands the internal developments and behaviors that permit us to survive. Furthermore, there are a number of major or impressive theories involving understanding mental health which we covered mostly, such as the following:

Analytical/developmental theories. Theories of development provide a framework for thinking about human growth, development, and learning, if you have ever wondered about what motivates human thought and behavior. Some of the philosophers are Freud, Jung, Erikson, and Kohlberg.

Behavioral theories. Behavioral psychology, similarly recognized as behaviorism, is a theory of education based upon the impression that all behaviors are attained through conditioning. Encouraged by well-known psychologists such as John B. Watson and B. F. Skinner, behavioral theories conquered psychology during the early half of the *twentieth century.* Philosophers such as Watson, Skinner, and Pavlov were effective theorists of such century.

Cognitive theories. Cognitive psychology is the *division* of psychology that studies mental processes including how individuals think, perceive, remember, and learn. As a portion of the greater ground of cognitive science, this branch of psychology is associated with other disciplines plus neuroscience, philosophy, and linguistics. The few famous philosophers of this study are Tolman, Piaget, and Chomsky.

Social theories. Social psychology looks at an extensive variety of social themes. Such includes group behavior, social perception, leadership, nonverbal behavior, conformity, aggression, and prejudice. It is significant to note that social psychology is not just about observing social influences. Social perception and social interaction are also vital to understanding social behavior. Well-known theorists are Bandura, Lewin, and Festinger.

Furthermore, if a person does not rest, he or she gets tired. If a person sees effects that are not there, he or she gets anxious. If a person uses plentiful drugs, he or she gets into legal distress. With such consideration, it is likely that these symptom-symptom influences are ingrained in actual everyday *biological, psychological,* and *societal developments.* This is astonishing, since it reveals that illnesses are not ill-understood transient beings, the countryside of which will have to be revealed by upcoming psychological, neuroscientific, or genetic studies. Consequently, a general mental health apprehension can be learned by simple understanding, such as the following:

- Biological factors, genes, brain chemistry
- Brain health, tumor, cancer
- Environmental concerns, accident, injuries
- Overall health maintenance, diet, exercise
- Life experiences, trauma, abuse
- Family history of mental health, and so on

However, a *simple understanding of brain development* is an essential part of overall health. For example, how does the brain take in all this information, process it, and cause a response? In a simple manner, the basic functional component of the brain is the neuron. A neuron is a specialized cell that can produce different actions because of its precise connections with other neurons, sensory receptors, and muscle cells.

A *typical neuron has four structurally* and functionally well-defined districts, such as the cell body, dendrites, axons, and axon terminals. The cell body is the metabolic center of the neuron. The nucleus is positioned in the cell body, and most of the cell's protein synthesis happens here. A neuron typically has numerous fibers named dendrites that extend from the cell body. These procedures typically division out and aid as the main device for receiving input from other nerve cells. The cell body likewise gives rise to the axon. The axon is frequently considerably longer than the dendrites; in some suitcases, an axon can be up to one meter in length. The axon is the portion of the neuron that is dedicated to transmitting communications away from the cell body and transmitting messages to other cells.

Approximately *large axons are bound by a fatty insulating substance called myelin*, which permits the electrical signals to travel down the axon at advanced speeds. Near its end, the axon splits into numerous fine branches that have focused swellings termed "axon terminals" or "presynaptic terminals." The axon terminals end near the dendrites of additional neurons. The dendrites of one neuron obtain the communication sent from the axon terminals of another neuron. The location where an axon terminal ends near a receipt dendrite is called the synapse. The cell that passes out information is named the presynaptic neuron, and the cell that accepts the information is called the postsynaptic neuron.

It is important to mention that the synapse is not a physical construction between the two neurons. There is no cytoplasmic assembly between the two neurons. The intercellular space between the presynaptic and postsynaptic neurons is termed the synaptic space or synaptic cleft. A typical neuron system is approximately one thousand synapses with other neurons. It has been assessed that there are extra synapses in the human brain than there are stars in our galaxy.

Additionally, *synaptic networks* are not motionless. Neurons form new synapses or reinforce synaptic associates in reply to life experiences. This dynamic alteration in neuronal networks is the foundation of education. Neurons interconnect using together electrical signals and chemical messages. Information in the procedure of an electrical impulse is passed away from the neuron's cell form along the axon of the presynaptic neuron in the direction of the axon terminals. When the electrical signal grasps the presynaptic axon terminal, it cannot cross the synaptic space, or synaptic cleft. As a substitute, the electrical alert activates chemical differences that can cross the synapse to affect the postsynaptic cell. When the electrical instinct grasps the presynaptic axon terminal, membranous pouches called vesicles transfer toward the membrane of the axon terminal. When the vesicles scope the membrane, they fuse with the membrane and free their contents into the synaptic space.

The *molecules contained* in the vesicles are chemical mixes named neurotransmitters. Each vesicle comprises numerous molecules of a neurotransmitter. The free neurotransmitter molecules float over the synaptic cleft and then bind to superior proteins, called receptors, on the postsynaptic neuron. A neurotransmitter molecule will bind only to an exact type of receptor. Hereafter, the binding of neurotransmitters to their receptors reasons that neuron to produce an electrical impulse. The *electrical impulse* then passages away from the dendrite ending near the cell body. Afterward, the neurotransmitter stimulates an electrical impulse in the postsynaptic neuron. It escapes from the receptor back into the synaptic location. Exact proteins named transporters or reuptake pumps transmit the neurotransmitter back into the presynaptic neuron. Once the neurotransmitter molecules are back in the presynaptic axon terminal, they can be repackaged into vesicles for release the next time an electrical impulse reaches the axon terminal.

Enzymes present in the synaptic space degrade neurotransmitter molecules that are not taken back up into the presynaptic neuron. The nervous system utilizes a diversity of neurotransmitter molecules.

Nonetheless, each neuron focuses on the synthesis and secretion of a solitary sort of neurotransmitter. Some of the predominant neurotransmitters in the brain contain glutamate, GABA, serotonin, dopamine, and norepinephrine.

Also, each of these neurotransmitters has an explicit supply and occupation in the brain. Mental health specialists base their analysis and treatment of mental illness on the indications that a person displays. The aim of these professionals in treating a patient is to find the signs that are interfering with the person's life so that the person can perform well. Study scientists, on the other hand, have a different drive. They want to absorb the chemical or mechanical changes that happen in the brain when someone has a mental disease. If scientists can regulate what occurs in the brain, they can utilize that information to progress better conducts.

Some early warning signs of mental concern might include the following:

- Eating, sleeping too much or too little (loss of balance)
- Pulling away from people and usual activities (low self-esteem, depressed)
- Having less energy (less desire or motivation)
- Feeling numb or as if nothing matters (disconnect)
- Physical discomfort, unexplained aches and pains (mind-body discomfort)
- Feeling helpless or hopeless (psychological, emotional)
- Smoking, drinking, or using drugs (for coping skills)
- Feeling confused, forgetful, on edge, angry, upset, worried, scared (emotional issues)
- Socially awkward, fighting with family and friends (social concerns)
- Experience persistent thoughts and memories (subjective experience)
- In developed cases, inability to perform daily tasks (disconnectedness)

Types of Mental Health

Although we are striving for a better understanding of brain to mind, each individual can experience different forms of mental health complications. Commonly, if individuals can distinguish what is a healthy mind, then they can contribute to what isn't healthy. A healthy mind is the absence of symptoms and dysfunction we described above. *Over the past decades*, scientists are reluctant to define mind as to have a much deeper meaning with humans' overall health development.

However, psychology offers positive models by distinguishing those behaviors, by characteristics of open-mindedness, compassion, and gratitude, which allow us to create logistical points to adopt the system of integration instead. There are psychosocial theories and application to education and for clinical practice. For example, these *four psychosocial theories deliberated* are self-efficacy, stress and coping, learned helplessness, and social support and have great power to guide the practice of health educators and clinicians as well as the process of health behavior change. What are other types of mental health conditions?

Anxiety Disorder

People with anxiety disorders respond to certain objects or situations with fear and dread. Anxiety disorders can include obsessive-compulsive disorder, panic disorders, and phobias. They have physical reactions to those objects, such as a rapid heartbeat and sweating. An anxiety disorder is diagnosed if a person has an inappropriate response to a situation, cannot control the response, and has an altered way of life due to the anxiety.

Anxiety disorders include the following:

Panic Disorder

Panic disorder is an anxiety disorder. It causes panic attacks, which are sudden feelings of terror for no reason. You may also feel physical symptoms, such as fast heartbeat, chest pain, breathing difficulty, and dizziness.

Panic attacks can happen anytime, anywhere, and without warning. You may live in fear of another attack and may avoid places where you have had an attack. For some people, fear takes over their lives, and they cannot leave their homes. Panic disorder is more common in women than men. It usually starts when people are young adults. Sometimes it starts when a person is under a lot of stress. Most people get better with treatment. Therapy can show you how to recognize and change your thinking patterns before they lead to panic. Medicines can also help.

Phobias

A phobia is a type of anxiety disorder. It is a strong, irrational fear of something that poses little or no actual danger. There are many specific phobias. Acrophobia is a fear of heights. You may be able to ski the world's tallest mountains but be unable to go above the fifth floor of an office building. Agoraphobia is a fear of public places, and claustrophobia is a fear of closed-in places. If you become anxious and extremely self-conscious in everyday social situations, you could have a social phobia. Other common phobias involve tunnels, highway driving, water, flying, animals, and blood. People with phobias try to avoid what they are afraid of. If they cannot, they may experience the following:

- Panic and fear
- Rapid heartbeat
- Shortness of breath
- Trembling
- A strong desire to get away

Treatment helps most people with phobias. Options include medicines, therapy, or both.

Behavioral Disorders

Behavioral disorders involve a pattern of disruptive behaviors in children that last for at least six months and cause problems in school, at home, and in social situations. Examples of behavioral disorders include attention-deficit hyperactivity disorder (ADHD), conduct disorder, and oppositional-defiant disorder (ODD). Nearly everyone shows some of these behaviors at times, but behavior disorders are more serious.

Behavioral disorders may involve the following:

- Inattention
- Hyperactivity
- Impulsivity
- Defiant behavior
- Drug use
- Criminal activity

Behavioral disorders include the following:

- ODD
- Conduct disorder
- ADHD

Attention-Deficit Hyperactivity Disorder (ADHD)

Attention-deficit hyperactivity disorder (ADHD) is the most normally diagnosed behavioral disorder of childhood. In any six-month period, ADHD affects an estimated 4.1 percent of youths ages nine to seventeen. Furthermore, boys are two to three times more likely than girls to develop ADHD. While ADHD is usually connected with children, the disorder can continue into adulthood. The three principal symptoms of ADHD are impaired capability to control activity level (hyperactivity), to fulfill responsibilities (inattention), and to constrain behavior (impulsivity).

Persons who have ADHD may exhibit predominantly hyperactive/ impulsive behavior, predominantly inattentive behavior, or a combination of both. ADHD is a problem of not being able to focus, being overactive, not being able control behavior, or a combination of these. For these problems to be diagnosed as ADHD, they must be out of the normal range of a person's age and development.

Causes: ADHD usually begins in childhood but may continue into the adult years. A combination of genes and environmental factors likely plays a role in the development of the condition. Imaging studies suggest that the brains of children with ADHD are different from those of children without ADHD.

Inattentive symptoms:

- Fails to give close attention to details or makes careless mistakes in schoolwork
- Has difficulty keeping attention during tasks or play
- Does not seem to listen when spoken to directly
- Does not follow through on instructions and fails to finish schoolwork or chores and tasks
- Has problems organizing tasks and activities
- Avoids or dislikes tasks that require sustained mental effort (such as schoolwork)
- Often loses toys, assignments, pencils, books, or tools needed for tasks or activities
- Is easily distracted
- Is often forgetful in daily activities

Hyperactivity symptoms:

- Fidgets with hands or feet or squirms in seat
- Leaves seat when remaining seated is expected
- Runs about or climbs in inappropriate situations
- Has problems playing or working quietly
- Is often "on the go," acts as if "driven by a motor"
- Talks excessively

Impulsivity symptoms:

- Blurts out answers before questions have been completed
- Has difficulty awaiting turn
- Interrupts or intrudes on others (butts into conversations or games)

No solitary reason of ADHD has been exposed. Slightly, a number of substantial risk influences affecting neurodevelopment and behavior expression have been concerned. Events such as maternal alcohol and tobacco use that affect the development of the fetal brain can increase the risk for ADHD. Damages to the brain from environmental poisons such as absence of iron have also been implicated. Scientists have observed the character of the neurotransmitter dopamine in the development of ADHD since this neurotransmitter plays a significant character in regulating movement, increasing motivation and awareness, and inducing insomnia.

The observation that ADHD is inclined to run in families strongly proposes that the illness has a hereditary factor. Children who have ADHD typically have at minimum one close relative who also has the condition. Inquiries of specific genes intricate in ADHD have absorbed on a dopamine receptor gene (DRD) on chromosome 11 and the dopamine transporter gene (DAT1) on chromosome 5. Continuing studies endure to observe these genes and others as influences in ADHD. Most likely, a mixture of numerous genes and environmental factors regulates whether an individual has ADHD.

Eating Disorders

Eating disorders involve extreme emotions, attitudes, and behaviors involving weight and food. Eating disorders can include anorexia, bulimia, and binge eating. Scientists have recognized convinced parts of the brain involved with anxiety, hunger and appetite, and alexithymia (the inability to feel and express emotions) for those with anorexia. A study found hypoactivation (slowing down) in the hypothalamus (the body's thermostat detecting hunger), amygdala (fear response region of the brain), and anterior insula (part of the brain responsible for interoceptive awareness plus body and emotions) for both members with active anorexia and weight-restored participants compared to healthy-weight controls before eating.

The education also recommended activation in the *hypothalamus*, *amygdala*, and anterior insula for those weight-restored were connected with hedonic (desire for favorite foods) and nonhedonic (hunger) features of appetite. It is thought that dysfunction in this region of the brain for those with anorexia may mirror the anxious response to the mere impression of food. And reduced activation in the anterior insula is accompanied with the incapability for self-awareness, such as being in a state of hunger, emotions, and other somatic sensations. A study examined the character of cognition (thoughts about eating) for appetite-connected activation in those with anorexia and initiated thoughts about food for those with anorexia linked to reduced activation in the cerebellar vermis and upsurge activation in the visual cortex. Furthermore, the study found those with anorexia fail to competently process information from the appetite regions of the brain and efficiently compose higher-order cognitions (thoughts). The most common eating disorders include the following:

Anorexia Nervosa

Anorexia nervosa is an eating disorder that makes people lose more weight than is considered healthy for their age and height. Persons with this disorder may have an intense fear of weight gain, even when they are underweight. They may diet or exercise too much or use other methods to lose weight. The exact causes of anorexia nervosa are not known. Many factors probably are involved. Genes and hormones may play a role. Social attitudes that promote very thin body types may also be involved. Family conflicts are no longer thought to contribute to this or other eating disorders.

The risk factors of anorexia include the following:

- Being more worried about, or paying more attention to, weight and shape
- Having an anxiety disorder as a child
- Having a negative self-image
- Having eating problems during infancy or early childhood
- Having certain social or cultural ideas about health and beauty
- Trying to be perfect or overly focused on rules

Anorexia usually begins during the teen years or young adulthood. It is more common in females but may also be seen in males. The disorder is seen mainly in white women who are high academic achievers and who have a goal-oriented family or personality.

To be diagnosed with anorexia, a person must

- have an intense fear of gaining weight or becoming fat, even when she is underweight;
- refuse to keep weight at what is considered normal for her age and height (15 percent or more below the normal weight);
- have a body image that is very distorted, be very focused on body weight or shape, and refuse to admit the seriousness of weight loss; and
- have not had a period for three or more cycles (in women).

People with anorexia may severely limit the amount of food they eat, or eat and then make themselves throw up. Other behaviors include the following:

- Cutting food into small pieces or moving them around the plate instead of eating
- Exercising all the time, even when the weather is bad, they are hurt, or their schedule is busy
- Going to the bathroom right after meals
- Refusing to eat around other people

- Using pills to make themselves urinate (water pills or diuretics), have a bowel movement (enemas and laxatives), or decrease their appetite (diet pills)

Other symptoms of anorexia may include the following:

- Blotchy or yellow skin that is dry and covered with fine hair
- Confused or slow thinking, along with poor memory or judgment
- Depression
- Dry mouth
- Extreme sensitivity to cold (wearing several layers of clothing to stay warm)
- Loss of bone strength
- Wasting away of muscle and loss of body fat

Binge Eating

Binge eating is when a person eats a much larger amount of food in a shorter period than he or she normally would. During binge eating, the person also feels a loss of control. A binge eater often

- eats five thousand to fifteen thousand calories in one sitting;
- often snacks, in addition to eating three meals a day; and
- overeats throughout the day.

Binge eating by itself usually leads to becoming overweight. Binge eating may occur on its own or with another eating disorder, such as bulimia. People with bulimia typically eat large amounts of high-calorie foods, usually in secret. After this binge eating, they often force themselves to vomit or take laxatives. The cause of binge eating is unknown. However, binge eating often begins during or after strict dieting.

Bulimia

Bulimia is an illness in which a person binges on food or has regular episodes of overeating and feels a loss of control. The person then uses different methods—such as vomiting or abusing laxatives—to prevent weight gain. Many (but not all) people with bulimia also have anorexia nervosa. Many more women than men have bulimia. The disorder is most common in adolescent girls and young women. The affected person is usually aware that her eating pattern is abnormal and may feel fear or guilt with the binge-purge episodes. The exact cause of bulimia is unknown. Genetic, psychological, trauma, family, society, or cultural factors may play a role. Bulimia is likely due to more than one factor. In bulimia, eating binges may occur as often as several times a day for many months. People with bulimia often eat large amounts of high-calorie foods, usually in secret. People can feel a lack of control over their eating during these episodes. Binges lead to self-disgust, which causes purging to prevent weight gain.

Purging may include the following:

- Forcing yourself to vomit
- Excessive exercise
- Using laxatives, enemas, or diuretics (water pills)

Purging often brings a sense of relief. People with bulimia are often at a normal weight, but they may see themselves as being overweight. Because the person's weight is often normal, other people may not notice this eating disorder.

Symptoms that other people can see include the following:

- Compulsive exercise
- Suddenly eating large amounts of food or buying large amounts of food that disappear right away
- Regularly going to the bathroom right after meals
- Throwing away packages of laxatives, diet pills, and emetics (drugs that cause vomiting).

Mood Disorders

Mood disorders involve persistent feelings of sadness or periods of feeling overly happy or fluctuating between extreme happiness and extreme sadness. Mood disorders can include depression, bipolar disorder, seasonal affective disorder (SAD), and self-harm. These disorders, also called affective disorders, may involve the following:

- Feeling sad all the time
- Losing interest in important parts of life
- Fluctuating between extreme happiness and extreme sadness

The most common mood disorders are as follows:

Depression

Depression is a serious medical illness that involves the brain. It's more than just a feeling of being "down in the dumps" or "blue" for a few days. If you are one of the more than 20 million people in the United States who have depression, the feelings do not go away. They persist and interfere with your everyday life.

Symptoms can include the following:

- Sadness
- Loss of interest or pleasure in activities you used to enjoy
- Change in weight
- Difficulty sleeping or oversleeping
- Energy loss
- Feelings of worthlessness
- Thoughts of death or suicide

Depression is a disorder of the brain. There are a variety of causes, including genetic, environmental, psychological, and biochemical factors. Depression usually starts between the ages of fifteen and thirty and is much more common in women. Women can also get postpartum depression after the birth of a baby. Some people get seasonal affective disorder in the winter. Depression is one part of bipolar disorder. There are effective treatments for depression, including antidepressants and talk therapy. Most people do best by using both.

Bipolar Disorder

Bipolar disorder is a serious mental illness. People who have it go through unusual mood changes. They go from very happy, up, and active to very sad and hopeless, down, and inactive, and then back again. They often have normal moods in between. The up feeling is called mania. The down feeling is depression. The causes of bipolar disorder aren't always clear. It runs in families. Abnormal brain structure and function may also play a role.

Bipolar disorder often starts in a person's late teen or early adult years. But children and adults can have bipolar disorder too. The illness usually lasts a lifetime. If you think you may have it, tell your health care provider. A medical checkup can rule out other illnesses that might cause your mood changes. If not treated, bipolar disorder can lead to damaged relationships, poor job or school performance, and even suicide. However, there are effective treatments to control symptoms: medicine and talk therapy. A combination usually works best.

Seasonal Affective Disorder (SAD)

Some people experience a serious mood change during the winter months, when there is less natural sunlight. This condition is called seasonal affective disorder, or SAD. SAD is a type of depression. It usually lifts during spring and summer. Not everyone with SAD has the same symptoms.

Some symptoms might include the following:

- Sad, anxious or "empty" feelings
- Feelings of hopelessness and/or pessimism

- Feelings of guilt, worthlessness, or helplessness
- Irritability, restlessness
- Loss of interest or pleasure in activities you used to enjoy
- Fatigue and decreased energy
- Difficulty concentrating, remembering details, and making decisions
- Difficulty sleeping or oversleeping
- Changes in weight
- Thoughts of death or suicide

SAD may be effectively treated with light therapy. But nearly half of people with SAD do not respond to light therapy alone. Antidepressant medicines and talk therapy can reduce SAD symptoms, either alone or combined with light therapy.

Suicide is a major health problem, and the global suicide mortality rate is recognized worldwide. Most suicides are related to psychiatric disease, with depression, substance use disorders, and psychosis being the most relevant risk factors. Nevertheless, anxiety-, personality-, eating-, and trauma-related disorders, as well as organic mental illnesses, similarly contribute.

Psychological studies have revealed that most people who have died by suicide have suffered from mental disorders. On the other hand, some individuals with mental disorders do not die by their own hand. The risk of suicide has been projected to be for numerous mental illnesses, such as depression, alcoholism, and schizophrenia.

Depression is a common thread, likewise known to be the most mutual disorder among individuals who die by suicide. Other risks *might* include family history of psychiatric disorders, male gender, suicide attempts, more severe depression, hopelessness, and comorbidity.

Self-Harm

Self-harm refers to a person's harming their own body on purpose. About one in one hundred people hurts himself or herself in this way.

More females hurt themselves than males. A person who self-harms usually does not mean to kill himself or herself. But they are at a higher risk of attempting suicide if they do not get help. Self-harm tends to begin in teen or early adult years. Some people may engage in self-harm a few times and then stop. Others engage in it more often and have trouble stopping.

Examples of self-harm include the following:

- Cutting yourself (such as using a razor blade, knife, or other sharp object to cut the skin)
- Punching yourself or punching things (like a wall)
- Burning yourself with cigarettes, matches, or candles
- Pulling out your hair
- Poking objects through body openings
- Breaking your bones or bruising yourself

Many people cut themselves because it gives them a sense of relief. Some people use cutting as a means to cope with a problem. Some teens say that when they hurt themselves, they are trying to stop feeling lonely, angry, or hopeless. It is possible to overcome the urge to hurt yourself. There are other ways to find relief and cope with your emotions.

Obsessive-Compulsive Disorder

If a person has OCD, they have repeated upsetting thoughts called obsessions. Individuals do the same thing over and over again to try to make the thoughts go away. Those repeated actions are called compulsions. Examples of obsessions are a fear of germs or a fear of being hurt. Compulsions include washing your hands, counting, checking on things, or cleaning. Untreated, OCD can take over your life. Researchers think brain circuits may not work properly in people who have OCD. It tends to run in families. The symptoms often begin in children or teens. Treatments that combine medicines and therapy are often effective.

Personality Disorders

People with personality disorders experience patterns of behavior, feelings, and thinking that can

- interfere with a person's life,
- create problems at work and school, or
- cause issues in personal and social relationships.

Personality disorders include the following:

Antisocial Personality Disorder

Antisocial personality disorder is a mental health condition in which a person has a long-term pattern of manipulating, exploiting, or violating the rights of others. This behavior is often criminal. The cause of antisocial personality disorder is unknown. Genetic factors and environmental factors, such as child abuse, are believed to contribute to the development of this condition. People with an antisocial or alcoholic parent are at increased risk. Far more men than women are affected. The condition is common among people who are in prison. Fire-setting and cruelty to animals during childhood are linked to the development of antisocial personality. Some doctors believe that psychopathic personality (psychopathy) is the same disorder. Others believe that psychopathic personality is a similar but more severe disorder.

A person with antisocial personality disorder may

- be able to act witty and charming;
- be good at flattery and manipulating other people's emotions;
- break the law repeatedly;
- disregard the safety of self and others;
- have problems with substance abuse;
- lie, steal, and fight often;
- not show guilt or remorse; or
- often be angry or arrogant.

Borderline Personality Disorder

Borderline personality disorder (BPD) is a mental health condition in which a person has long-term patterns of unstable or turbulent emotions. These inner experiences often result in impulsive actions and chaotic relationships with other people. The cause of BPD is unknown. Genetic, family, and social factors are thought to play roles.

The risk factors of BPD include the following:

- Abandonment in childhood or adolescence
- Disrupted family life
- Poor communication in the family
- Sexual, physical, or emotional abuse

This personality disorder tends to occur more often in women and among hospitalized psychiatric patients.

Symptoms. Persons with BPD are often uncertain about their identity. As a result, their interests and values can change rapidly. They also tend to view things in terms of extremes, such as either all good or all bad. Their views of other people can change quickly. A person who is looked up to one day may be looked down on the next day. These suddenly shifting feelings often lead to intense and unstable relationships.

Other symptoms of BPD include the following:

- Intense fear of being abandoned
- Cannot tolerate being alone
- Frequent feelings of emptiness and boredom
- Frequent displays of inappropriate anger
- Impulsiveness, such as with substance abuse or sexual relationships
- Repeated crises and acts of self-injury, such as wrist cutting or overdosing

Exams and Tests. BPD is diagnosed based on a psychological evaluation that assesses the history and severity of the symptoms.

Treatment. Individual talk therapy may successfully treat BPD. In addition, group therapy can sometimes be helpful.

Medications have less of a role in the treatment of BPD. But in some cases, they can improve mood swings and treat depression or other disorders that may occur with this condition.

Outlook (Prognosis). Outlook of treatment depends on how severe the condition is and whether the person is willing to accept help. With long-term talk therapy, the person often gradually improves.

Possible complications:

- Depression
- Drug abuse
- Problems with work, family, and social relationships
- Suicide attempts and actual suicide

Psychotic Disorders

People with psychotic disorders experience a range of symptoms, including hallucinations and delusions. An example of a psychotic disorder is schizophrenia. Hallucinations—hearing or seeing things that are not real, such as voices. Delusions—believing things that are not true. However, these symptoms can occur in people with other health problems, including bipolar disorder, dementia, substance abuse disorders, or brain tumors. Psychotic disorders include the following:

Schizophrenia

Schizophrenia is a severe, lifelong brain disorder. People who have it may hear voices, see things that aren't there, or believe that others are reading or controlling their minds. In men, symptoms usually start in the late teens and early twenties. They include hallucinations, or seeing things, and delusions such as hearing voices. For women, they start in the midtwenties to early thirties. Other symptoms include the following:

- Unusual thoughts or perceptions
- Disorders of movement
- Difficulty speaking and expressing emotion
- Problems with attention, memory, and organization

No one is sure what causes schizophrenia, but your genetic makeup and brain chemistry probably play a role. Medicines can relieve many of the symptoms. Nonetheless, it can take several tries before you find the right drug.

Suicidal Behavior

Suicide causes immeasurable pain, suffering, and loss to individuals, families, and communities nationwide. Suicide is the second leading cause of death among fifteen- to twenty-four-year-olds. Suicide is preventable, so it's important to know what to do.

Warning signs of suicide. If someone you know is showing one or more of the following behaviors, he or she may be thinking about suicide. Don't ignore these warning signs. Get help immediately.

- Talking about wanting to die or to kill oneself
- Looking for a way to kill oneself
- Talking about feeling hopeless or having no reason to live
- Talking about feeling trapped or in unbearable pain
- Talking about being a burden to others
- Increasing the use of alcohol or drugs
- Acting anxious or agitated; behaving recklessly
- Sleeping too little or too much
- Withdrawing or feeling isolated
- Showing rage or talking about seeking revenge
- Displaying extreme mood swings

Trauma and Stress-Related Disorders

Post-traumatic stress disorder (PTSD) can occur after living through or seeing a traumatic event, such as war, a hurricane, rape, physical abuse, or a bad accident. PTSD makes you feel stressed and afraid after the danger is over. It affects your life and the people around you.

PTSD can cause problems like the following:

- Flashbacks, or feeling like the event is happening again
- Trouble sleeping or nightmares
- Feeling alone
- Angry outbursts
- Feeling worried, guilty, or sad

PTSD starts at different times for different people. Signs of PTSD may start soon after a frightening event and then continue. Other people develop new or more severe signs months or even years later. PTSD can happen to anyone, even children. Medicines can help you feel less afraid and tense. It might take a few weeks for them to work. Talking to a specially trained doctor or counselor also helps many people with PTSD. This is called talk therapy.

Mental coordinate may be contingent on an excellence of openness to living in the moment that may be crucial for the therapist's own stance and serve as a deliberate goal for the process of treatment itself. Of note from the neuroscience works are initial studies propose that mindful meditation exercise, as one example of a receptive mental state, may truly lead to enhanced growth of the middle prefrontal regions as well as preserved neural tissue in these regions with aging.

The three goals of developmental psychology might be to describe, explain, and optimize human development. For instance, to describe human development, it is necessary to focus both on typical patterns of change which is normative development and on individual difference in patterns of changes. Although there are typical routes of development that humans will follow, no two persons are exactly alike. Two siblings are not the same, nor do we ever confuse them. Which one of you reminding me which. Developmental psychologists are also learning to explain the changes they have observed in relation to normative processes and individual differences. However, it is often easier to define development than to explain how it occurs. Developmental psychologists hope to enhance development and smear their theories—practice for serving individuals in applied circumstances, like parents develop secure attachments with their children, etc.

Moreover, *constructivism* is a subject of *learning theory* in which goal is placed on the knowing and experience of the learner. This often is on the social and cultural factor of the learning process. Educational psychologists discover the individual constructivism through Piaget's theory of *cognitive* development that is from social constructivism. Also, Lev Vygotsky's work on sociocultural learning, describing how interactions with adults, more capable friends, and cognitive tools are internalized to form human *mental constructs*. Vygotsky's theory and other educational psychologists industrialized the significant notion of instructional scaffolding. What scaffolding proposal in the social or information environment is provision for learning that is gradually withdrawn as they become internalized. As they say, it takes a village to raise a child. This means including scientists, psychiatrists, psychologists, mindfulness, teachers, and educational systems.

Consequently, to understand the characteristics of learners in childhood, adolescence, adulthood, and old age, educational psychology advances and applies theories of human development, often represented as stages through which persons grow as they mature. *These developmental theories revealed changes in mental abilities (cognition), social roles, moral reasoning, and beliefs about the nature of knowledge. Motivation is the reason for people's actions, desires, and needs.* Motivation is also one's *direction to behavior*, or what causes a person to want to repeat a behavior. Although an individual is not motivated by another individual because motivation comes from within, still we get our sparks from the eye of others. Motivation can be conceived of as a cycle in which thoughts influence behaviors, in which behaviors drive performance.

There is no doubt, *performance affects human thoughts*, and the cycle begins again. Each stage of the cycle is composed of many dimensions including attitudes, beliefs, intentions, effort, and withdrawal which can all affect human motivation. Most psychological theories hold that motivation exists purely within the individual. Nevertheless, sociocultural theories express motivation as an outcome of participation in actions and activities within the cultural context of social groups. We have many books written already. However, this is not a repeat of the cycle of writing journey journals; but with motivation, we might consider movement toward schools, education, and our development. The highest order of needs is for self-fulfillment, including recognition of one's full potential, areas for self-improvement, and the opportunity for creativity. Even at a working environment, to successfully manage and motivate employees, the natural system posits that being part of a group is necessary. Since structural changes in social order, the workplace is more fluid and more adaptive.

Let's buckle our seat belt for the *discovery of our other brain* that might sound less realistic, but if we have figured life from the sum point of being not whole, we have not lived as a whole. Discovering the other brain is the discovery of truth for the absence of happiness, love, health, and success. Human might still to think the first organ to form in the embryo is the beating heart. In fact, the nervous system is the first bodily organ to emerge. The fatal nervous system serves as the cornerstone upon which the entire embryonic body will be built. How does that help people flourish? It is all about way of thinking, knowing, mindfulness, awareness, and making greater decisions, isn't it? Consequently, are we smart or unwise? Another way of saying it is some of us are more curious learners. Some of us might be less motivated to adapt to and learn from anything there is to learn, to just be open minded. Although we are in the twenty-first century, we still don't have the hundred percent definition of human development and brain-to-mind integration; however, we are getting close. This book might explore today's brain from all angles of science to physics to spirituality, beliefs, consciousness, mindfulness, and so on. The same as educators, doctors, caregivers, and parents focus on delivering core content. Nonetheless, it's the way that students or learners *interact* with that *content*, and the learning skills they develop, that'll define the quality of their education and best prepare them for a successful life. Teaching can be vocabulary experience, and learning requires not only a good listener, but an aware interrupter, as teachers do not teach meaning.

Chapter 2

Human Brain Anatomy:
Neuroscience, New Century

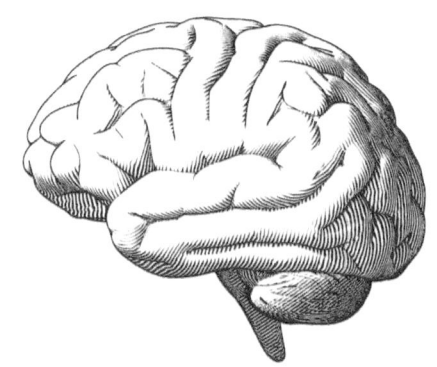

Integration of Brain with Its Parts

The nervous system has one role by sitting inside our head. This is referred to as our brain. The distribution of neuronal activity inside our head has interconnected via linkage throughout our brain. These are the cells, neurons, and glial cells, where micro systems surround within the membranes. Even though these cells are open and interconnected within and among other cells through the body, the cluster of cells means the nuclei link up to form the center. Those neurons link to distinct nuclei, center and region of one to another, then form circuits. These clusters of neurons can be interconnected within two sides of our hemisphere. Our nervous system is made up of layers of networking mechanisms which are open subsystems generating their assembly and functions from other larger open systems.

The integration of which that resources the brain inside our head has its own organization of operation. Could it be true our neuronal firings come from mind originally What does it really mean when we say neuronal firing? Could it be the basic cells to the nature of this activity? Our neurons are becoming active and link through the flow of energy. This happens in the form of electrochemical energy transformations. However, at this point, we can generalize that our brain activity is the flow of electrochemical energy. Perhaps this activity can be measured and changed with a magnetic electrical device. Thus, we can say this energy system is real to this point of our learning journey. When this energy flow within our brain carries a symbol, then this means given information. Scientists call this neural representation, which means the neurons represent something other than themselves. This is the activity of the brain (neurons and nervous system). What about our mind? Such activities for our mind are called mental representation. We see the difference between neuron representation to mental representation. How our brain activity (neuron firings) links to our personal life experience, our thoughts, our emotions, our mind, is a big topic, and there are many evidence and research, but still not clear enough. Deeper into our book journey, we will explore the consciousness, awareness, metaphysics, and our personal experiences from enlightenment to the universe, to see if we could link our brain to mind and consciousness as a whole aspect of being.

Let's look at what *modern science* has said. The stance of modern science is that the neuronal firing leads to our mind. However, we have learned so far that our nervous system and energy information flow are not happening within our head alone, but it's throughout the body. Our neurons are integrative like a spiderweb through our entire body. At some point, we learned the fundamental purpose of our brain integration with our heart, our lungs, our emotions, and even our intestines. Therefore, to speak back to scientists, we may say the energy flow and our information distribution are not a system inside the skull alone but widely spread. For example, the burning sensation on your toes is a whole body-and-mind experience. Also, the mind receives its information and energy flow not just from our skull or our body but beyond our physical life. This information can be the outcome of social experience between us and among others throughout the universe.

There is also the *consciousness aspect of the mind* that gives this whole experience of integration a sense of awareness. Our attention (awareness) affects our experiences that affect the neuron firings which shape our brain development. Being aware or conscious is doing just that. Could it be possible then consciousness or awareness itself would trigger energy distribution? For example, when taking a picture, the integration of mind-to-brain stimulation is essential to where we put the camera's lens. The lens of the camera depends much on who controls it. It's less on seeing; it's more on the witness of seeing. Consciousness is the sea to an infinite potential for creating possibilities which become actualities. In other words, observation moves the energy from the uncertainty to the certainty ground. Perhaps that's how something arrives in our mind as a form of energy flow and soon becomes thought or remembering something becomes memories. Energy itself also manifests as potential for open possibilities to probability for creating that actuality.

Energy is not only part of us, but *interconnected within the universe.* If we think it this way, then our mind or consciousness becomes part of this natural system that serves a self-organizing system. Likewise, this energy system we all become aware and part of brings us to the interconnectedness system, from me to we. We are connected not only to our subjective experiences with our families and friends, but through natural energy and whichever to be considered as a mystical sense of the generator of diversity to the open plane from which we all arise into being. This would link us back to the fact that not only the brain-mind extends beyond skull, but consciousness also extends beyond our physical abilities. The integration of the neuronal regions looks as if to associate with our consciousness which is called neural correlation of consciousness. However, it's still a mysterious and magical experience of being aware. We will explore our consciousness through the book journey. It's good enough to start with general knowledge of the brain-mind-consciousness integration here. Viewing the mind as relational is not something new. The mind has been explained by modern scientists to some degree in the nature of brain activity, which our brain is a social organ. Thus, it functions in time of socializing. We already learned enough to understand the ingratiating of our whole system, not just brain to mind. This organization depends on each part—health, development, experience, consciousness, awareness, and function.

Therefore, the mind can't be the sole function of the brain alone as our subjective experience shapes our mental abilities, our neurons, and how we think. Could it be possible then we found the mind's location? Could it be possible the mind location is the integration of its relationship?

- Mind between brain and its structural parts (embodied).
- Mind between brain and body (our organs) function.
- Mind between brain and our subjective experiences (our personal journey).
- Mind between brain and our relationship (others, families, friends, cultures).
- Mind between brain and our belief system and faith.
- Mind between brain and nurturing environment (community, plants, diversity, animals, education, work) and universe as a whole.
- Mind between brain and our consciousness (awareness) system.

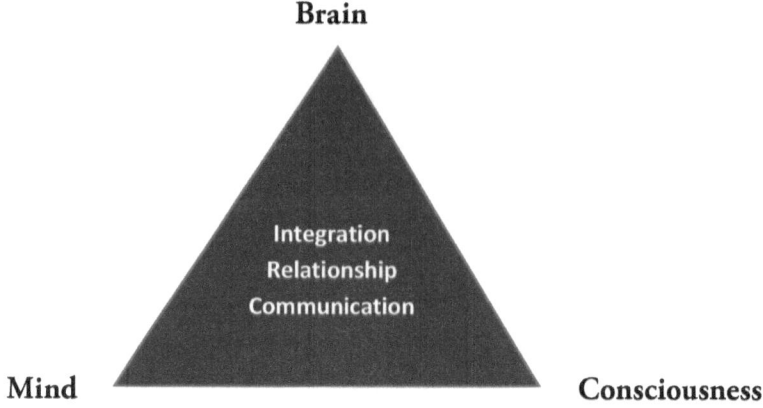

Brain

Integration
Relationship
Communication

Mind   Consciousness

Mind location is the integration between

This actually works well for the "location" of our mind and its connection to our brain—as the brain simply creates a physical structure from the outside. Could it be then possible our infinite mind is the process of a "higher energy" system? *That has no boundaries to physical activity, social or physical brain stimulation, brain, or our skull? This is somehow a complex system of self-regulated, self-organized, driven-energy-flow, information-processor, embedded, conscious, aware, embodied, relational, interpersonal, and interconnected as a whole. Wow, that sounds completely true to its nature and nurture of the brain-to-mind-consciousness system of our development.*

Based on what we have acknowledged, it can be the process of energy and information flow which is infinite. Therefore, the brain to mind is a self-organizer organ, which we call energy and information flow, which passes through our system and depends on a self-organized structure. Maybe that's why we have been told our mind has a mind of its own. Well, it can be true that our brain is a self-organizing system of development that has the all parts and functions to create and adopt what we pass through. By the same token, the all-natural energy system has the same habit. For example, the human body is not proficient in growing grass in the same way that our cosmos is not programmed to grow hair. Our body does need its nurture to the point we stimulate the growth for body hair, but the role of implementation has been there to its nature's course. As much as the impact of the sun and water, soil has its role in growing grass. The notion of earth for growing plants is a natural cosmic system. It's best to keep in mind to be open minded to reflect on our needs for classifying them to better understand them and let the self-organizing system to carry on with its job. To interfere with any nature course of development, we might end up interfering with their natural organization of development. This can be human development, consciousness, or cosmos to the universe.

Too often we are given the answer to remember rather than to solve. Well, this is one way to learn but not the only way. I generalized—in very simple manner about the brain parts and we learned enough about our brain structure. The importance of learning how humans can become aware of their whole brain-mind. Every one of us is unique to the history. Life began around 3.5 billion years ago. Human creatures first appeared about 650 million years ago. Life progression can be seen inside the human brain. Our modern-shaped human brains may have only come into existence about forty thousand years ago, based on many research. The rounder, bigger brain shapes that researcher's perspective when people started heading out of the cave, developing tools, language, and self-awareness. Does this mean our brain shrinks over time? What about our mind?

And *now based on scientists' experience*, they've pinpointed when they believe we grew into our modern skulls. Our modern cortex has great influence over the first brain that was shaped by evolutionary transformation to develop ever-improving abilities such as parenting, bonding, communicating, cooperating, and importantly loving one another. The human brain has been called the most complex object in the known universe, and in many ways it's the final frontier of science. It's fascinating, a hundred billion neurons, close to a quadrillion connection among them, and we don't still fully understand a single cell. To look even closer, it is made up of more than 100 billion nerves that communicate in trillions of connections called synapses. The integration of the whole functional brain defines the healthy brain. The cortex is divided into two hemispheres which are connected by the corpus callosum. As humans developed, the left hemisphere came to focus on sequence, linguistic, visual-spatial processes. The integration of two sides needed humans to have healthy functional abilities.

The brain is made up of many specialized areas; that is the art of this integration:

- The cortex is the outermost layer of brain cells. Thinking and giving movements begin here. For example, setting goals, actions, shapes emotions by guidance or inhibiting the limbic system (PFC). The anterior cingulate cortex (ACC) steadies attention and monitors plans and helps integrate thinking and feeling.
- The brain stem is between the spinal cord and the rest of the brain. Simple functions such as breathing and sleep are controlled by stem of the brain. The brain stem sends neuromodulators such as norepinephrine and dopamine throughout our brain in order to get us ready for action and keep us energized.
- The basal ganglia are a group of structures centrally located in the brain. The basal ganglia coordinate messages between multiple other brain areas. They are involved with rewards, stimulation seeking, and movement. Ganglia are massive tissues.
- The cerebellum is at the base and back of the brain, responsible for the function of coordination and balance.

Likewise,

- The insula senses the internal state of our body, including gut feelings and empathy experiences, located on the inside of the temporal lobes on each side of human head.
- The thalamus is the major relay station for sensory information.
- The corpus callosum passes information between the two hemispheres of the brain.
- The limbic system, central to emotional and motivational, includes the basal ganglia, hippocampus, amygdala, hypothalamus, and pituitary gland.

- The hippocampus, from new memories, detects threats.
- The amygdala responds to emotional changes.
- The hippocampus regulates and drives attention to being hungry or sex.
- The pituitary gland makes endorphins, triggers stress hormones, and stores and releases oxytocin.

The brain is also divided into several lobes:

- The frontal lobes are responsible for problem-solving and judgment and motor function.
- The parietal lobes manage sensation, handwriting, and body position.
- The temporal lobes are involved with memory and hearing.
- The occipital lobes contain the brain's visual processing system.

The brain is surrounded by a layer of tissue called the meninges. The skull (cranium) helps protect the brain from injury.

A Typical Neuron

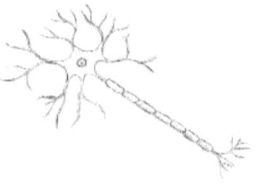

Discovering neurons might be the first step in the direction of brain education. What are neurons? The basic building blocks of human nervous system are neurons. They interconnect among each other via minor junctions termed *synapses*. In spite of numerous categories of neurons, their elementary design is similar. How neurons connect is through electrical impulses, though some cells give out spikes called dendrites which obtain neurotransmitters from other neurons. Neuron fire together, and they wire together. Neurons accept millisecond by millisecond all the excitatory and inhibitory indications and regulate somewhat to fire or not. If neurons fire, an electrochemical wave ripples down its axon. The fiber spreading near the neurons also directs signals. This activity issues neurotransmitters into its synapses with receiving neurons. Thus, the decision is either inhibiting them or exciting them to fire an exchange.

Nerve indicators are sped up by myelin which is a fatty matter that protects axons. There are three modules of neurons: afferent neurons, efferent neurons, and interneurons. The afferent neuron would carry sensory information, for instance, from hand to brain, letting it know the body is touching something hot. The brain would then produce this information and use efferent neurons to tell the arm muscle to contract and move the hand away. Afferent neurons are the ones that carry the information from tissues and organs into the central nervous system (CNS), while efferent neurons transport signals from the CNS to the effector cells. On the other hand, interneurons connect neurons within the CNS.

The gray matter of the human brain is composed largely of the cell's bodies of neurons. There is also a white matter which is made up of axons and glial cells. The gray matter includes regions of the brain involved in muscle control and sensory perception such as seeing and hearing, memory, emotions, speech, decision-making, and self-control. The gray matter experiences development and evolution through childhood and adolescence. New studies using cross-sectional neuroimaging have revealed that by around the age of eight, the volume of gray matter begins to decline. However, the density of gray matter appears to upsurge as a child develops into early adulthood. Males tend to exhibit gray matter of increased capacity but lower mass than that of females. Also, glial cells execute a metabolic support function like wrapping axons in myelin and recycling neurotransmitters. It's astonishing that neuronal cell bodies are like 100 billion on-off switches associated with the atonal wire–involved network inside the human head. Can neurons change? A recent study displays how neurons can be intensely changed from one category into another from within the brain and how neighboring neurons identify the reprogrammed cells as different and adapt by changing how they interconnect with them.

Neuroscientists held that the current work establishes that *synaptic networks* among neurons are not made aimlessly. The brain is much more sophisticated, and different neurons have habits to regulate the behavior of neighboring circuits in their own exclusive way to eventually change how much inhibition, for instance, they receive from their synaptic partners. The consequences are significant for discovering the guidelines by which neurons in the brain are strengthened in the first place. Nonetheless, they may also deliver a way to comprehend how to rewire the brain in the setting of a malfunctioning, pathological circuit. Furthermore, developed neurons never divide: that is their general rule. They do not undergo cell division. In most situations, neurons are manufactured by special types of stem cells.

A category of glial cells, named astrocytes, has also been understood to turn into neurons. In humans, neurogenesis mostly ceases throughout adulthood. Nevertheless, in two brain zones, the hippocampus and the olfactory bulb, there is indication for substantial numbers of new neurons. The brain is the central organ of the human *nervous* system and when combined with the spinal cord makes up the CNS To generally understand the brain is to understand the simple parts of the brain to begin with, such as it consists of the cerebrum, the brain stem, and the cerebellum. These three parts control most of the activities of the body, from processing, integrating, and coordinating the information that is received from the sense organs to making decisions.

In a simple manner, the brain obtains information through our five senses: sight, smell, touch, taste, and hearing. It accumulates the communications in a way that has meaning for us and can supply that information in our memory. The brain panels our thoughts, memory and speech, movement of the arms and legs, and the function of many organs within our body. As we mentioned, the CNS is collected of the brain and spinal cord. The *peripheral nervous system* is composed of spinal nerves that subdivide from the spinal cord and cranial nerves that branch from the brain.

Cerebrum

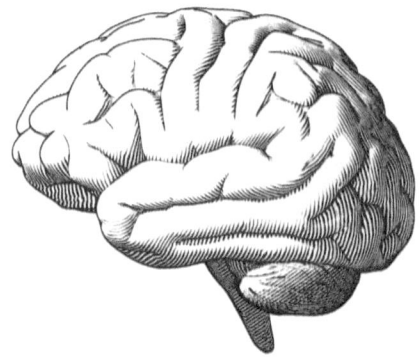

The brain is composed of the cerebrum, cerebellum, and brain stem. What is our cerebrum? The cerebrum is the largest part of the human brain. It is the major part of the brain and is composed of right and left hemispheres. It accomplishes advanced roles like interpreting touch, vision, and hearing, as well as speech, reasoning, emotions, learning, and fine control of movement. A deep groove has divided the cerebrum into nearly exactly similar left and right hemispheres. The cerebrum cortex is the outer part of the cerebrum that is made up of gray matter organized in layers. Underneath the cortex is the white matter of the brain. The neocortex is the major portion of the cerebral cortex.

The neocortex has six neuronal layers. The rest of the cortex is of allocortex, which has three or four layers. The hemispheres are connected by five commissures. The surface of the brain is doubled into edges and grooves. These parts got their name usually conferring to their location, for example, the frontal gyrus of the frontal lobe. Each hemisphere is predictably separated into four lobes, namely, frontal lobe, parietal lobe, temporal lobe, and occipital lobe. There is integration among each part of the human brain. Each lobe is associated with one or two particular functions, though there is another function that extends among them.

Cerebellum

The *cerebellum* is located under the cerebrum. Its function is to coordinate muscle movements, maintain posture, and maintain balance. The cerebellum part of the brain has three parts: an anterior lobe, a posterior lobe, and the flocculonodular lobe. The anterior and posterior lobes are associated in the middle by the vermis. Underneath between the two lobes is the third lobe that is called the flocculonodular lobe. The cerebellum is positioned at the back of the cranial cavity which is lying beneath the occipital lobes. This is disconnected by the cerebellar tantrum that is a sheet of fiber. The cerebellum is collected of an inner medulla of white matter and an outer cortex of gray matter.

The cerebellum's anterior and posterior lobes appear to play a character in the coordination and smoothing of complex motor movements. The flocculonodular lobe plays a role in the maintenance of balance. Any growth benign or malignant might affect the coordination or balance of human development to some degree. (I personally dealt with such benign growth for years. When education becomes one with personal experiences, it gives birth to pure knowledge. Another reason why I write books on brain education is my life experience.

The medial longitudinal fissure has divided the human cerebrum in two cerebral hemispheres: the right and the left hemispheres. The left side of the forebrain mostly represents the right side of the body, and the right side of the brain represents mostly the left side of the body. This contralateral organization includes both executive and sensory functions. They are merged by a bundle of fibers called the corpus callosum that transmits communications from one side to the other. Each hemisphere panels the opposite side of the body. If a stroke happens on the right side of the brain, the left arm or leg may be weak or paralyzed. Not all functions of the hemispheres are communal. Overall, the left hemisphere controls speech, comprehension, arithmetic, and writing. The right hemisphere controls creativity, spatial ability, artistry, and musical skills. The left hemisphere is central in hand use and language in about 92 percent of people. The cerebrum has gross and many subdivisions. As a result, it's important to acknowledge that this unit lists the purposes that the cerebrum as a whole serve since it is a major part of the brain and controls emotions, hearing, vision, personality, and much more.

The human motor function of the body gets its direction conscious wise or volitional via the cerebrum. The frontal lobe motor and motor cortex areas are responsible for the functions and plans. Our visual, auditory, gustatory, and olfactory information and somatosensory are the primary sensory areas of the cerebral cortex that receive and process. These brain districts synthesize sensory information into our perceptions of the world combined with connotation cortical areas. The olfactory bulb takes up a great area of the cerebrum in most vertebrates. The olfactory bulb is accountable for the sense of smell.

Neurons in the *olfactory* bulb direct their axons straight to the olfactory cortex. This system of olfactory sensory is exclusive as outcome. Any harm to the olfactory bulb results in a loss of olfaction, the sense of smell. Aside from our sense of smell, parts of the cerebral cortex are mainly attributed to speech and language. The motor portions of the language are attributed to Broca's area inside the frontal lobe, while speech sense of understanding is attributed to Wernicke's area which is located at the temporal-parietal lobe junction.

As we refined throughout the chapters integration of all brain parts needed so the brain function as a whole. Thus, these two regions are interconnected by a large white matter tract, the arcuate fasciculus. Any harm to *Broca's* area will result in expressive aphasia which is nonfluent aphasia, whereas damage to Wernicke's area of this part will result in receptive aphasia which is also called fluent aphasia. Let's take a break and look at our hippocampus and its responsibilities. Human explicit or factual (declarative) memory processors are attributed to the hippocampus and connected regions of the medial temporal lobe.

The importance of the integration of this part makes our memory, aside from the *basal ganglia* which involve implicit or procedural memory, such as complex motor behaviors. In addition, the interconnected areas of the cortex, especially the dorsolateral prefrontal cortex, as well as the hippocampus are involved in human short-term or working memory. What makes humans not the sum of being but whole is the interconnectedness of self (body, mind, soul) and the world around us.

Misinterpretation of one or another is the important part of education system to illuminate for development determinations. Let's look at the cerebrum regions of our brain development and its relevant resources of responsibility to the whole brain function. The cerebrum is a gross division with many subdivisions and also subregions. It is important to learn that this section lists the functions that the cerebrum as a whole serves. As we mentioned, this location, the cerebrum, is a major part of the brain that is controlling much more of our functions, such as our emotions, hearing, vision, and personality.

Frontal lobe

- Personality, behavior, emotions
- Judgment, planning, problem-solving
- Speech: speaking and writing (Broca's area)
- Body movement (motor strip)
- Intelligence, concentration, self-awareness

Parietal lobe

- Interprets language, words
- Sense of touch, pain, temperature (sensory strip)
- Interprets signals from vision, hearing, motor, sensory, and memory
- Spatial and visual perception

Occipital lobe

- Interprets vision (color, light, movement)

Temporal lobe

- Understanding language (Wernicke's area)
- Memory
- Hearing
- Sequencing and organization

Language

Overall, the left hemisphere of the brain is accountable for language and speech and is termed the *dominant* hemisphere. The right hemisphere acts a large part in understanding visual information and spatial handing out. In about one-third of individuals who are left-handed, speech function may be positioned on the right side of the brain. Left-handed individuals may need distinct testing to regulate if their speech center is on the left or right side prior to any surgery in that area. *Aphasia* is a disorder of language disturbing speech production, comprehension, reading, or writing, due to brain damage—most frequently from stroke or trauma. The category of aphasia rests on the brain area damaged.

Broca's area lies in the left frontal lobe. If this area is injured, one may have trouble moving the tongue or facial muscles to produce the sounds of speech. The individual can still read and comprehend spoken language but has struggle in speaking and writing (e.g., forming letters and words, doesn't write within lines)—named Broca's aphasia.

Wernicke's area lies in the left temporal lobe. Damage to this part causes Wernicke's aphasia. The person might speak in long sentences that have no meaning, add unnecessary words, and even make new words. They can make speech sounds; however, they have difficulty understanding speech and are consequently oblivious of their errors.

Cortex

The surface of the cerebrum is called the cortex. It has a folded presence with peaks and valleys. The cortex comprises 16 billion neurons (the cerebellum has 70 billion = 86 billion whole) that are prearranged in precise coatings. The nerve cell bodies color the cortex gray-brown that's how generous its name—gray matter. Underneath the cortex are extended nerve fibers (axons) that link brain parts to each other—called white matter. The folding of the cortex upsurges the brain's external area, permitting more neurons to suitable inside the skull and qualifying advanced functions. Each fold is named a gyrus, and each groove between folds is called a sulcus. There are names for the folds and grooves that help describe exact brain regions.

Deeper into Structures

Trails called white matter tracts attach areas of the cortex to each other. Communications can hand over from one gyrus to another, from one lobe to another, from one side of the brain to the other, and to structures deep in the brain.

Hypothalamus. This is positioned in the base of the third ventricle and is the principal regulator of the autonomic organization. It establishes a character in governing behaviors such as hunger, thirst, sleep, and sexual response. Likewise, it regulates body temperature, blood pressure, emotions, and secretion of hormones.

Pituitary gland. This sits in a small pocket of bone at the skull base named the sella turcica. The pituitary gland is associated with the hypothalamus of the brain by the pituitary stalk. Known as the master gland, it panels additional endocrine glands in the body. It conceals hormones that regulate sexual development, promote bone and muscle growth, and reply to pressure. The hormones of the pituitary gland aid in controlling the purposes of other endocrine glands. The pituitary gland has two parts: the anterior lobe and the posterior lobe, which have two very distinct occupations. Additionally, the hypothalamus directs signals to the pituitary to issue or inhibit pituitary hormone assembly. The pituitary gland is frequently called the master gland since its hormones regulate other portions of the endocrine organization, specifically the thyroid gland, adrenal glands, ovaries, and testes. However, the pituitary doesn't completely track the demonstration. The pituitary gland is only about one-third of an inch in diameter, which is about as large as a pea and situated at the base of the brain. Subsequently, their purposes are so tangled, it's no wonder that the hypothalamus and pituitary are situated close to each other. They're essentially associated with the pituitary stalk or, additionally theoretically, the infundibulum.

The pituitary glands are complete of the anterior lobe and posterior lobe. The anterior lobe provides and releases hormones. The posterior lobe does not produce hormones per se—this is done by nerve cells in the hypothalamus—yet it does issue them into the circulation.

Pineal gland. This is situated behind the third ventricle. It aids in controlling the body's inner clock and circadian rhythms by secreting melatonin. It has approximately part in sexual development. The pineal gland is a small pea-shaped gland in the brain. The purpose isn't completely unspoken. Researchers do distinguish that it provides and adjusts some hormones, like melatonin. Melatonin is greatest recognized for the character it acting in regulating sleep patterns. Sleep forms are also named circadian rhythms. The pineal gland likewise plays a character in the guideline of female hormone levels. This may disturb fertility and the menstrual cycle. This is because in part to the melatonin shaped and expelled by the pineal gland.

Thalamus. This assists as a relay position for nearly all information that arises and goes to the cortex. It is involved in pain sensation, attention, alertness, and memory. The thalamus is a small assembly inside the brain situated just directly above the brain stem among the cerebral cortex and the midbrain and has extensive nerve networks together. The main purpose of the thalamus is to communicate motor and sensory signals to the cerebral cortex. It also adjusts sleep, awareness, and wakefulness. The brain is composed of ventricles or fluid-filled spaces. The thalamus is the third ventricle. It is a part of the brain termed the diencephalon and is one of the major assemblies consequent from the diencephalon through embryonic development. The thalamus sits at the top of the brain stem close to the center of the brain, from where nerve fibers develop toward the cerebral cortex. The thalamus is divided into two prominent bulb-formed sizes of around 5.7 cm in length and situated symmetrically on separate sides of the third ventricle.

The *thalamus* is complete with blood *by four branches* of the posterior cerebral artery, specifically the polar artery, paramedian thalamic-subthalamic arteries, and thalamogeniculate arteries aside from the posterior choroidal arteries. Within the thalamus sit myelinated nerve fibers termed lamellae. This distinct the construction into specific parts. Dissimilar assemblies of neurons make up other parts such as the periventricular, the nucleus limitans, and the intralaminar elements collectively called the allothalamus. The allothalamus varies in construction from the main part of the thalamus called the isothalamus.

Basal ganglia. These comprise the caudate, putamen, and globus pallidus. These nuclei work with the cerebellum to coordinate fine motions, such as fingertip movements. The basal ganglia state to a group of subcortical nuclei inside the brain accountable principally for motor control, motor learning, executive functions, and emotional behaviors. Additionally, they perform a significant character in reward and reinforcement, addictive behaviors, and habit development. The basal ganglia are situated at the base of the forebrain (cerebrum). The basal ganglia are a cluster of subcortical nuclei profound to cerebral hemispheres. The major constituent of the basal ganglia is the quantity striatum that encompasses the caudate and lenticular nuclei, the subthalamic nucleus (STN), and the substantia nigra (SN). These constructions intricately synapse onto each other to endorse or provoke movement.

Divisions of the basal ganglia. The major subcortical brain assembly of the basal ganglia is the striatum with a capacity of roughly 10 cm. It is a heterogeneous construction that obtains afferents from several cortical and subcortical assemblies and developments to numerous basal ganglia nuclei. Inside the striatum, there are two key partitions: dorsal striatum (DS) which mainly intricate in regulator over conscious motor movements and executive purposes. This dorsal striatum (DS) entails the caudate nucleus and the putamen. This is a white matter. The nerve tract in the dorsal striatum splits the caudate nucleus and the putamen. Aside from this, the ventral striatum is accountable for limbic purposes of recompense and dislike. It comprises the nucleus accumbens and the olfactory tubercle, interior and exterior segments of globus pallidus, subthalamic nucleus (STN)—a lens-shaped cell cluster that makes up the major part of the subthalamus, and substantia nigra (SN), which is a long nucleus positioned in the midbrain yet measured functionally as part of the basal ganglia. This is due to its mutual networks with other brain stem nuclei. It contains two mechanisms, the pars compacta and the pars reticulata. These mechanisms have dissimilar associates and practice dissimilar neurotransmitters.

Limbic system. This is the center of human emotions, learning, and *memory.* Comprised in this organization are the cingulate gyri, hypothalamus, amygdala (emotional reactions), and hippocampus (memory). The limbic classification is the part of the brain involved in our behavioral and emotional responses, especially when it comes to behaviors we need for survival like feeding, reproduction, caring for our young, and fight-or-flight responses. The *structures of the limbic system* are hidden deep inside the brain, beneath the cerebral cortex and above the brain stem. The thalamus, hypothalamus, and basal ganglia are similarly elaborate in the movements of the limbic classification; yet two of the main assemblies are the hippocampus and the amygdala.

The hippocampus, similar to other assemblies in the brain, originates as a pair, one in each hemisphere. Connections completed in the hippocampus likewise aid individual subordinate memories with numerous senses. The hippocampus is also significant for spatial direction and the capability to circumnavigate the world. Moreover, the amygdala is a collection of cells near the base of the brain. There are two, one in each hemisphere or side of the brain. This is where emotions are given meaning, remembered, and attached to associations and responses to them (*emotional memories*). When individuals feel endangered and afraid, the amygdala automatically activates the fight-or-flight response by sending out signals to release stress hormones that prepare your body to fight or run away. As we explored within the book, this response is triggered by emotions like fear, anxiety, aggression, and anger.

Memory. This is a complex procedure as we explored throughout this book. A brief review of the memory is that it includes three phases: encoding (deciding what information is important), storing, and recalling. Different ranges of the brain are involved in different categories of memory. The brain has to pay attention and review in command for an occasion to move from short-term to long-term memory, called encoding.

Short-term memory. Correspondingly called working memory, it arises in the prefrontal cortex. It stores information for about one minute, and its volume is limited to about seven items. For instance, it allows you to dial a phone number someone just told you. It also interferes throughout reading, to remember the sentence a person has just read and, consequently, to make sure that the next paragraph sounds logical.

Long-term memory. This is processed in the hippocampus of the temporal lobe and is triggered when a person wants to memorize something for an extended time. This memory has limitless content and period scope. It encompasses individual memories as well as evidence and statistics.

Skill memory is administered in the cerebellum, which spreads information to the basal ganglia. It supplies instinctive learned memories like washing hands, riding a bicycle, or brushing teeth.

Ventricles and cerebrospinal fluid. The ventricles of the brain are a collaborating network of cavities filled with cerebrospinal fluid (CSF) and located within the brain parenchyma. Or the brain has hollow fluid-filled cavities named ventricles. Inside the ventricles is an assembly called the choroid plexus that makes clear colorless CSF. CSF streams within and around the brain and spinal cord to help cushion it from damage. This mixing fluid is continually being absorbed and refilled. There are two ventricles deep within the cerebral hemispheres called the lateral ventricles. The third ventricle attaches with the fourth ventricle through an extended thin tube termed the aqueduct of Sylvius. From the fourth ventricle, CSF flows into the subarachnoid space where it washes and cushions the brain. CSF is recycled by distinct constructions in the superior sagittal sinus called arachnoid villi. An equilibrium is upheld among the amount of CSF that is absorbed and the amount that is shaped. A disturbance in the organization can source a buildup of CSF, which can cause expansion of the ventricles (hydrocephalus) or source a collection of fluid in the spinal cord (syringomyelia).

Skull. The determination of the bony skull is to shield the brain from damage. The skull is shaped from eight bones that fuse together along suture lines. These bones embrace the frontal, parietal (two), temporal (two), sphenoid, occipital, and ethmoid. The face is molded from fourteen paired bones counting the maxilla, zygoma, nasal, palatine, lacrimal, inferior nasal conchae, mandible, and vomer. Furthermore, inside the skull are three distinct areas: anterior fossa, middle fossa, and posterior fossa.

Cranial nerves. The brain interconnects with the body through the spinal cord and twelve pairs of cranial nerves. *Although we achieved the term of interconnected brain, mind, body from deep acknowledgment within this book, the cranial nerves are another example of such networking.* Ten of the twelve pairs of cranial nerves that regulate hearing, eye movement, facial sensations, taste, swallowing, and movement of the face, neck, shoulder, and tongue muscles are instigated in the brain stem. The cranial nerves for smell and vision are invented in the cerebrum. The twelve cranial nerves, in order from I to XII are olfactory nerve, optic nerve, oculomotor nerve, trochlear nerve, trigeminal nerve, abducens nerve, facial nerve, vestibulocochlear nerve, glossopharyngeal nerve, vagus nerve, spinal accessory nerve, and hypoglossal nerve. The vagus nerve (X) has many branches and is responsible for tasks including heart rate, gastrointestinal peristalsis, sweating, and muscle movements in the mouth, including speech, and keeping the larynx open for breathing. Furthermore, cranial nerves are the nerves that arise straight from the brain (including the brain stem). By contrast, spinal nerves appear from segments of the spinal cord. Cranial nerves transmit information among the brain and parts of the body, principally to and from districts of the head and neck.

Cranial nerve anatomy and terminology. Spinal nerves arise consecutively from the spinal cord with the spinal nerve neighboring to the head (C1) developing in the space above the first cervical vertebra. The cranial nerves develop from the CNS above this level. Each cranial nerve has a pair and is present on both edges. The totaling of the cranial nerves is built on the direction in which they arise from the brain, front to back (brain stem). The terminal nerves, olfactory nerves (I), and optic nerves (II) emerge from the cerebrum or forebrain; and the residual ten pairs emerge from the brain stem that is the lower part of the brain. The cranial nerves are measured mechanisms of the peripheral nervous system. Nevertheless, on an organizational level, the olfactory, optic, and terminal nerves are more precisely measured parts of the CNS. The Roman numeral, name, and main function of the twelve cranial nerves are as follows:

Number	Name	Function
I	Olfactory Smell	
II	Optic Sight	
III	Oculomotor	moves eye, pupil
IV	Trochlear	moves eye
V	Trigeminal	face sensation
VI	Abducens	moves eye
VII	Facial	moves face, salivate
VIII	Vestibulocochlear	hearing, balance
IX	Glossopharyngeal	taste, swallow
X	Vagus	heart rate, digestion
XI	Accessory	moves head
XII	Hypoglossal	moves tongue

- The olfactory nerve (I): This contributes to the sense of smell; it is one of the few nerves that are proficient in revival.
- The optic nerve (II): This nerve carries graphic information from the retina of the eye to the brain.
- The oculomotor nerve (III): This panels greatest of the eye's movements, the constriction of the pupil, and upholds an open eyelid.
- The trochlear nerve (IV): This is a motor nerve that innervates the greater oblique muscle of the eye. This wheels rotational movement.
- The trigeminal nerve (V): This is accountable for sensation and motor function in the face and mouth.
- The abducens nerve (VI): This is a motor nerve that innervates the lateral rectus muscle of the eye. This panels lateral movement.

- The facial nerve (VII): This directs the muscles of facial expression and is involved in the conveyance of taste sensations from the anterior two-thirds of the tongue and oral cavity.
- The vestibulocochlear nerve (VIII): This is accountable for transmission of sound and equilibrium (balance) information from the inside ear to the brain.
- The glossopharyngeal nerve (IX): This nerve obtains sensory information from the tonsils, the pharynx, the middle ear, and the rest of the tongue.
- The vagus nerve (X): This is accountable for numerous responsibilities, including heart rate, gastrointestinal peristalsis, sweating, and muscle movements in the mouth, counting speech and keeping the larynx open for breathing.
- The spinal accessory (XI): This is a nerve that is responsible for specific muscles of the shoulder and neck.
- The hypoglossal nerve (XII): This is a nerve that is responsible for the tongue movements of speech, food manipulation, and swallowing.

Meninges. The meninges sits to the membranous coverings of the brain and spinal cord. Or the brain and spinal cord are enclosed by three coatings of matter called meninges, from the outermost layer inward. There are three layers of meninges: the dura mater, arachnoid mater, and pia mater. These coverings have two main purposes: deliver a helpful outline for the cerebral and cranial vasculature and substitute with cerebrospinal fluid to defend the CNS from mechanical injury.

Dura mater. The dura mater is divided into several septa. One of these, the flax cerebri, is a sickle-shaped barrier sitting between the two hemispheres of the brain. Additionally, the tentorium cerebelli offers a robust, membranous roof over the cerebellum. A third, the falx cerebelli, develops downward from the tentorium cerebelli between the two cerebellar hemispheres. Also, dura mater is a sturdy, thick membrane that carefully lines the inside of the skull. Its two layers, the periosteal and meningeal dura, are fused and distinct only to form venous sinuses.

Arachnoid mater. The arachnoid mater is named for its spiderweb-like appearance. It is a thin, transparent membrane surrounding the spinal cord like a slackly fitting sac. Another way of describing it is a slim, weblike membrane that shelters the whole brain. The spiderlike is made of flexible tissue. The space among the dura and arachnoid membranes is named the subdural space.

Pia mater. The pia mater is fastened by astrocyte procedures. It is positioned very near the brain surface and shelters all exterior surfaces of the CNS. The term "pia mater" resources tender matter. It is a collection of subtle connector tissues and has numerous small blood vessels. The pia mater is the solitary coating that grips firmly to the brain and follows all of its convolutions. Cerebral arteries and veins travel in the subarachnoid space, totally enclosed by pia mater. The pia mater also originates near the cerebral blood vessel divisions where they infiltrate the brain surface and ultimately grasp its internal assemblies. The pia mater embraces the external part of the brain subsequent its folds and grooves. The pia mater has numerous blood vessels that spread deep into the brain. The space among the arachnoid and pia is named the subarachnoid space.

Blood supply. Blood is passed to the brain by two paired arteries: internal carotid arteries and vertebral arteries. The internal carotid arteries source most of the cerebrum. The vertebral arteries stream the cerebellum, the brain stem, and the bottom of the cerebrum. After transitory through the skull, the right and left vertebral arteries connect together to form the basilar artery. The basilar artery and the internal carotid arteries interconnect with each other at the base of the brain named the circle of Willis. The communication among the internal carotid and vertebral-basilar organizations is a significant protection chin of the brain. If one of the main vessels becomes blocked, it is likely for collateral blood flow to come across the circle of Willis and prevent brain damage. The venous circulation of the brain is very diverse from that of the rest of the body. Typically, arteries and veins track together as they source and drain exact parts of the body. Nevertheless, this is not the circumstance in the brain. The main vein collectors are cohesive into the dura to form venous sinuses—not to be confused with the air sinuses in the face and nasal district. The venous sinuses gather the blood from the brain and permit it to the internal jugular veins. The greater and inferior sagittal sinuses drain the cerebrum; the cavernous sinuses drain the anterior skull base. All sinuses ultimately drain to the sigmoid sinuses that depart the skull and form the jugular veins. These two jugular veins are fundamentally the only drainage of the brain.

Cells of the brain. The brain is made up of two types of cells: nerve cells (neurons) and glial cells. Brain cells make up the functional tissue of the brain. The rest of the brain tissue is structural or connector (as another form of integration) termed the stroma which comprises blood vessels. The two key categories of cells in the brain are neurons, also known as nerve cells, and glial cells, also known as neuroglia.

Neurons are the emotional cells of the brain that regulate by collaborating with other neurons and interneurons in neural circuits and larger brain webs. The two key neuronal modules in the cerebral cortex are excitatory projection neurons and inhibitory interneurons. They are around 70–80 percent neurons and 20–30 percent inhibitory interneurons. Neurons are often assembled into a nucleus where they typically have roughly alike networks and functions. Nuclei are associated with other nuclei by traces.

Glia are the supporting cells of the neurons and have many roles not all of which are obviously understood. Glia is assembled into macroglia of astrocytes, ependymal cells, and oligodendrocytes, and much small microglia. Astrocytes are known to be accomplished of communication with neurons linking a signaling process similar to neurotransmission called gliotransmission.

Nerve cell. The neuron transports information through electrical and chemical indications. A neuron is made up of three basic parts: the cell body, or soma; the branching dendrites that receive signals from other neurons; and the axon, which sends signals out to surrounding neurons through the axon terminal. When a neuron fires an action potential, electric and chemical signals spread from the axon of one neuron to the dendrites of another neuron across a small gap called the synapse.

Glial cell. Like neurons, glia are significant cells of the nervous organizational system. Scientists used to think that glia were like glue, only for holding the neurons in place. The name *glia* is Latin for glue. Nevertheless, the glial cells are not just brain glue. In circumstance, glia actively contribute in brain signaling and are essential for the healthy function of neurons. Unlike neurons, glial cells cannot fire action potentials to communicate messages, but that does not mean they are inactive. Glia interconnect to each other and to neurons using chemical signals and can even respond to many of the same chemicals that neurons can, such as ions and neurotransmitters. This means that glia can overhear the neurons to help reinforce the communications that are passed among them. There are many types of glial cells in the brain. The three important glial cell types are as follows:

Oligodendrocytes—a superior type of glial cell recognized as an oligodendrocyte that wraps around the axons of neurons, creating what is recognized as the myelin sheath. Like insulation around an electrical wire, oligodendrocytes insulate the axon and help neurons pass electrical signals at incredible speed and over long distances.

Microglia—the brain's immune cells, protecting it from invaders and cleaning up debris. They also prune synapses. Microglia are the immune cells of the central nervous system. They move around within the brain and continually interconnect with other glia.

Astroglia—or astrocytes are the caretakers. They control the blood brain barrier, permitting nutrients and molecules to interrelate with neurons. They regulate homeostasis, neuronal defense and repair, and scar formation and also affect electrical impulses.

Astrocytes

Astrocytes are star-shaped cells that surround neurons and provide neuron functions. Astrocytes support neurons in signaling to other neurons by passing chemicals from one neuron to another. Though microglia are the main immune cells of the brain, astrocytes can also aid microglia when the brain is in distress.

Brain Stem

Our brain stem is the posterior part of our brain. The brain stem is joined and structurally continuous with our spinal cord. The brain stem lives beneath the cerebrum. Its three parts are midbrain, pons, and medulla oblongata. It is located in the back—the base (clivus) ends at the foramen magnum part of the skull. The brain stem demonstrates the great role of the nervous system. For example, ten of the twelve pairs of cranial nerves emerge straightly from the brain stem. The brain stem contains nuclei of many cranial and peripheral nerves. It is likewise involved in the regulation of numerous vital processes. For example, it plays a role in breathing, regulation of eye movements, and balance.

Almost all nerve tracts, which transmit information to and from the cerebral cortex to the rest of the body, travels through the brain stem. Also, the main motor and sensory supply to the neck and face is provided by the brain stem. Out of a human's twelve pairs of cranial nerves, ten are coming from the brain stem. The brain stem is an important part of the brain-body organization *(interconnectedness system of development)* since the nerve integration of the motor and sensory systems from the main part of the brain passes to the rest of the body via our brain stem. *This interconnectedness includes the corticospinal tract, the dorsal column-medial lemniscus pathway, and the spinothalamic tract. On the other hand, our brain stem has influence on our regulation of cardiac and respiratory function as well as regulates the central nervous system. Human sleeping cycle regulation and consciousness maintenance is another important role of the brain stem. Thus, to look at a few basic functions of the human brain stem, we may include heart rates, breathing, sleeping, and eating.*

We learned the three parts of our brain stem. The midbrain from the Greek point of view is a portion of the central nervous system. This is associated with our vision, hearing, motor control, sleeping and waking, arousal, and alertness aside from our temperature regulations. Midbrain is one part of which and has its own three parts. The midbrain's three parts are the tectum, tegmentum, and ventral tegmentum.

- *Tectum* means roof in Latin that forms as a roof or ceiling in a region of the brain, notably the dorsal part of the midbrain. The human tectum is accountable for auditory and visual reflexes.
- *Tegmentum* in Latin means covering and forms the floor of the midbrain in an overall area within the brain stem. It is situated between the ventricular organization and the distinctive basal or ventral structures at each level. The tegmentum is the position of numerous cranial nerve (CN) nuclei.
- The *ventral* tegmental zone is Latin for covering. The ventral tegmental position is in the midbrain among several other main fragments. Ventral is a collection of neurons situated adjacent to the midline on the floor of the midbrain.

The second part of brain stem is the pons. The human pons is positioned between the medulla oblongata and the midbrain. The pons transmits signals with its tracks from the cerebrum to the medulla to the cerebellum. The pons likewise coordinates events of the cerebellar hemispheres. The pons is responsible for carrying the sensory signals to the thalamus. The pons location houses the respiratory pneumotaxic center and apneustic. This makes up the pontine respiratory group in the respiratory center. The pons is placed in the brain stem and builds between the midbrain and the medulla oblongata and in front of the cerebellum. Moreover, the pons itself can be broadly divided into two parts: the basilar part, which is the ventral part of the pons, and the pontine tegmentum, which is the dorsal part. Since we learned about the pons's response to signals, it's significant to distinguish that pons comprises nuclei that relay signals from our forebrain to our cerebellum.

In addition, the nuclei are accountable for respiration, sleeping, swallowing, bladder control, tasting, facial expression, and sensation, including eye movements and postures. The third part of the brain stem is the medulla oblongata. The medulla location is in the brain stem's anterior and partially inferior to the cerebellum. It has the shape of a cone neuronal mass. The medulla's responsibility is for autonomic functions, for example, vomiting or sneezing. The medulla deals with the autonomic functions of our breathing, heart rate, and blood pressure.

This is because the medulla holds the cardiac, respiratory, vomiting, and vasomotor centers. How blood travels to the medulla is through a number of arteries. These arteries are as follows:

- Anterior spinal artery
- Posterior inferior cerebellar artery
- Direct branches of the vertebral artery

The medulla itself can be thought of as being in two parts:

- The upper open part
- The lower closed part

Brain Interconnectedness

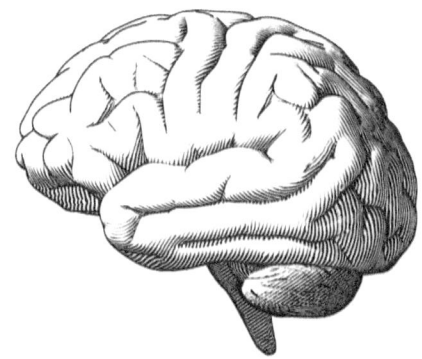

Doubt for a moment, we pause the story of nature and nurture and just accumulate the intelligence of a well-developed brain and its system; we will arise to accept the notion of interconnected brain, body, and mind on its own term. Each of our body systems is interconnected and reliant on each other. Our heart that is part of our circulatory system does not beat unless the brain, which is part of our nervous system, tells it to. The skeletal system is reliant on the digestive system for upsurge in size and strength. The muscular system requests breathing and cardiovascular organizations to source energy in the form of oxygen and nutrients. Consequently, its revenues altogether the arrangements for human growth and development.

Microanatomy means a department of anatomy dealing with the structure, composition, and function of tissues. Thus, what is the microanatomy of the human brain? To simplify it even further, the human brain is primarily composed of neurons, glial cells, neural stem cells, and blood vessels. Now the neuron types include interneurons, pyramidal cells including Betz cells, motor neurons, and cerebellar Purkinje cells. A human (adult) has a billion neurons and non-neuronal cells. Out of these neurons, 19 percent are located in the cerebral cortex. The other major estimate is 80 percent are located in the cerebellum.

The human brain is contained in and protected by the bones of the head called skull. The cerebrum is the largest part of the human brain. The adult human brain weighs on average about 1.2–1.4 kg (2.6–3.1 lb.) which is about 2 percent of the total body weight. Although women's brain might slightly be smaller than men, neurologically speaking, there are no differences between the sexes shown to correlate in any way with IQ or other cognitive performance. Also, it is vital to say that the size of the brain and a human's intelligence are not related. Studies tend to indicate a small to moderate relationship between brain volume and IQ.

From the great psychoanalyst Carl Jung toward the new century the understand of mind, brain, left more room to accept and grow further. Moreover, the idea of wholeness for humans depends on the aptitude to our own shadow. The medical definition of the brain (without mind or consciousness) might lie in understanding the brain in a scientific view. Such explanation might be that the brain is the portion of the central nervous system that is located within the skull. It functions as a primary receiver, organizer, and distributor of information for the body. It has a right half and a left half, each of which is called a hemisphere.

Years ago, the answer to one of the thorniest questions in evolution— how did *Homo sapiens* progress language, musical aptitude, and other exclusively human characters?—may at last be around. The answer may lie in an earliest brain construction thought to coordinate body movements, conferring to a brash theory on brain evolution that has expanded assistance from new research. The theory embraces that modern human progressed when extents of the cerebellum, the part of the brain just above the brain stem that controls movement, and frontal parts of the higher cortex are both prolonged.

At the time, elementary influences between them also extended, establishing an exceptional circuit. This prolonged circuit, which does not originate in other cardinals or vertebrates, may have been caused by a transformation in one or more genes that support the emerging brain. The fragment of the brain that stretches humans' motor dexterity is enflamed to give them mental skills. Studies using a new technique for tracing circuits in the primate brain initiate straight *nerve cell networks* between a part of the cerebellum that is recognized to have progressed comparatively recently and a part of the higher cortex that is intricate in memory. Motor regions lie externally in this circuit, secondary to the concept that the cerebellum does more than coordinate movements.

Some scientists contend that the cerebellum's solitary function is to regulate movement. It may perform a role in cognition. Nonetheless, it would encompass visualization movements to advance definite motor presentation or captivating actions that necessitate muscle movements. *Centuries ago*, from 1949, after conducting electroencephalographic copies with psychosomatic diseases had become influenced that the emotional components of these disorders were seated in deep brain structures that he termed the visceral brain (and renamed the limbic system in 1952), that involved the hippocampus, amygdala, and cingulate gyrus. Subsequently altogether mammal own variations of these structures, studies determined that they are phylogenetically ancient and that the emotional replies they produce are solitary diffusely regulated by such newer, human structure as the neocortex.

Human sentimental behavior endures to be conquered by a moderately crude and primitive organization. The goal of theories' reviews is to identify initial steps toward understanding current neuroscientific brain development findings in the framework of definitive developmental theories of cognitive development. Studies classify difficulties which arise when neuroimaging studies are considered without taking into account the prior conclusions from classic developmental theories. Astonishingly slight progress has been made in the direction of understanding in what way brain development affects mental growth through child development.

Research aims at the connecting and integrating current human neuroscientific brain maturation discoveries with the theoretical thinking of theorists in the behavioral institution of studying cognitive development. Developmental explore in the ground of internal regulator and self-regulation assists as a reference fact for understanding the relation between brain maturation and mental evolution. Education shows how a deeper appreciation of *structural and functional neural development can be gained from considering the traditional theoretical frameworks.* That arrange the typical improvement in developmental neuroscience that can trust more the knowledge from developmental experimental psychology.

Aside to that developmental reproductions of cognitive development this can be embarrassed and expressed with further accuracy on the foundation of knowledge of differential organizational and functional brain maturation. Developmental neuroimaging studies have had countless influences on thinking about developmental variations in behavior. Schoolbooks on cognitive development are now joining brain development as supplementary clarifications for developmental progresses in an extensive area of skills. Neuroscientists are speculating about how brain development results in deviations in cognitive function.

In spite of this common curiosity, the two research ranges (developmental psychology and neuroscience) might be still separated and an opening remainder between the knowledge of brain development and cognitive development. Could it be possible the developmental neuroimaging studies are inclined to be more data-determined slightly than theory-motivated? It is not uncommon that developmental changes in cognitive function are understood as the humble maturation of a single brain circuit, overlooking the long history of cognitive theorizing about the development of thought and behavior.

Similarly, it is not unusual that developmental changes in realms such as working memory are explained in terms of the typical stage of intelligent development though disregarding the significant improvements that have been made in relating these functions to brain maturation, which could oblige the present accessible developmental theories. Taken together, previous studies which have used working memory patterns have stated that the brain districts that are significant for these occupations in adults are differentially communicated in childhood and adolescence. However, the paradigms are frequently relatively humble and do not agree for a straight examination of deviations in storage capacity.

Like the dispensation of information in working memory, and the communication with competing information in working memory. Hence, a challenge for forthcoming research is to advance experimental paradigms constructed on developmental theory that tolerates for the exam of different neural development record.

Consequently, what theoretical framework can studies use to understand the neuroimaging discoveries? There is perhaps no theory available which aids this goal. Nonetheless, there are theories accessible which agree for a direct recording between cognitive theories and brain development paths. The practical development of the human brain might, for instance, be connected to developmental theories in a testable method using the neural maturation accounts put forward. This concept was developed to offer a biological framework for the development of early attention classifications.

According to studies, cognitive abilities arise through three possible directions of neuroanatomical development, namely, maturational development (the growth of other brain areas), collaborating specialization (changes in interactions among brain parts that were previously partly active), and skill learning (the outlines of activation of cortical areas change through the gaining of new skills). Nonetheless, this model was established to explain the perinatal and experience-dependent changes in the first two years of life. These routes of neuroanatomical development could likewise be used as an initial theme for reviewing additional progressive levels of cognitive development like working memory.

These maturation accounts can be interpreted in initiation patterns detected in ventrolateral PFC, dorsolateral PFC, and superior parietal cortex. For example, the additional enrolment of dorsolateral PFC in working memory manipulation studies could be understood in terms of the maturational account then similarly in relations of the collaborating specialization account. In distinction, the qualitative alterations in brain initiation among children and adults funding the skill of learning account. Even though all the three theoretical potentials can account for experiential changes in the brain activation that reasons in favor of the interactive specialization. Forthcoming studies can test whether this developmental route accounts for developmental information better than the maturational and skill education account.

The interconnected human biology not only refers to the connectedness of each individual to its body part, but to everything there is—from the interpersonal brain to the infinite mind and from self-identity to open-ended being. As we already clear our way to acknowledge, humans are still a work in progress This might be another answer or a definition to our development journey: an open-ended being. From the origin of life to human nature is a bundle of characteristics. Human development includes ways of thinking, feeling, and acting, which humans are said to have naturally. Our emotions such as primary emotions directly reflect the changes in states of mind (close relationship). It's through emotional experiences that we understood life's meaning. Emotions serve as meaning to information we attain, where that is how range of differentiated process become integrated (become aware).

The story of nature needs nurture is an essential part of the learning experience of this book journey. Therefore, the definition of brain continues—open-minded. Moreover, we learned how synaptic linkages are created by both genes and by experience. Interpersonal experiences form new connections among neurons by how genes are activated. In addition, we traveled to how proteins are produced and how interconnections are established within our neural networking system. The brain has self-regulatory circuits that may directly contribute to enhancing how the mind regulates the flow of its two important elements: energy and information. Despite being aware of our mind, many different definitions exist to what mind is. However, there are better results to today's approach of the mind that can be an embodied process. The responsibility of such is to maintain this flow of energy and information.

Furthermore, "information" that has a close relationship with where, why, how, when, and what serves the purpose of our knowledge and defining our "personal brain." This maintaining process might also be at the heart of our mental life. During brain development, the core processes (speed, spread, control) are the first manifestations of the systems. Hence, they are mainly action and perception bound. As we pointed out, the core relationships are integration systems. Thus, core processes are inferential traps within each of the systems that respond to informational structures with core specific interpretations that carry "value" or *meaning* to the human species. This operating system, its rules, and its processing skills are systems of human mental actions to which they are used to purposefully contract with "information and relations" in each level of the brain structures.

On the other hand, we initiate the importance of human genes which have been subject to recent selective sweeps, since humans perform an active, constructive role in codirecting their own development and evolution. Findings and experimental evidence often favor a general process, rather than a modular account, of cognition. The important feature of the scientific developing mind and integrated classification that ought to be exported to the rest of intellectual life is the search for explanations.

Hence, that is not to just say that history is one damn thing after another, that stuff happens, and there's nothing we can do to explain why, yet to relate phenomena to more basic or general phenomena and to try to explain those phenomena with still more basic phenomena, as we already cleared these findings. We have repeatedly seen what happened in the sciences, where, for instance, biological phenomena were explained in part at the level of molecules, which were explained by chemistry, which was explained by physics, and so on. There's no reason that this *process of explanation* and the birth of integration can't continue. The emphasis has been on the human brain and mind which studies have crammed nearly every related discipline: evolutionary biology, neuroscience, psychology, linguistics, and artificial intelligence.

Each research, from bottom to top and back to front, tells us there is a path leading through science, philosophy, history, and religion, that we people are physical objects. There is much to learn, to understand our *biological history*, brain, and conscious mind. So many philosophers have walked that path toward life itself, brain journey consciousness. Many authors described consciousness as something like the product of multiple, layered computer programs running on the hardware of the brain while readers felt that they had shown how the brain creates the soul. Others thought that they missed the point entirely.

To look back, we revealed that another definition is that organisms are open systems that maintain homeostasis, are composed of cells, have a life cycle, undergo metabolism, can grow, adapt to their environment, respond to stimuli, reproduce, and evolve. However, several other definitions have been proposed; and there are some borderline cases of life, such as viruses, etc.

The definition of life has long been a challenge for brain development, mind, consciousness to scientists and philosophers, with many varied definitions put forward. *This is partially because life is a process, our development, our experience, our mind, our time, our consciousness, not a substance. This continuous process versus the product definition.* It's clearly complicated by a lack of knowledge of the characteristics of living entities, if any, that may have developed outside of humans' planet—Earth. The philosophical definitions of life have also been put forward, with identical concerns on how to differentiate living things from the nonliving. The most current definitions in biology are illustrative. Life is considered a characteristic of something that preserves, reinforces its existence in the given environment, and exhibits most of the following traits.

Furthermore, looking into the *phenomenon of life* can be processed in several ways: first, life as it is known and studied on planet Earth; second, life imaginable in principle; and third, life by hypothesis, which might exist elsewhere in the universe. Would it make sense, if one thinks at present of the origin of the life, one might as well think of the *origin of matter*? Well, the two problems are in some fact curiously connected. As expected, modern astrophysicists do think about the origin of matter. In addition, we went deeper—to there is much evidence that is convincing to the point thermonuclear reactions, either in stellar interiors or in supernova explosions, give rise to all the chemical elements of the periodic table. This rise is more massive than hydrogen and helium.

Some thermonuclear reactions are more probable than others. With such review, we can conclude we are an "open-ended being" through which the universe is gazing at and exploring itself. In other words, humans are a vibrant part of what the whole universe is doing in the same way that rain is a function of what the whole storm is doing. Humans are an inextricable portion of the reality process. This may or may not have begun or ended with the big bang. We also consist of the same atoms as everything else. For this point, we are the universe, and definitely each of us is distinct from everything else. The idea of humans coming into this world might be vague. The idea that humans came out of it, as grass from the soil, is a better explanation maybe.

The *interconnected life, neurons, universe,* and each human are an expression of the whole realm of nature, a unique flow of the total universe. What the interpersonal brain is referring to is one's unique self-identity, which is separate from that of any other individual, develops through the process of energy-information scheme, *awareness,* and *education.* This is an ever-continuing system and can be measured as both a goal and a lifelong process of human development. The interpersonal brain upheld the same ground as individuation, as an important human lifelong goal.

Can it be a fact that civilization is the product of the cerebral cortex? The domain of intuition and critical analysis? Would our brain part be essential to our daily activities? The neocortex where humans have their ideas, inspirations, where we read and write, where we create music or solve mathematics. It is the distinction of the human species. Can it be this part of our brain is the seat of humanity? The neocortex is where matter is transformed into consciousness. After all, it consists more than two-thirds of the human brain mass. There is no doubt that we are our brain, and our brain is who we are. *When talking about the brain and its anatomy, where does the location of the mind come to place?* Philosophy of mind studies such concern as the problem of understanding consciousness and the mind-body problem.

From the past to the twenty-first century, still the relationship between the brain and the mind is a significant challenge. This is the challenge of philosophical and scientific points of view. This is due to difficulty in explaining how human mental activities like thoughts and emotions can be implemented by physical structures of the brain—such as neurons and synapses. Therefore, what might be a core aspect of the human mind? *The mind and its relational process are embodied, so it regulates the flow of energy and information.* Will go even deeper throughout this book. There have been doubts about the possibility of existing physical explanation of thought that drove most philosophers to dualism, when the mind comes into question.

Thus, philosophy of mind is a branch of philosophy that studies the nature of the mind. The mind-body understanding is a model issue in philosophy of mind. Contempt, other issues such as the hard problem of consciousness, and the nature of mental states, the human mind is challenged. The structures of the mind that are looked at include mental events, mental functions, mental properties, consciousness, the ontology of the mind, the nature of thought, and the relationship of the mind to the body.

From research to imaging, still the brain is not fully understood, and research is ongoing. We are living with the brain every day, and we are still puzzled by it every day. The idea of there being two or more selves in a single body sounds crazy. Most of our greatest philosophers and psychologists have recognized the essential multiplicity of the human mind. As we explored, from Plato's time, he saw the human psyche as a three-part affair consisting of self, spirit, and appetite. Furthermore, Freud in the twentieth century endured the idea of ego and superego models; the knowledge of horizontal splits between human consciousness and unconscious mind. And the notion of powerful entities within the unconscious mind. In parallel with this, neuroscientific investigation strongly suggests that there's no essential self to be found in the human brain.

The more we learn about this amazing organism, the more we see humans are bundles of learning and biological processes of responding in and out. Could it be possible if the mind contains a changeable conglomeration of the small mind—fixed reaction, talents, flexibility of thanking depending on consciousness functions as human needs? Can mindfulness play a role in operating such? Would it be better to change education of *attention* to education of *consciousness* and mindfulness? After all, being mindful means having control over your brain, and attention whereas needed. Neuroscientists with researchers from allied disciplines study how the human brain works.

Neuroscience research has expanded considerably in recent decades. Neuroscience has made accomplishments in several important ways to the forefront of both scientific and public interests. Several scientific accomplishments occurred such as the development of fMRI BOLD neural imaging; the discovery of neural plasticity, critical periods of neural development; the development of second-generation antidepressants and antipsychotics; the discovery of genetic mutations responsible for Huntington's disease and ALS; the discovery of neural origins and impacts of alcoholism; and physiological impacts on the brain of the children's early experience.

To go over the brain activity, we defined that the brain is reliant on possible interconnections of neurons that are associated together to reach their goals. Neurons are the collected of a cell body, axon, and dendrites.

What dendrites are often great number of branches that obtain information in the form of signals from the *axon terminals of other neurons.* Neurons join at synapses to form pathways and involvement neural networks. This activity among them is determined by the procedure of neurotransmission. Can it be true that the brain consumes up to 20 percent of the energy used by the human body, more than any other organ? In our blood, glucose is the primary source of the energy for cell and function for many tissues. Although the human brain makes up only 2 percent of the body weight, it receives 15 percent of the cardiac output. The brain mostly uses glucose for energy. If glucose is lacking, as can happen in hypoglycemia, it can result in loss of consciousness.

Let's bring our attention to neuroglia. Let's take a look at what this is or does. Neuroglia are also called glial cells or simply glia. They are non-neuronal cells in the central nervous system (brain and spinal cord) and also the peripheral nervous system. Their function is to preserve homeostasis, form myelin, and deliver provision and protection for our neurons. The few categories of glial cells are astrocytes, oligodendrocytes, ependymal cells, radial glial cells, and microglia. The largest glial cells are astrocytes. Our white blood cell is called mast. This cell interacts in the neuroimmune system in our brain.

Mast cell work is to maintain the blood-brain barrier, especially in the brain area where the barrier is absent. Mast cells in the central nervous system are present in a number of brain structures and in the meninges. Likewise, they provide neuroimmune responses in inflammatory conditions. Similarly, take a look at cerebrospinal fluids in our brain deeper. What is cerebrospinal fluid (CSF)? CSF is a clear, colorless body fluid found in our brain and spinal cord. How is this fluid found in our body? Cerebrospina is produced by the ependymal cells, which is in the choroid plexuses of the ventricles of the human brain. This is also absorbed in the arachnoid granulations. So why do we have the fluid anyway? CSF acts as a pillow for the brain for providing the basic mechanical and immunological protection for our brain and our skull. At hospitals, doctors take a sample of CSF via lumbar puncture to understand the intracranial pressure or to indicate diseases such as infections of the brain and surrounding meninges infections.

In addition to clear and colorless CSF, our body depends on blood circulation. Cerebral circulation is the movement of blood through its network arteries and our veins feeding the brain. It is the responsibility of arteries to deliver oxygenated blood, glucose, and nutrients to the brain. Then our veins carry deoxygenated blood back to our heart while removing the carbon dioxide. Aside from carbon dioxide, it removes lactic acid and different metabolic products too. Therefore, as part of an *interconnected structure, the human brain is depending on its blood supply like all other organs.* The cerebral circulatory system has many safeguards as a result. This is called the autoregulation of the blood vessels. Any failure of these safeguards can cause a stroke. How the brain relieves its blood supplies is normally divided into anterior and posterior segments. However, the two main pairs of arteries are internal carotid arteries and vertebral arteries. You might have heard about the blood-brain barrier before.

Subsequently, what do you think this means to you inside your brain-body? Well, the *blood-brain barrier* is highly tending to the semipermeable membrane barrier. What it does is it separates the circulating blood from the brain and extracellular fluid from the central nervous system. Our brain's largest arteries provide blood to the smaller capillaries. To keep our brain safety in mind, the smallest blood vessels in our brain are lined with cells joined by tight junctions. This prevents the fluids from seeping in or leaking out to the same amounts they do in other capillaries. This actually creates the blood-brain barrier.

As part of an interconnected organization, let's take a brief look at what part of our brain controls the *movement* of our muscles. The *motor system of the brain is accountable for the generation and control of our movement.* The generated movements travel from the brain via our nerves to the motor neurons in our body. This panels the movement of the muscles. Importantly, the corticospinal tract is responsible for carrying movement from the brain to the spinal cord, torso, and limbs. Cranial nerves are responsible for carrying movements related to eyes, mouth, and face. The motor cortex is responsible for our gross movement. This includes locomotives and movement of our arms and legs. This is divided into three parts: the primary motor cortex. This part is found in the prefrontal gyrus. This section is devoted to the movement of different body parts by support and regulation of two more areas, lying anterior to the primary motor cortex: premotor area and supplementary motor area. The motor cortical homunculus is accountable for our hands and mouth. This concerns he finer movement.

The motor cortex is similarly in control for our impulses. Impulses travel with the corticospinal region with the front of the medulla and cross over at the medullary pyramids. Subsequently, they travel down to the spinal cord, generally joining interneurons and in turn connecting to lower motor neurons inside the gray matter. Hereafter, they convey our impulse to move the muscles themselves. The cerebellum and basal ganglia of the brain are accountable for the fine, complex, as well as coordinating our muscle movement. Our muscle tone, our posture, and our movement initiate control from the connection between the cortex and basal ganglia.

To take a brief look at which part of the brain is essential for the *sensory abilities*, we should look at *cranial nerves* then. The human sensory nervous scheme is involved in the reception and dispensation of the sensory information. How it manages is the information is established first through the cranial nerves at that time through tracts in our spinal cord and directly at the center of the brain exposed to the blood. In addition, the brain similarly receives and interprets the information from our senses: vision, smell, hearing, and taste. Similarly, from the skin by touching permit information to the brain. The *skin* directs to the brain information about fine touch, pressure, pain, vibration, and temperature. The sensory cortex is positioned near the motor cortex and has ranges associated with our sensation from different body parts. On the other hand, *vision* is the aptitude to interpret our surroundings though using light in the visible spectrum that is replicated by the substances in the environment.

Consequently, the insight we obtain is called *visual perception, our sight, vision.* The sensory inducement of light into an electrical nerve indication is done by a photoreceptor in the retinas transduced. This is directed to the visual cortex in our occipital lobe. Each right side of the retina gives a visual to the left side of the retina. Human vision has much to do on how we distinguish ourselves and the environment around us. It's vital to recognize how we see things or what we see can convert the problem of our visual perception. What we see might not simply be a translation of retinal stimuli. What visual processing does to generate what is actually seen still has its problems. Now, what is going on with hearing or its aptitude aside of our other sense.

The human *hearing perception* is the ability to perceive sounds. This happens by sensing any vibrations, any changes in the pressure of the surroundings via our ears. Sound can be heard through any solid, liquid, or gaseous matter. Hearing is one of the traditional five senses. Our motion for balance is generated by the movement of a liquid inside our ears. Likewise, transmitted vibration is produced by the ossicles for sound. Hence, it produces a nerve signal which passes via auditory vestibular nerves and so on. The human sense of smell is generated by the receptor cell. This is located in the epithelium of the olfactory mucosa which is in the nasal cavity. How this information passes through our olfactory nerve is by comparatively permeable part of the skull, where this nerve directs to the neural circuitry of the olfactory bulb from where the information is approved to our olfactory cortex.

Our *taste* is produced by the *receptor* on the *tongue*. This passes to our facial and glossopharyngeal nerves then into our solitary tract in the brain stem. Well, if you are wondering what is olfaction, it is a chemoreception. This forms our sense of smell. It also has many other purposes, such as detecting hazards, pheromones, or food. Integration of other senses needs to form the sense of flavor.

This interconnectedness of our whole brain plays a superior role in human daily life. One dysfunction part leading another part of the brain undeveloped in some point, thus result as *misunderstanding of many disabilities*. Brain is accountable for "how we function daily."

The *autonomic functions* of the brain comprise the regulation. This correspondingly means rhythmic control of the heart rate and rate of breathing and maintaining homeostasis. What's *autonomic nervous*? The autonomic nervous organization is a division of the peripheral nervous system. The autonomic nervous system provides smooth muscle and glands, hence stimulating the regulation of the internal organs. This arrangement is a regulator system that normalizes our important daily bodily functions, such as heart rate, digestion, respiratory rate, pupillary response, urination, and sexual arousal.

The brain organ and its bodily parts are one network of organization, constructed on its own well-being, thus brain-body-interpersonal definition. The *vasomotor* center of our medulla is responsible for influencing our blood pressure and heart rate. This supports the cause of arteries and our veins to somehow constricted at rest. The *baroreceptors* in aortic bodies in the aortic arch generate information about blood pressure. This passes to the brain with the afferent fibers of the vagus nerve. Also, the *carotid sinus*, carotid bodies near our carotid artery, plays a big part in information about pressure changes that passes through our nerve, joining the glossopharyngeal nerve. Once this information travels to our solitary nucleus in the medulla, signals from here influence the vasomotor center to alert vein and artery constriction consequently.

The brain controls our *rate of breathing by respiratory* centers that are situated in the medulla and pons. It's hand-in-hand control and connection of brain to body function. Our respiratory center has three main respiratory assemblies: neurons, two in the medulla and one in the pons. The respiratory center panels the respiration. How? By constructing motor indications that are passed down the spinal cord with the phrenic nerve to the diaphragm and also with additional muscles of respiration. The human *spinal nerve* is a mixed nerve that conveys the signals of sensory, and autonomic among the body and spinal cords. Humans have four respiratory centers, the dorsal respiratory group in the medulla that sources the feeling of breath in and obtains the sensory information from the body.

By the same token, the *ventral respiratory* group influences with breathing out. The respiratory centers likewise sense blood carbon dioxide and pH. The pneumotaxic center in the pons influences the period of each of our breath and so on. The *hypothalamus* portion of the brain panels our body temperature, hunger, thirst, fatigue, and sleep. This district is in charge of significant features of parenting and attachment behaviors. The hypothalamus has more responsibility to guide certain metabolic processes as well as the autonomic nervous scheme. The hypothalamus has a larger purpose on combine and secretes certain neurohormones. As we went over it prior, this is known as releasing hormones or hypothalamic hormones. The hypothalamus is situated in a brain structure that has distinct nuclei and less anatomically distinct zones which are found in all our vertebrate nervous systems.

Let's turn out attention deeper into the *language function*. This function is carried out in the cerebral cortex. The wider network of cortical regions contributes to the language. It gives us significant understanding in our brain development.

The study of *neural mechanisms* that are responsible for our comprehension, languages, and production is called neurolinguistics.

This interdisciplinary area inducements its theories of practice from neuroscience, cognitive science, and neuropsychological points. The procedure of "how humans speak" is the way we communicate with each other. This *communication* is the skill of learning words and ideas and using our feelings. This is not just brain stimulation but our experience through the environment. That's how the brain forms and comprehends what language is. This ability distinguishes humans from other species. Despite daily use of conversations, very little is known about this, and there is huge a scope for research on it.

Language processing concerns the way humans use words to communicate ideas and feelings and how such communications are administered and understood. It is how the brain creates and understands language. Most recent theories reflect that this procedure is accepted out entirely by and inside the brain; however, environmental factors perform a role in the development of language dispensation. The function of this cortical area of the brain is symbolic representation, although we know the existence of different forms. There are many other parts to contribute toward language development, and there are two ranges that are considered more valuable for communication skills. These two areas are Wernicke's area and Broca's area. Both of these parts are located in the left side of the dominant hemisphere of our brain.

In addition, there are *nondominant hemisphere, cortical thickness, and prefrontal areas* of the cortex; and the communication between the hemispheres is a relevant contribution to our learning languages. Humans using their emotions has something to do with the responsibility of the amygdala, mid and anterior insula cortex, prefrontal cortex, and orbitofrontal cortex. Consequently, how we define our feelings has a two-step process, from combining evoke following by our feelings (psychological) and our expressions, autonomic responses—actions. There is evidence that shows the *basal ganglia* can contribute to happiness or perhaps our cingulate cortex activity production to sadness.

The human brain comprises a predefined instrument that is the foundation for the achievement of all languages. Correspondingly, the brain can be supposed as a kind of programmed engine ready to be constructed. This configuration originates from meetings with the perceived world through the senses and hence the corresponding language pattern procedures. The understanding of universal grammar is somehow equivalent to the nature of math and science and can be better understood through the following reasoning. It would seem that the derived classification of physics, geometry, and several other mathematical structures fit flawlessly into the authenticity of the inner workings of the world.

Furthermore, such perfect acceptable universal grammar is a phenomenon that few academics and philosophers, including *Albert Einstein*, find problematic to believe could merely be coincidence. Subsequently, all humans share the same basic brain structures which house the language aptitudes and that are the result of natural selection. Hence, there are profound resemblances among all languages, although they don't arise in the outline of grammar. As we went deep into the structure of the brain and its functions, there is no doubt the human brain contains the elementary structures required to absorb any language.

This innate cognitive structure could also explain why mathematics and logic are universally acknowledged and not culturally qualified. Language is an ability unique to humans and likewise shaped by evolution and instinct to explain the precise problem of communication between social gatherers. Language is more process over to its creation. It is the free creation from social gathering. Its laws, rules, grammars, and principles are fixed; yet the method in which the ideologies of generation are used is free and enormously diverse. Even the explanation and use of words encompass a procedure of free formation.

The best description one can give to language is it is an *organized intermediate of communication* whether it is a vocal or printed natural language, sign language, implicit language, or formal programming language. Languages are categorized by two basic foundations: syntax (grammatical rules) and semantics (meaning). In some languages, the meaning might differ reliant upon a third influence named context of usage. Reliant on limitations and difficulty present in the grammar, languages categorized a place in the hierarchy of formal languages. Alan Turing also had a contribution to language development; the formation of Turing machines can distinguish and resolve different kinds of problems and languages.

Languages describe problems. For instance, there is a language of all strings made up entirely of 1s—some members of this language would be "1," "111111," "111111111," etc. One could make a *Turing machine* to compute these strings. For example, write a program that just types the Turing machine, write a 1 each time it changes to the right and have it so the machine continuously transfers to the right. Another way of saying it is if a language is familiar, there are strings not in the language for which the Turing machine may not pause. The method in which the human brain produces grammatical-syntactic and lexical-semantic purposes has been widely discussed in neurolinguistics. The distinctness and selectivity of the illustration of syntactic-morphological possessions in the dominant frontal cortex and the representation of the lexical semantics in the temporo-parietal cortex have been investigated.

Furthermore, *the brain's aptitude to acclimatize to its environment explains* how we become focused to the sounds of our *innate tongue*. All infants are born with the capability to distinguish between the speech sounds of different languages yet ultimately become adjusted to the inputs they hear the most; neural traits conforming to native phonemes is wired, while those consistent to foreign sounds are trimmed. For bilinguals, this opening of "universal" sound processing stays open longer based on their experience to richer language environments. This means the inputs that the brain receives form how individuals experience the world around them. Just as exercise can change the body, so can mental activity, such as learning and using language, shape the physical constructions of the brain.

When *two neurons rejoin to a stimulus* (such as a word), they commence to form chemical and physical paths to each other, which are wired or deteriorated depending on how often they are co-activated. This procedure of neurons that fire together and wire together is the foundation for all learning and is reproduced in the development of gray matter and white matter. The bilingual brain is continuously equipped to procedure words from all known languages—increasing the number of alleged linguistic competitors. Over a period, bilinguals can become specialists at regulating these competitors, to the fact where the brain areas that monolingual trust on to determination within-language competition (e.g., the anterior cingulate cortex) display less initiation for bilinguals unless they need to manage competition across languages.

Throughout *the twentieth century, the foremost model for language processing* in the brain was the *Geschwin-Lichtheim-Wernicke* model. This is based principally on the analysis of brain-injured patients. However, due to developments in intracortical electrophysiological recordings of monkey and human brains, as well noninvasive systems such as fMRI, PET, MEG, and EEG, a dual auditory pathway has been discovered. In agreement with this standard, there are two pathways that attach the auditory cortex to the frontal lobe, each pathway secretarial for dissimilar linguistic parts. The *auditory ventral stream* trail is accountable for sound acknowledgment and is accordingly recognized as the auditory "what" pathway.

The *auditory dorsal stream* in both humans and nonhuman primates is accountable for sound *localization* and is hence identified as the auditory "where" pathway. In humans, this pathway is also accountable for speech production, speech replication, lip-reading, and phonological working memory and long-term memory. In harmony with the "from where to what" model of language evolution, the reason the ADS is considered with such a comprehensive choice of purposes is that each designates a different phase in language evolution. There is a moderately small study on the neurology of reading and writing.

Most of the studies achieved deal with reading rather than writing or spelling, and the common of both kinds emphasizes merely the English language. In terms of spelling, English words can be separated into three groups—regular, irregular, and novel words. Regular words are those in which there is a regular, one-to-one communication among graphemes and phonemes in spelling. Irregular words are those in which no such communication happens. Nonwords are those that display the predictable orthography of regular words but do not transmit meaning, such as nonce words and onomatopoeia.

A matter in the cognitive and neurological study of reading and spelling in English is whether a single-route or dual-route standard best defines how well-read speakers are able to read and write all three categories of English words conferring to recognized standards of orthographic precision. Single-route models suggest that lexical memory is used to supply all spellings of words for repossession in a single procedure. Dual-route models suggest that lexical memory is working to produce irregular and high-frequency regular words, while low-frequency regular words and nonwords are handled using a sublexical set of phonological instructions.

We understood the general purpose of the human brain—it's development. Knowing about the function of the major region of the brain can help us to focus our attention on ways that will create the desired linkage among them. For example, the brain is responsible for our *cognition*. Our brain is much involved in countless cognitive processes that constitute our cognition as a whole. How we control our behavior—selecting a best behavior, filtering information, setting goals, and so on—is part of the *cognition process* and executive functions.

How we hold information till we process them is the responsibility of working memory. Working memory is a cognitive system with limited space. It's important to know short-term memory is different from working memory. For instance, short-term memory can be used to recite to remember a phone number. This duration is believed to be in a few seconds. Moreover, our brain stem receives input from the body and sends back down again to regulate the basic process, for instance, the function of our heart and lungs and controlling the energy levels of our body via regulating heart rate and respiration.

Similarly, the *brain stem shapes* the energy levels of the brain areas above it, the limbic and cortical regions. The brain stem controls our states of arousal, predicting if we are full, hungry, or not; if we are relaxed or driven by sexual desire; or if we are sleeping or awake. Clusters of our neurons located in brain stem come to activate when certain conditions need mobilization of energy distribution throughout our body and brain. This is also known as fight to fight-freeze array of responses is accountable for our survival. Importantly the brain stem is a fundamental facet of our motivational system. This aids us in satisfying our basic needs for life, such as food, shelter, and safety.

Let's *remind ourselves* the importance of other parts of our brain and its *interconnectedness* to the whole. The limbic regions lie deep within the brain. This part works closely with the brain stem and the body proper to create not only our basic drives but also our emotions. The limbic region evaluates our *feelings* that give us understanding or meaning to our emotions. Since the limbic regions assist us in evaluating our *emotions*, this also directs us through *relationships*, and we become attached to one another.

In addition to our heart, we are head wired to connect with one another. The limbic regions support to generate several different forms of memory of particular experiences of our emotions that gave texture and color to that experience. This is located to either side of the central hypothalamus and pituitary. Two specific clusters of neurons have been intensively studied: the amygdala and the hippocampus. The amygdala is shaped like an almond, and this area might respond to fear and instantaneous survival awareness.

Sometimes we may act on our *experiences* that we build through our past emotions, and we act on it at any given moment without being aware of it. For instance, seeing a longer rope, you may scream away from it, feeling of a snack experience in the past saved in this region. In order for us to become more aware of our feelings inside our head and consciously attend and understand them, then we need to link these subcortically created emotional states to our cortex. My son, who is twelve years old, loves the idea of how our brain regions have shapes, allowing him to easily memorize them and link their functions. For instance, our hippocampus is shaped like a seahorse —cluster of neurons. And its name sounds like hippo. This region work is much interconnected *linkage together* the widely separated area of the brain— form our *perceptual* regions to our *repository* for fact to our *language* area.

I was drawn to the human brain since a young age, to its unforgiveness and to its caring. This three-pound ball of fat in nature it is power and it is mysteries, as much as it is weak. Just five minutes without oxygen, and it loses its function. Early astronomers' research has voyaged as far as to the heavens for many answers, but in the human brain, there resides enough mystery—potential to have content and explore Galileo.

Founded on research, the neocortex has the same number of neurons as a galaxy has stars: 100 billion.

If we look at the entire physical cosmos, the human brain is a tiny part of it. Nonetheless, isn't it the most perfect tiny organized part? It's important research for neuroscience, understanding human potential, because that is where *psychology meets biology*. Looking back as far as the 1800s, scientists steered several experiments meant to examine how people observe the world via their individual bodies (self-identity). It is reflective that we use our sensory organs—our eyes, and ears and nose—to take in and understand the world around us.

Interestingly, a person's *exclusive nervous system* develops over the course of their life cycle in a way that *resembles the evolution* of nervous systems in animals across vast periods. The human nervous system begins developing even before a person is born. It commences as a simple bundle of tissue that forms into a tube and outspreads along the head-to-tail plane, becoming the spinal cord and brain. Approximately, twenty-five days into its development, the embryo has a diverse spinal cord, hindbrain, midbrain, and forebrain. It has often been cited that the brain studies itself, that humans are uniquely capable of using the most sophisticated organ to comprehend the most sophisticated structure. Advances in the study of the brain and nervous system are among the most stimulating findings in all of psychology. In the future, research involving neural activity to multifaceted, actual world attitudes and behaviors will assist us to understand human *psychology* and better arbitrate in it to service society.

To settle, the brain is more in relationship *(how-to relationship)* with our body than its main connectors to our body. It's more *embodied (with all our organs)* over *enskulled (just inside the head)*, and it's *embedded (social networking)*. In addition, our brain is not just the brain activity of neuron firings or structure for maintaining our well-being; our brain is the soul integration of *social networking* for processing what are the rules in today's world. Each of us is accountable for our own activities based on our brain-to-mind development and understanding which plays as *cause* and *effect* to the world we live in.

This definition of mind-brain as natural integration as a whole, not sum, as individuals (self) is a best way to discover brain-to-mind and learning experiences which eventually leads to self-identity. With that said, we generally agreed that the mind is that which enables humans to have their *personalized awareness and intentionality* toward their environment, as well as to recognize and respond to operate and to have consciousness, including thinking and feeling. Overall, the mind is complex and rich. Our subjectivity, consciousness, and mental relations are not identical with brain activity. Thus, keep an *open mind (open-ended brain definition)* to these statements as we move along. Let's not discourage the findings of modern science but explore them deeper.

Chapter 3

The Development of the Mind

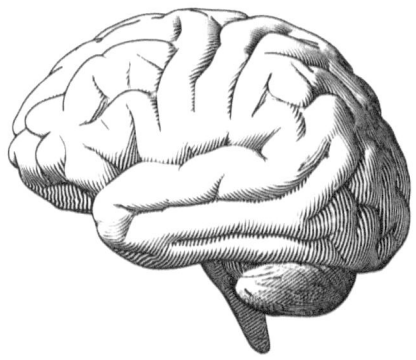

Mind and Brain Integration

The Physical Mind

Theory of mind is not a clearly definable concept. It remain less shining light, thus its continuum: on incipient self-awareness to full awareness, rudimentary theory of mind to full theory of mind and addition to or consciousness conjecture. Aside to theory of the mind and reality as well as denial in human working its place over many generations. With more intelligent social activities and education comes the experience of risks from denying the practical reality or anxiety resulting from awareness of morality, as well as, possibilities for suicidal thoughts, depression, PTSD, many mental health concerns, and pathological lying due to unusual combinations. Since humans are the final product in our evolutionary transition, creating the ability to balance the situation for breeding is necessary.

Looking at the brain cortex during the functional imaging of stimulation metallization can contribute to some point on human mental states to others. We cannot conclude this as seat of the theory of mind but might add intriguing that the prefrontal cortex is involved in the optimism bias, in which this region of the brain sends updated signals to the amygdala that is a deeper structure to fear response as addition to other responsibilities. We might be able to speculate rarely that coincidentally theory of mind and denial of reality emerged because they become physically integrated in the prefrontal cortex and amygdala during the evolutionary development of the human brain as one aspect of its definition. Mind over matter is one thing; mind over reality is another reason humans crossed the evolutionary psychological barrier of living knowing their mortality by mental abilities and denying reality. Although science and any other theories have contributed to developing mind, evolutionary development is still the past, which is the beginning of beginnings—has been the *continuum.*

Evolution would not consent an organ to burn much energy without usage. Therefore, the brain is continually active even during sleep. The brain is a buzzing hive of activities as a contributing system of development. This development journey has brought humans to many questions on how life or the universe emerged. How did consciousness begin? History might've proven track of times and human development to some degree. However, when it comes to *consciousness*, it might remain a mystery.

Consciousness is not some newly acquired potential to human and cosmic principles, but an indispensable working component of the living system—manner of function. For example, a simple communication of saying hello to you involves so many brain stimulations. However, who is it that knows my greeting? How do you know? Where's this knowledge of knowing coming from? What does knowing really mean to you? *It's then we search deeper into our brain, mind, and consciousness.* *We have defined the brain function to its parts, but where is the mind's location?* Can't be this notion of knowing is the essential part of the mind? Some use the term "mind" to refer to intellect, thoughts, reasoning, contrasting mind to heart, or emotions. Can't it be the mind—the whole subject—felt experience for just being alive? It's not this unaccompanied or that definition, but truly "everything" from our thoughts, emotions, intellect, relationships, experience, culture, belief, and connection *(neural network)* to others and the universe. *The mind also refers to our consciousness.* The experience of being aware of all there is and the felt sense of being alive. The experience of knowing within awareness. The true sense that does not see self but the witness to what self has seen.

From our learning journey, we have discovered being human is more than a brain; we won't be complete with body parts alone. *The self is not bound by skull nor skin.* In addition, the mind is neither a ephemeral entity nor brain functions. Can it be then the property of the neuronal system which is based on language in the conscious brain? If we look at language itself, it's clear that it is not a system of animal communication, but only human brain response. The system to which guides itself and makes its awareness reflective. Syntax is not the property of language, but it is arranged by the spatiotemporal of our real-life lesson that language is obliged to reflect.

Human language, unlike animals, is endorsed by devoted off-line neural circuits that are lateralized to the left side of our brain. Its output is located in endogamy, which is responsible for modifying the organism's behavior which contributes to decision-making of the brain. Damage to this circuit leads to impaired speeches. If we have to compare our language with animal communication, we would find that they are not on the same development continuum but are unique in their own kind. Separately, our human ability to process precepts via words brings us a cognitively balanced world of representations which, though distorted, empowers us to speak and think. Language is the implement of reflection and communication and disconnects the brain from having to respond in an online fashion, in addition to opening the door for it the world of the mind. For instance, the ability to name or call out the word "cat" and to draw our attention to it enables our brain to specify many things about the cat. Whose cat that is, the color, gender, place, etc., come to mind as forms of *thoughts* or sources of *experiences*. Evolution and human experience are an essential agency, almost a gift given in nature that creates new possibilities and phenomena.

The journey to the heart of being human on this planet starts with our mind. The mind is the essence of our fundamental nature. Some call this our essence, some core, spirit, or soul. The mind is a term that includes consciousness, perception, thinking, judgment, language, and memory. It is usually referred to as the term of an entity's thoughts and consciousness. The mind is aware of imagination, recognition, and appreciation and is responsible for processing feelings and emotions. I can say a changed mind is a changed brain. From the brain stimulation point of view, when neurons fire together, they wire together.

Our mind that creates new activities shapes our brain development. This is also a good learning skill to reach inside our brain to create more healthy experiences and happiness. The mind is designed to generate behavior that would have been adaptive in general, from our ancestors' environment. From evolution to natural selection, the mind works as an information processor to a goal-pursuing mechanism. Although each mental state and behavior has its own quality and personality to direct desire (self-identity/individuality), what really evolved was the mind.

The mind is not a single organ or single definition, but the *integration* of a much greater organization of organs which we can think of as psychological and mental modules. Humans have proven their intelligence via evolution, from culture to language, to biology, physics, water or fire, silence, and so on. As we explained earlier, the integration of brain to body and brain to mind, aside to the mind of others, we have discovered under the microscope the lairs of communication and the complexity of everyday world. Also, through history and research of neuroscientists, we can conclude all parts of the cerebral cortex look alike at some point to the brain of different animals. Can it be possible then that mental activities are same? As we learned, human language is unique to animal communication. Therefore, the birds migrate, the bees make honey, the ants farm, the spiders web, and the humans speak.

There are millions of other species in our earth with a different set of cognition programs. To understand the brain of humans or animals, it's not much hassle to distinguish between the parts. However, what makes the brain especial is how we see, think, feel, and act. This special thing of *the brain is not information receiving, but information processing. If we refer to information as bite or symbols, then we have discovered maybe matters or neurons in the brain.* They symbolize things in the world as they signal by these things that our organ perceives them. If the bite of matter that continues each time bumps to another bites that too continues symbol in just the right way these symbols would communicate to one new belief that will correspond to another symbol jolting into another and so on to new confidence that are rationally connected. As we read prior, from a young age, a simple experience (interpersonal experience) will lead to build a greater experience in adulthood.

The *computational theory* of mind agrees to have certainty and desire in our behavior as way of contributing them to the physical evolution process of our universe. *Evolutionary thinking can be a well funder to careful reverse engineering.* Almost none of human biological phenomena is accidental, but antecedents. In response to the integration scheme of the whole, a human small group from which we all descended, a rewiring of the brain took a place. This has been the contribution to our knowledge of complex thoughts, mental state, planning, interpretations, and so on—which are from our interpersonal experience and relationships.

The mind empowered by the motor writing of the speech areas where the brain gets its access to parts—itself that the off-line mechanisms of language were able to reach. This has been a success to humans over other species. It's the result of *integration of self-generated* experiences in our world that is accompanied by an awareness of activity self which is part of the experience and relationship of *development continuum (open-ended brain definition). What this integration means is the information-human experience cannot be inseparable from the original generation of the mind.*

The mind also is a source category for imagination. It is the product of the mind that has generated much inventories, science, medicine, and space discovery, which the insight is the essential information for this success and survival constitute of an evolutionary system of significant.

From Darwin's evolutionary psychology to revolution in evolution, biology explained much of mechanisms of thoughts, emotions in terms of information and computation. Biology endows humans with their five senses aside to drive of fear, hunger, intellect for learning; on the other hand, biological evolution has been teaching us through cultural evolution that differs from society to society. It brings balance between nature and nurture development. *Biology* is essential as culture is particularly part of human nature's behavior. *Evolution* was a great experience as part of our history to what is relevant to our development integration, not a soul answerable to human behavior, genes, or development—of course.

Human history has provided decent and bad evolution updates, since the human brain has the inclination for both. Hence, instead of generating wrong memory of past relationships, today, forming a logical understanding to what we can do to adapt a new experiences for new generations. We arrived to the scientific age aside to interpersonal journey. To value our understanding is to try to explain things, for instance, to explain human behavior is a complex interaction of integration between the genes, the brain, the science within blood circulation (biochemical), the nurture development (families to society), and the psychology of the individual due to nature and nurture. Likewise, review, revise, and resume are essential fragments of our brain stimulation to the accountability of the education scheme. It's much wiser to take what has been given from *interpersonal communication* and achievement of *subjective experience* and build on it. Keeping one thing in mind, science and ethic are different, but they are a self-contained system. Despite human freewill, the mind involves universal thinking. Therefore, the journey of this book has been free of any belief system.

Our mind is our *mental life* and a noisy parliament of competition and growing up. Attachment theory, patterns of relationships, and interpersonal communication have a much deeper structure to the brain and stimulation of neurons—adapt to explore and how to learn not just importantly till age five but for the long life ahead. Children defy their parents from the moment they were born to confound all life expectancy thereafter. Does this mean we are accountable for others (neural networking)? Do our activities and actions speak louder than we can predict (embedded neuron)? Would this make us not much of a bystander? We might be at least to some point. From then we learned how the mind is possible and how our mind today is a unique human development. One aspect of the mind is being the function of a system that contains information and energy flow. This information and energy flow is created by our attention that is an essential feature of the mind which has neuronal firing activities.

However, this system is not embodied alone and stretches beyond our skulls as we learned through the evolutionary process at some points. *The mind is within the body (skull-based), between ourselves, others, perhaps other entities, and the universe in which we live. Information and energy flow is generated by our daily attention. This energy and information is an essential part of our mind. This leads directly to the activation of our neuronal firings. Pay attention next time, where your attention goes, there your neuronal firing flows. As the outcome of this neuronal firings, our genes get stimulated and empower any of the neuroplastic changes needed to be originated. Recall this growth of our new neurons. Also such neuronal firing shaping the synapses, laying down of myelin and modification of epigenetic regulators. Consequently, it's easy to comprehend the mental procedures of energy and information flow forms the physical development and assets of the brain at the levels of its molecules and anatomical part. As a result, the mind can change the physical nature of the brain—both its function and its structures.*

This mind-brain experience has been an issue for generations. Can it be easier now to see the mind uses the brain structure, body (our organs), and our relationship between ourselves (personal experiences or subjective experiences) and between others (family friends, the universe, other entities, environment) to create a "self-organization" compound organization? Which this creates each moment to moment of are life, and shapes our experiences of the mind in now time. Well, it's obvious the brain stimulation cannot hide or secret the mind, as much as the breast tissues cannot deny milk production. If we look into the mind as a form of verb-information processor, we may find what this information transformation encompasses.

From the importance of integration of our whole brain to body, we comprehend each region integration of neuronal firing patterns converts our minute-to-minute experiences into our memories. For instance, in the hippocampus, this development takes place gradually during early years and continues to grow new connections and new neurons through adulthood. The more we grow to adulthood, this form of emotional and *perceptual memories* takes profiles into our *autobiography collections*. It will lay the *foundation* for our abilities to recall the story of the *snake we experienced*. Similarly, this ability (integration) depends on the development of the highest part of our brain, the cortex.

We exposed the location of our cortex: the outer layer or bark of our brain. This is also named new mammalian or neocortex. This is due to expending with appearance of primates and with emergence of human being. The more elaborate the frontal portion of the cortex, the more *conceptual experience* that gives us insight into our inner world. This region has intricate firing patterns that represent the three-dimensional world beyond the bodily functions. This *frontal region cortex* creates neuronal firing patterns that show its own representation. It's happening in a more *aware* way of thinking about things. For example, it *permits* us to take a *pause* to think what we should think, imagine, or distinguish between our face or experiences. As long as we determine how much to think, we will appreciate having this region as a form of our whole integration system.

The next time when start thinking, paying attention and how much attention is required is the best way to not be neurotic nor lost in the lobes of the cortex valley. Our cortex shows as folded complex hills and valleys. The *posterior cortex* is responsible for our *physical experience* through our *five senses*, keeping track of the location and movement of our physical body through touch-motion perception, for example, riding motorcycles or bicycles knowing that our senses moves within during turn or twist of the road or parking in small spots.

Moreover, distinct groups of neurons control our legs, arms, hands, fingers, and facial muscles. These neuronal groups extend to our spinal cord where they cross over so that we make our right-side muscles work by activating our left motor area. The same thing happens with our touch, which is located deeper in the brain in the area of the parietal lobe, somatosensory.

From the *integration* of our *development* and brain regions, we sense the physical world by our *premotor strip*. This region consents to plan our *motor actions*. This region enables us to interact with our *external* environment. Despite our physical movement and bodily survival and emotional function, we may explore more on the abstract and symbolic forms of information flow. The integration of information flows sets us humans apart from other species. The *prefrontal realm* is responsible for representation of concepts such as time, sense of being, and mortal judgment. *Meanwhile, we understood the interconnectedness of our region and its influence as a whole. When we put something in front of the mind, we are activating this region with other regions of our brain, for instance, our visual experience from our occipital lobe.* We also generate an image from our memories as we talk about the experience of the rope and snake.

The middle *frontal region* of the brain is an essential part of a healthy life. This is the important aspect of our development that regulates functions from shaping bodily processes to overseeing brain stem activities and creating *awareness* of thinking what we should think as well as moral judgment and empathies This region connectedness makes it possible to *create pathways to our social development with other brains in the world (embedded social network)*. Let's pathology wise look into the connected regions of the middle prefrontal region. This region creates links to separate and differentiate neuronal regions such as the cortex, the limbic areas, the brain stem inside the skull, and the nervous system within. In addition, it sends and receives signals from these parts and back from our *social environment*. The balance of such and such of this integration has made it clear for our whole brain to body functions. Consequently, what will go wrong when integration is off? Canwe function as the sum of our whole? Might be, but not fully. For example, when intelligent is in place, we think well as way of everything into our brain works for us to some degree. When one region is off, then we feel not ourselves to some point.

Losing our mind can be one example. Especially when mother of two or more children, lose patience sometimes. This might be due to children not cooperating or not eating right or homework concerns. How we deal with this has much to do with our mind riding the wave of our (mis)firing brain. This dysfunction of our brain activity can be due to any certain conditions, such as the limbic lava from the fiery emotional centers below our cortex, just beneath the middle prefrontal regions might have some concerns. This can lead to not eating or sleeping well.

Our middle frontal cortex is where to calm down our emotions. Reactive limbic and brain stem layers stop from being able to regulate all the energy fired up. Thus, the coordination and balance are disrupted. The middle cortex of the prefrontal region is responsible for coordinating the activity area of the nervous system that enables bodily functions like our heart rate, respiration, and digestive system. The two important parts of our nervous systems, the sympathetic and parasympathetic, are the main causes of our control and excel coordination to offer balance. Not only for our self-work but to be reasonable and attuned with others. *This emotional balance puts us at ease with self and others.*

This middle prefrontal region's function is to bring us back to clarity and focus inside out. It gives us that *awareness to pause* before we go to the extreme on our emotions or create action as a result. As we mentioned above, once we experienced the snake, we might fear anything that resembles the snake. However, the middle prefrontal region has direct connections down into the limbic area and makes it conceivable to inhibit the firing of the *fear-creating amygdala.* We can always overcome this by using our *cortex to calm down.* Also using our empathy will drive us to other human minds understanding the situation differently from their perspective in addition to our own inner mind. The integration of brain development is essential to what we do or say, as studies show that if the frontal cortex is damaged, we may become amoral. The frontal cortex guides us through our own stages of being.

It is the bigger interconnectedness of its own part to its function and our body inside out. This region receives information throughout the interior of the body, such as heart and intestines, to give us understanding of what to do or not. When we were a young child, our parent might have told us that our headache has nothing to do with our stomach pains. They have a way of separating these two organs as far as they may look. But they were good at *gut feeling* to some point, which makes sense now. Well, as much as we get our attention and activities from our brain, as much as we get overwhelmed by understanding this organ. More than one hundred billion interconnected neurons in such small closed space.

As we mentioned in the first chapter, *humans are complex beings. If we were too simple, we weren't figuring all these out.* Especially how complex we are is our average neurons have ten thousand concoctions linking them to other neurons. The brain is so complicated that we can't figure its own game. Our brain complexity gives us almost infinite choices for how our mind will use those firing patterns to itself. These patterns can be seen through images during brain scans. The scan shows simple blood flow to certain regions. Therefore, it shows clear when oxygen increases, and increased blood flow to given areas of the brain hints that neuron are firing there. Focusing our attention to past experiences or an important event impacts neuron firing. As we said, where our attention goes, there our neurons flow.

The next time you find yourself mad about something, you might know the blood flow increases to irritate the amygdala and less blood flow to the prefrontal. What is amazing is that the power to direct our attention is within us, to shape our brain firing patterns which shapes the architecture of our brain itself, especially when we learned the parts and patterns of our brain activity and development. Keep repeating our patterns and the physical properties of firing neurons will correlate with our subjective experiences. That is our mental health. This process goes hand in hand. Our day-to-day mental activity affects our neurons as much as our neuron firing has its own effects.

The connection between the brain and the mind is essential to our life journey. It's more like when we want to drive our car, we learn to drive it with our awareness of mind to do properly and with our coordinating and balancing brain stimulation. This is a good exercise for taxi drivers, *building specific locations of the brain* for remembering addresses and street signs. Knowing this, we can *simply focus our mind to build the specific muscles of the brain, by reinforcing brain-to-mind connections, establishing new circuits, and linking them together.* When we build our muscles, we try to flex them. However, when we try to build our brain, we use our *attention to stimulate the firing in the neuronal group.*

Our brain has no muscles. Its recognized clusters of neurons form different groups like nuclei, parts, areas, zones, regions, circuits, and hemispheres. The brain chemicals are another way to look at the brain health, communication, messengers, and its function. If we look into communication, we may study the neurons in our brains in a variety of ways. When we have an experience, for instance, our neurons become active. The long side of the neuron—the axon—has a flow of ions in and out of its encasing membrane which works similar to electrical belongings. To the end point of the axon, this electrical flow guides to the release of a chemical neurotransmitter. *This happens in the small space of the synaptic which joins our firing neurons to the near postsynaptic neurons. This action either activates or deactivates the neurons. If it's reasonably right, our neuronal firings can guide to build synaptic connections. Our brain is taking notes from our experiences as one way to know us well enough from the womb (self-identity and interpersonal brain definition). Consequently, if we generate a better rational condition for our neurons, then we focus our attention to our emotional arousal and our repetition. That's how we build synaptic linkages between neurons by experiences.*

If we think of the mind as the movement of information, this information is through our nervous system. On a physical level, these are all the electrical signals running back and forth. Similarly, most of this is happening below the conscious awareness. As a thought travels through the brain, neurons fire together in distinctive ways. This is based on the specific information being handled. In addition, those patterns of neural activity change the neural structure. *In addition, during early development, our brain becomes mature starting from the brain stem. Once we step in to the world, our limbic area is almost developed. However, the neurons of the cortex take the connection among themselves. As a result, they leave an open space to explore and experience, which is an important part of teaching and learning stages of development.*

The first year of growing up journey, the majority of proliferating of synapses develops. The connection that was missing between neurons builds itself through *genes* and its percentages and our experiences to some point. The reason I have mentioned this is our genes and the chances to percentages of development journey also determine along. For instance, personalities might be nonexperience things. This can be the influence of our genes to some degree. Having a laid-back personality or being shy or the opposite can be the work of genes before we were born.

We may blame our neuronal propensities for such development, or we may not. This is because our experience and relationship with the world inside out has its own role for development (the story of nature needs nurture). Thus, we may change our personalities as a result. According to this, if we were bitten by a snake at an early age, we may be frightened when we come across snakes, even if they might not be threatening to you. Perhaps any resemblance to the shape of a snake might bring the frightening experience to life. By the same token, with any positive experiences, you may feel the pleasure by seeing them.

Since we understood our coping abilities and our brain chemical combined with our experience, we can determine our abilities to change for the better. Self-directed experience is essential to learning and creating more neuronal firings. Our experience can influence the myelin (the fatty sheath around the axon) and neuronal stem cell. It's great to learn the capacity to change our brain much depends on our experience, and it's called neuroplasticity. Next time, be creative with your attention knowing these colorful thoughts will increase neuroplasticity that will stimulate to release neurochemicals, which eventually leads to building synaptic connections between our activated neurons.

Research has shown early *childhood experiences* change the long-term *regulation* of our *gene's mechanism inside our nuclei of neurons. This process is called epigenesis.* As a result, we might speak to our genes with every thought we create *(nature needs nurture).* The fast-growing field of epigenetic is showing that who we are is the *product* of the things that happen to our life journey. *The good news is genes are actually switched on or off depending on our life experiences. Our life doesn't alter the genes we were born with. What changes is our genetic activity. This means the hundreds of proteins, enzymes, and other chemicals that regulate our cells.* Can it be possible that only 5 percent of gene variations are thought to be the direct cause of health issues? Still, that leads to another 95 percent of our genes to connect to disorders acting as an influencer. This can be influenced by our life factors or other ways.

As much as we can form our physical appearance, for instance, if we desire to go with blond hair, genes cannot stop you to go ahead and color your hair blond. We can shape genes inside too. Our *biology doesn't* spell our *destiny* and can't control our genetic makeup. Instead, the genetic activity is largely influenced by daily thoughts, attitudes, and perceptions. We are coming back to our fullest understanding of interconnectedness or integration of our mind-body.

One best method is to think with an educated brain and a meditative mind. Meditation without prior knowledge of the brain's overall health is just as I described each (e.g., stages to regions and regulations) is almost like jumping out of a plane without a parachute. This practice puts us in contact with the source of the *mind-body system.*

As a result, we give our thoughts direct access to beneficial genetic activity which can also affect how well the cells function through the genetic activity inside the cells. Accordingly, we have educated the brain. When we focus our attention, then we create neural firing patterns which permit connection to the disconnected areas to integrate. Consequently, our synaptic connections build, our brain becomes integrated, and our mind understands adaptation. The brain is part of the visible, triangle world of the body. The mind is part of the invisible, transcendent world of thought, feeling, attitude, belief, and imagination triangle.

The brain organ *mostly integrates with the mind, consciousness,* and overall relationships that complete our well-being triangle of life journey. Let's pathologies this information into more exceptional relevant experience and through what science, theories, and our development have given us one step further. We mentioned about the physical aspect of the brain—its function, integration with bodily organs (heart, lungs, etc.). Let's see if we can locate the physical aspect of the mind. This brings us to the integration of its relationship and its location.

1. Mind between brain and its structural parts (embodied).
2. Mind between brain and body (our organs) function.
3. Mind between brain and our subject's experiences (our personal journey).
4. Mind between brain and our relationship (others, families, friends, cultures).
5. Mind between brain and our belief system and faith.
6. Mind between brain and our consciousness (awareness) system.

Brain

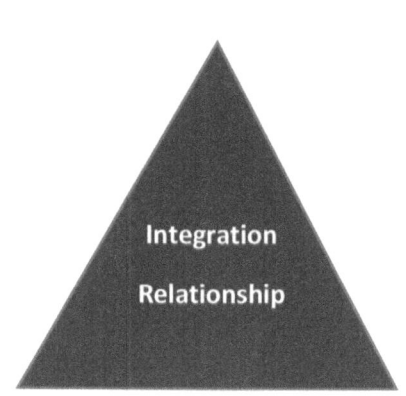

Consciousness Mind

The interconnected brain, mind, consciousness, and its location

The mind, our thoughts, and our feelings interrelate with the physical nervous system to stimulate how we reply to experiences through our lives (relationship). What we propose and pay consideration to guides and adjusts electrical and chemical signals so that physical variations can be perceived with scans that degree such activity, like blood flow in the brain (connectedness). Another way of saying this is the mind-body, or brain-body, connection is the link between a person's thoughts, feelings, and behavior and his or her physical symptoms. Find out the role that this connection plays in our overall development, for example, all physical symptoms have an emotional element.

The feeling of pain is physical, psychological, and emotional. The emotional cortex is the part of the brain which contracts with emotions, and this gets activated when the bodies face a tense state, regulating the fight, flight, or freeze response. The fight, flight, or freeze response causes the body to issue stress hormones, which can yield physical symptoms. *Furthermore, if we look deeper into mind and brain connection, we will conclude:*

1. Mind between brain and its structural parts (embodied)

The interconnectedness or integration means linking differentiated parts together so they work as a whole. We explored much the integration of the brain, and to some point in consciousness. Likewise, we learned our mental activities such as emotions, thoughts, inner subjective experiences of being alive, felt and embodied sense, and memories are directly shaped by our body's whole state. Especially, when we think or when our mental life taking place, changes appears in the circuits and synapses of the brain inside our head—aside throughout the whole body by the distributed nervous system (NS). For instance, we choose to write with our hand, but we comprehend with the brain-mind. We learned the mind is energy and information that is not just inside our head alone, but throughout our bodily system.

Our attention integrates with our neural firings, as opposed to where our attention goes where our energy flows. *Experience means neural firing.* When neurons fire together, then the genes located in their nuclei become active, which means the creation of new proteins *(relationship).* Thus, our mind changes our brain development to some point and affects our overall health. *The mind is a regulatory organization for the energy flow and information.* First, the mind observes information and energy flow. Second, the mind interprets the patterns and direction of the flow. Each of us has a different mind; our thoughts, feelings, memories, and attitudes are also a different set of regulatory patterns. The core aspect of mind develops in memory, attachment, emotions, our life narrative experiences *(interpersonal brain).* It's somehow clear that the physical nature of the brain is related to the subjective nature of the mind.

2. Mind between brain and body (our organs) function

It's vital to remember that the activity of what we call brain is not limited to our skull alone. Our heart nerves that process as complex information that is connected and relay to brain. Our energy is the capacity to carry out the activity such as movement of fingers to grab a pen and by the same token thinking of what we may write or read as our neural utilizes energy. *Anything we write or read is a form of information that is interpreted by the mind that gives us meaning (the importance of education on development).* For instance, when thirsty, the meaning of being thirsty is to drink water. The same if we can understand the meaning of hungry, pain, cramps, headache, stomachache, sadness, excitement, and so on has interconnected with our mind. This is how the mind creates information from the flow of energy and how this becomes motivation and effort of energy in a new manner.

Understanding this system of energy flow and information helps us understand mental experiences, which is essential to our subjective experience of life. Because we learned enough about the mind is a regulatory process that is monitoring and modifying information. In addition, the development of nerve cells throughout our body starts from the womb.

The cells that are formed as the outer layer of the embryo fold inward to become our spinal cord. From here, clusters of these cells start to gather at one end of our spinal cord to become the skull-encased brain.

Other neural tissues become woven with our skin, our heart, our lungs, and our intestines. Similarly, some of this neural extension creates parts of our autonomic nervous system. This permits us to keep our balance, whether we are awake or asleep. Other connections of sensory nerves come to us via five senses that permit us to perceive the physical world. The integration is a clear, not a complex, system between brain to mind and bodily system. Therefore, *it is the location of our mind.* Next time when you heard the phrase of get feel or a heartfelt story, you will draw the connections between.

3. Mind between brain and our subjective experiences (our personal journey)

As we stated above, experience means neural firing. When neurons fire together, then the genes located in their nuclei become active, which means the creation of new proteins. The brain shapes its structure with each experience that comes to mind from very early age. A subjective experience states to the emotional and cognitive influence of our experience as opposed to an objective experience which is the real event of the experience. While something objective is tangible and can be experienced by others, subjective experiences are *produced by the individual's mind.* While quite real to the person feeling a subjective experience and often thoughtful, it cannot be objectively measured by others, for example, if we are all having a subjective experience whenever we are experiencing pain.

While we as individuals can identify and feel the specific components of the pain, no one else can fully measure or feel our own subjective experience of our own pain (interpersonal). The possible reality that is, our mind is not merely brain activity but something more, something that is fully *embodied,* not just enskulled, and also something that is deeply *interpersonal.* This can be possibly our interior sense of meaning, our *interpersonal connections,* and our experience. As we looked in the brain structure, we understood *experience affects the formation of the connections (synapses) among neurons to establish pathways for the different hierarchies of brain function.* These pathways govern or control our intellectual, emotional, psychological, physiological, and physical responses to what we do every day. Hence, we find our mind between each layer of our subjective experience, from feelings to memories, events to places, family to friends or situations.

Experience-based brain (interpersonal experience and self-identity) and biological development in the early years differentiates neuron functions and establishes major neurological pathways. This can set trajectories that affect the capability, health, and well-being of individuals through the life cycle. The billions of neurons in the brain have the same genetic coding. Nevertheless, as the brain develops through *experience* in early life, neurons distinguish through precise gene initiation. In detail via brain structure, the development of the limbic hypothalamus pituitary adrenal (LHPA) pathway in early life has long-term effects on behavior and cognition. We used many expressive terms for behaviors that relate to the function of the LHPA frontal brain pathway, for example, attention-deficit hyperactivity disorder (ADHD).

And the story of Jack and his fellow classmates (environment affects). This seems to be a product of the communication between the environment and genetic susceptibility, besides between the LHPA and frontal brain pathways. Environmental factors that contribute to ADHD in susceptible persons comprise condition and delivery difficulties, prematurity, and a dysfunctional family atmosphere. Hereafter, being in relationship is not solitary fundamental to well-being and contentment yet is similar somewhat for which humans are wired neurologically. Outcomes from studies on the networks among the development of the brain and individual psychology exhibit that in addition to our neurological tendency for social connectedness and empathy, interpersonal relationships essentially touch the structure and functioning of the brain, which in turn influences a person's emotional, social, and *mental development.*

One of the foremost statistics in this area is that *relationships* are not just significant to us emotionally or *subjectively* but that *relationships influence the development of the mind* as outlined in the flow of energy and information. The definite assembly of the brain *(integrated brain-mind)* is set up to permit connection with each other. The mind truly develops not just from one's own brain *(embedded)*, the neurophysiological, but through connections with (relationship within relation) the brains of those with whom we are in relationship—mainly by our *early experience of relationship with parents.* That is, interpersonal communications profile the hereditarily planned maturational information that regulates the development of the nervous system (NS).

Early life experience contributes much to our interpersonal journey, yet there are five (teamwork, repair, coherent narrative, emotional communication, and reflective discussion) *interpersonal processes* which are serious in the optimal determining of brain development *(how relationship).* A person's experience of these interpersonal processes with each parent—one's early attachment experience—impacts all following relationships, counting our romantic relationships.

4. Mind between brain and our relationship (others, families, friends, environment cultures)

Everyday stimulus, from the social activities (family friends, culture) is capable of generating a response in the nervous system (NS). The impression behind "When I see it, I will believe it," is a term meaning we all have a "mind of our own." Despite we explored that, the brain to mind is a self-regularity and self-organized system, can we say "the mind has minds of its own"? What about the impression behind "make me care"? This means somewhat for which *humans are wired neurologically.* The input from other minds does add up to our daily activities (the *embodied minds and the minded bodies).*

Friendship infuses the human social landscape. These bonds are vital that disrupting them leads to health complications, and difficulties forming friendships appear in neuropsychiatric conditions, such as autism and depression. A neuroethological method smears behavioral, neurobiological, and molecular techniques to clarify friendship in relation to its underlying mechanisms, development, evolutionary origins, and biological purpose.

Recent studies associate a communal group of neural circuits and neuromodulatory pathways in the development, maintenance, and manipulation of friendships across humans and other animals. We maintain that understanding the neuroethology of friendship in humans and other animals carries us more rapidly to perceive deeply what it *means to be human*. From an early age (babies) to the older life cycle (elderly), *psychosocial embedding in interpersonal relationships* is central for survival *(neuronal networking)*. Inadequate social stimulation affects cognitive and memory performance, hormone homeostasis, brain gray/white matter connectivity and function, as well as resilience to physical and mental diseases.

Cognitive psychology has tried to understand the functioning of the mind through computational models, which provide an important basis for the study of this concept. Unlike behavioral currents and psychoanalysis, cognitive psychology relies on *mental processes* to study the *mind scientifically*. Hence, we can relocate the physicality of the mind in a person's set of *intellectual* or *mental* faculties. The human mind refers to the group of cognitive psychiatric processes that include functions like *perception (mindful of environment, family dynamic, friends, culture), memory (remembering, early age, evolution), reasoning (the understanding reason behind the energy and information flow)*, etc. Therefore, depending on how the neurons are activated and connected (integration of whole) to the different parts of the brain, our mental skills will be more or less efficient.

Our basic mental or cognitive skills are the basis of how the mind works. Throughout our lives, we continue to develop these skills according to *genetics and experiences* lived. *Neuroplasticity* makes it thinkable for the brain to adapt to the needs of the environment, which means it depends on how a person stimulates his or her cognitive skills. The mind also sometimes refers to the *conscious experience* of being in the world, the "first person" world of felt perceptions, urges, emotional reactions, and imagined wonderings (e.g., the pain of a pinprick or dreams of what might be). Third, the term "mind" also relates to what people are doing, ways of investing effort and attention (between self and others). Over a hundred million years ago, our ancestors passed on three fundamental approaches for survival.

Such as, the development of adapting separation. Physically and emotionally separation from mental state to between themselves. Likewise, with this adaptation comes constancy in order to balance, discovering opportunities to fight or to reject. The countryside of this development has been effective, although it might not be easy. For the contribution of development *journey the neuron network* evolved to generate pain, stress *experiences* within different conditions. The change of one circumstance can bring unfriendly experience. This condition happens as a natural way of *interconnectedness*. Furthermore, the human parietal lobes of the brain are located in the upper back of the head. This left lobe might be helpful for many to be distinct from the world, and the right lobe indicates where they *locate self in the environment (neural networks)*. That is where the thought of "I am different" (self-identity) comes to perform the character.

5. Mind between brain and our belief system and faith

The early experiences and daily situations can influence the way individuals *think* about self and others (embedded) and how to make sense of the world in your present life. These experiences are inclined to formulate the core of the belief system which is generally global and absolute in nature. From birth, parents, culture, and environments heavily influence our thinking (mind) and beliefs. It is the belief arrangement that *generates perception, emotions, values, habits*, and human *reactions* to *stimuli*. The first seven years of a child's life is the most crucial stage of development. Hence, in these years, the child's elementary foundation of perception is laid. After the age of seven, the *subconscious mind is reprogrammed by life experiences*. We gain knowledge from others, things we hear, we read, or any other external influences that we are exposed to *(nature that nurtures)*.

Beliefs tend to not occur in isolation; beliefs network with one another, affecting one another, and together form a system *(the interconnected being and world)*. Consequently, belief and human faith classifications get evolved; such information via experience flow occurs to each chapter of the mind as part of this development in command to confirm the endurance of human beings. Astonishingly, belief systems have the power to command the course of persons' lives. Such beliefs are advanced as a child and branch out into adulthood. As mentioned previously, the core of the belief system won't continue in isolation.

Hence, they tend to network and support each other. A change in one's belief/faith will distress the system as a whole (the interconnected system). If it is a core belief, a change potentially leads to the disruption of the arrangement. If a traditional belief changes, other fragments of the scheme will have to reposition in instruction to reconstruct the coherence of the organization.

It is scientifically demonstrated that when individuals change their perceptions, beliefs, and faith, they send entirely different communications to the cells and reprogram their expression. Individuals can reprogram the pessimistic cells to be more positive through implementing optimistic thinking performance like mindfulness and gratitude, for permanent results *(experience brain based and neuroplasticity).* Hereafter, if individuals try to change the circumstances and improve the situation, they must modify the current perception of reality by changing the belief system (changing mind is changed brain and heart, so to speak).

Beliefs are fundamentally the administrative principles in life that deliver route and meaning in life. Beliefs are the preset, prearranged screens to our *perceptions* of the world (external and internal). *Beliefs are like interior guidelines to the brain* on how to characterize what is happening, when a person correspondingly believes something to be accurate. In the absence of beliefs or helplessness (faith or hope) to tap into them, individuals feel disempowered. Thus, the foundations of beliefs include environment, events, knowledge, past experiences, and visualization (it is a mindset).

Beliefs are not just mental premises but are intertwined with emotions (conscious or unconscious). Research findings have frequently keen out that the *emotional brain* is no longer limited to the traditional areas of the hippocampus, amygdala, and hypothalamus. The sensory contributions individuals obtain from the environment experience a filtering procedure as they travel across one or more synapses, eventually accomplishing the extent of higher dispensation, like the frontal lobes. There, the *sensory information* arrives to conscious awareness. The minds to capture inner and outer *perceptions have higher brain abilities.* For this reason, the question that arises in this context might be does the integration and acceptance of these perceptions consequence in the formation of beliefs? Is the institution of such beliefs contingent on proof demonstrations? The proofs might be the perceptions, which we can directly see, or having a scientific proof or tradition or faith. Beliefs are established as stimuli customary as reliable evidence and deposited in the *memory.* These perceptions are comprehensive and recognized into belief. Accordingly, they impact the cognitive and emotional valuation, addictiveness, rejoinders to false positives, and determined ordinary defensive responses which the whole brain function is obligated in steadying the belief and in returning to the environmental organization.

6. Mind between brain and our consciousness (subconscious) system

The mind is made up of two parts: the conscious mind and the subconscious mind. It has been originated that the subconscious mind is 95 percent accountable in the way that a person responds to the external environment, from which the five senses obtain the stimuli. Our conscious mind, which is the seat of the rational regulator, has only a 5 percent character in dispensing the stimuli and determining how to respond. This subconscious mind is formed by individual beliefs increased through the life cycle.

Consciousness is the awareness of the self in space and time. It can be distinct as human awareness of both internal and external stimuli. Researchers that study states of human consciousness and modifications in perception in command to comprehend how the body works to produce conscious awareness. Consciousness differs in both arousal and content, and there are two types of conscious experience: the phenomenal, or in the moment, and access, which recalls experiences from memory. There are many studies on the definition of consciousness.

For example, developmental psychologists assess consciousness not as a single entity, but as a *developmental procedure* with probable advanced *stages of cognitive (mind between brain and consciousness)*, moral, and spiritual quality. Social psychologists cite consciousness as a product of a cultural stimulus having less to do with the individual.

Neuropsychologists' interpretation of consciousness is *as ingrained in neural systems and organic brain structures* (interconnected mind, brain, consciousness network). Cognitive psychologists base their consideration of consciousness on computer science. Sigmund Freud separated human consciousness into three levels of awareness: the *conscious, preconscious,* and *unconscious.* Carl Jung viewed that a human being is inwardly whole but that most people have lost touch with the important parts of themselves (self-identity, self-awareness). The determination of life is individuation (self-identity), which is *the process of* integrating *the conscious with the unconscious, synergizing the many components of the psyche (integration as a whole).* It has been argued that consciousness is influenced by other parts of the mind.

These include unconsciousness as a personal habit, being unaware, and intuition. Phenomena related to semiconsciousness include awakening, implicit memory, subliminal messages, trances, hypnagogia, and hypnosis. While sleeping, sleepwalking, dreaming, delirium, and comas may signal the presence of unconscious processes, these processes are seen as symptoms rather than the unconscious mind itself. Carl Jung's view on the collective unconscious is common to all human beings and is responsible for a number of deep-seated beliefs and instincts, such as spirituality and sexual behavior. Sometimes referred to as the objective psyche, it raises the idea that a segment of the deepest unconscious mind is genetically inherited and is not shaped by personal experience.

The unconscious mind (or the unconscious) consists of the processes in the mind which occur automatically and are not available to introspection and include thought processes, memories, interests, and motivations. Many neuroscientists have pointed out that brain cells fire away almost as much in some states of *unconsciousness,* meaning deep sleep as they do in the wakeful *conscious state* (brain-conscious networking). *In some parts of the brain, can identify neurons associated with conscious experience*, while other neurons don't seem to have any effect on it. There are also cases of a very low level of brain activity. For example, during some near-death experiences and comas, when consciousness may not only continue, but even become more intense.

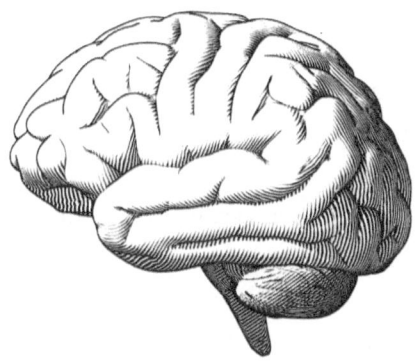

The Developing Mind

The brain is the dominant processing component of the body (embodied) and plays a significant character in interpreting the content of the mind (thoughts, feelings, attitudes, beliefs, memories, imagination) into multifaceted outlines of nerve cell firing and chemical release. Such multifaceted patterns of nerve cell firing and chemical release are called neurosignatures. Hence, they confidentially affect the physiology and biochemistry of the human body. Theory of mind (ToM) is a widespread phase from the ground of psychology as a valuation of an individual human's gradation of capacity for empathy and consideration of others. ToM is one of the forms of behavior that is characteristically displayed through the minds of mutually neurotypical and atypical individuals.

Meaning, that being the ability to attribute—to another or oneself—mental conditions like beliefs, intents, desires, emotions, and knowledge. ToM as an individual competence is the knowledge that others have beliefs, desires, intentions, and perspectives that are diverse from one's own (self-identity and interpersonal mind-brain). Holding a practical ToM is measured vital for success in a person's everyday social communications and is used when inferring others' behaviors. Deficits can occur in persons with autism spectrum illnesses, genetic-based eating condition, schizophrenia, and ADHD. ToM is a concept to that extent as the output like thoughts and feelings of the mind is the individual thing being straight observed. Thus, the presence of a mind is contingent. The belief that "others have a mind" is termed ToM since each individual can only perceive the presence of "their own mind" through contemplation.

Hence, no one has direct access to the mind of another, so its reality and how it works can only be conditional from the explanations of others. It is characteristically presumed that others have minds corresponding to one's own; and this statement is founded on the mutual, social communication, as observed in joint attention, functional use of language, and being mindful of others' emotions. Some Theory of mind ToM agrees one to trait thoughts, desires, and intentions to others, to forecast and explain their actions and to suggest their purposes. As formerly distinct, it empowers one to comprehend that mental states can be the source of—and consequently be used to explain and predict—the behavior of others (mind within—with others). Being able to trait mental conditions to others and thinking of them as grounds of behavior recommends, in part, that one must be able to perceive the mind as an originator of representations. If an individual does not have a comprehensive ToM, it may be a mark of cognitive or developmental weakening.

ToM seems to be an inborn potential capability (nature and nurture) in individuals that necessitates social and other experiences over several years for its full development. Furthermore, into the interconnected organization of the whole, a topic of mutual attention to psychologists and academics is the spontaneous flow of thoughts (energy, information flow) when the individual is awake yet not elaborate in cognitive demands. Such dispute, characteristically raised question as the notion of consciousness which is known in the psychological literature as mind-wandering. A natural and self-governing flow of thoughts and feelings arises (the flow of energy and any information given at that moment) when individuals are conscious (aware, mindful), but not intricate in cognitive demands; such term is "mind-wandering" (MW).

The rising position of cognitive neuroscience and the growing use of its brain imaging approaches have permitted the observation of the brain networks underlying MW. In fact, using PET images and fMRI, it was discovered that resting brain activity (MW) involves many areas in the medial prefrontal cortex, the posterior cingulate cortex, and the inferior parietal lobule. Furthermore, it was suggested that the hippocampal formation played a character even if its participation endured debatable. The default mode network (DMN) is connected to the incidence of MW or task-unrelated thought. In distinction, the frontal-parietal network (FPN) and visual network (VS) are intricate in responsibilities with external stimuli. However, it is not clear how these practical network communications fund these two different procedures—MW and on-task—particularly with respect to individual differences in the MW experience.

Moreover, MW was escorted by a large number of transitional nodes, which expressed a multiplicity of brain districts. Interestingly, the purposeful connectivity of the FPN and VS is strongly associated with individual behavioral presentation, thus the individual dissimilarity of MW, which infers the importance of other complementary large-scale brain networks. Over the past eras, the psychological and neuropsychological narrative has steadily confirmed that ToM classically advances during the preschool and school-age period and that it experiences continuous changes across the life span. In specific, this capability, which is very significant for social features of life, undergoes important changes both on the behavioral and on the neural level in effective and ineffective neurocognitive aging. As such information respects the most current indications concerning the neural foundation of MW, a metalogical evaluation. Such information concentrating on the initiation of the DMN alone may be overly reductive for a comprehensive explanation of the neural basis of spontaneous thought. In detail, studies acknowledged numerous areas, among which those that characteristically fit in to the DMN (such as the medial prefrontal cortex / anterior cingulate cortex) and a sequence of regions outside the DMN (like the secondary somatosensory cortex and the insula).

Consequently, in the present study, researchers investigate the neural basis of MW following as a whole-brain approach (i.e., looking also at parts beyond just the DMN). What draws the line between MW or mindfulness is the interconnected system of a whole. A remarkable feature of the human cognitive organization is its capability to arrange itself (self-organized and self-regulated) for the performance of precise responsibilities through suitable alterations in perceptual range, response biasing, and the online preservation of appropriate information. Hence, the procedures behind such flexibility, raised to *communally as cognitive control.* Cognitive control procedures are frequently assembled into *controlled* and *automatic.* Controlled processes are comparatively gentler and are employed consciously. Automatic processes are fairly rapid and are drafted subconsciously.

Characteristically, controlled procedures depend on *working memory* and automatic procedures straight admission *long-term memory* without connecting working memory. Frequently, in the development of learning in a new mission, students start out trusting on controlled processes and with time and repetition depend more on automatic processes. While controlled and automatic developments are often contrasted with each other, they can occur in corresponding and accompaniment of each other. In medical education, these processes are often referred to as *types* or systems 1 and 2. Type 1 reproduces the automatic, default, but powerful mode of processing that attracts a generation of experiences in long-term memory. Type 2 reproduces the grouping of resource-intensive, executive purposes including working memory and attention. A common misapprehension is that one procedure or system is better matched to comprehensive responsibilities than the other. The *prefrontal cortex* (PFC) has been documented as one of the greatest vital brain districts accountable for cognitive control, thoughts, and actions. Progressive practical imaging has provided tools needed for the delicate valuation of functional brain activities and also practical irregularities in numerous brain areas.

From the cognitive control system to the *quantum mechanics explanation* of life (brain, mind, consciousness system of whole) is a continuum definition. Furthermore, scientists respect quantum mechanics as unconnected to our consideration of how the brain works. Still, it's not hard to see why Penrose's theory has increased devotion. Artificial intelligence specialists have been forecasting some type of computer brain for years, with little to show so far. And for all the recent developments in neurobiology, we appear no closer to resolving the mind-brain problem than we were a century ago. Even if the human brain's neurons, synapses, and neurotransmitters could be entirely planned—which would be one of the great achievements in the history of science—it's not vibrant that we'd be any nearer to amplifying in what way this three-pound mass of wet tissue produces the immaterial world of human thoughts and feelings. Something seems to be missing in present theories of mind or consciousness. Other philosophers have ventured that consciousness may be a *fundamental property of nature* present outside the known laws of physics. Others— often registered *mysterians*—claim that subjective experience is simply beyond the capacity of science to explain. Other theories, for instance, Penrose's, potentials a deeper level of explanation that consciousness is not computational; and it's beyond anything that neuroscience, biology, or physics can now explain. Hence, we need a major revolution in our considerate of the physical world in command to accommodate consciousness.

The most possible place, if we're not going to go outside physics, is in this big unfamiliar—namely, making logic of quantum mechanics. This draws on the elementary possessions of *quantum computing*. These bits (qubits) of information can be in multiple states. For example, in the on or off position, at the same time, such quantum states occur instantaneously—the superposition—before merging into a solitary, almost prompt, calculation. Quantum coherence arises when a whole system of electrons act together in one quantum state.

Much studies, including Penrose's, argue that human consciousness is nonalgorithmic (in mathematics and computer science, an *algorithm* is a limited sequence of well-defined, computer-implementable directions, characteristically to solve a class of problems or to achieve a computation) and hence is not proficient in being modeled by a conventional Tuning machine which includes a digital computer. Yet *quantum mechanics* plays a vital role in the consideration of human consciousness. Most of the theory is spent reviewing, for the scientifically minded consistent subjects such as Newtonian physics, special and general relativity, the philosophy and limitations of mathematics, quantum physics, cosmology, and the nature of time. Besides, how each of these bears on his developing theme: that *consciousness is not algorithmic*. Other studies, including Hoffman's studies of consciousness, note on *visual perception* and *evolutionary psychology* which exploit *mathematical models* and psychophysical trials. For example, subjects include facial attractiveness, the recognition of shape, the perception of motion and color, the evolution of perception, and the mind-body problem.

Additionally, other studies, including Hameroff's, state that quantum coherence happens in *microtubules, protein structures inside the brain's neurons*. Microtubules are tubular structures inside eukaryotic cells (part of the cytoskeleton) that perform a character in defining the cell's shape, as well as its movements, which includes cell division—separation of chromosomes throughout mitosis. Microtubules are the quantum device. In neurons, *microtubules* assistance regulate the strength of synaptic networks, and their tubelike shape might shield them from the surrounding noise of the larger neurons. The microtubules' symmetry and lattice structure are of specific attention to many studies, including the Penrose theme.

The *mind-body problem* is a debate regarding the *relationship* between thought and consciousness in the human mind, and the brain as part of the physical body. It is dissimilar to the interrogation of how mind and body function chemically and physiologically, as that question presumes an interactionist explanation of mind-body relationships. This question arises when mind and body are considered as separate, grounded on the principle that the mind and the body are fundamentally diverse in nature. The problem was addressed by Rene Descartes as far as in the seventeenth century, resulting in Cartesian *dualism*. Dualism preserves an inflexible distinction between the dominions of *mind and matter*.

Monism sustains that there is only one unifying reality, substance or essence, in relations of which everything can be explained. Each of these classes comprises numerous alternatives.

The two key methods of dualism are substance dualism. This grasps that the mind is molded of a dissimilar type of substance not administered by the laws of physics. Aside, the property of dualism, which embraces those mental possessions linking conscious experience are the fundamental properties.

Likewise, the fundamental properties are recognized by an accomplished physicist. The three main forms of monism are physicalism, which grasps that the mind contains matter systematized in a precise method; *idealism*, which embraces that only thought accurately exists and matter is simply a depiction of mental processes; and *natural monism*, which holds that both mind and matter are features of a separate essence that is itself identical to neither of them. Furthermore, *psychophysical parallelism* is a third possible substitute concerning the relation between mind and body, between *communication* (dualism) and *one-sided action* (monism).

The mind-body problem happens since we naturally want to include the mental life of conscious organisms in a wide-ranging scientific consideration of the world. On the one hand, it seems understandable that everything that transpires in the mind is contingent on or is something that occurs in the brain. On the other hand, the significant structures of mental states and actions, landscapes like their intentionality, meaning their subjectivity and their conscious experiential quality appear not to be understandable merely in relations of the physical process of the organism. This is not just as we have not yet collected sufficient experiential information: the problem is theoretical. We cannot at present visualize a clarification of color perception, for instance, which would do for that phenomenon what chemistry has done for combustion—a description which would tell us in physical relationships.

Likewise, without remains, what the experience of color perception is. Logical examinations of the individual structures of the mental states that are intended to get us over this hurdle normally contain unlikely procedures of reductionism, behavioristic in stimulus. The question that comes to mind is whether there is another way of delivering mental phenomena into a combined conception of objective reality, without depending on a fine standard of objectivity which rejects everything that makes them stimulating. Other philosophies including Aristotle (Greek philosopher) communal Plato's view of multiple soul and additionally enlightened a hierarchical procedure, which is equivalent to the characteristic functions of plants, animals, and people, meaning a nutritive soul of growth and metabolism that all three share, such as a perceptive soul of pain, pleasure, and desire that only people and other animals share, yet the faculty of reason that is unique to people only. In this view, a soul is the hylomorphic form (being compound of matter and form) of a viable organism, in which each level of the hierarchy officially supervenes upon the substance of the previous level.

For such theory, including Aristotle, the first two souls, based on the body, perish when the living organism dies, while remaining an immortal and become continuous intellective part of the mind. For Plato, though, the soul was not reliant on the physical body. He believed in metempsychosis (philosophy that refers to transmigration of the soul), the migration of the soul to a new physical body. It has been considered a form of reductionism by some philosophers. If we view the branches of *ontology* is the philosophy that studies perceptions such as existence, being, becoming, and reality. It includes the questions of how entities are assembled into basic categories and which of these beings happen on the most fundamental level. Ontology is sometimes referred to as the *science of being* and goes to the major subdivision of philosophy known as metaphysics (examines the fundamental nature of reality the relationship between mind and matter and between substance and attribute and potentially actuality).

Ontologists often try to regulate what the categories or highest kinds are and how they form an organization of classes that delivers an encompassing classification of all entities. Frequently anticipated classes include substance, properties, relations, states of affair, and events. These groups are branded by fundamental ontological concepts, like particularity and universality, possibility and necessity. Ontology dualism makes dual promises about the nature of existence as it relays to mind and matter and can be separated into three different types: *Substance* dualism asserts that mind and matter are fundamentally separate kinds of foundations. *Property* dualism suggests that the ontological difference lies in the differences among properties of mind and matter (as in interconnected). *Predicate* dualism views the irreducibility of mental predicates to physical predicates.

Other concepts of mind or consciousness are the models for the mental processes. Many educational backgrounds claim that some of the most puzzling paradoxes of consciousness arise because we grip too long to a habit of thought, a habit that usually keeps us out of trouble. There is no question that where there is a conscious mind, there is also an opinion of interpretation. Nonetheless, what transpires when we close in on the viewer and attempt to discover this point of view inside the *brain*? There is no solitary detail in the brain where the information funnels in, where it all comes together for *central processing*. Hence, such has some far-from-understandable and fairly counterintuitive significances.

Descartes thought hard about this problem, but the brain did have a center: the *pineal gland*, meaning for an individual to be mindful of something, traffic from the senses had to reach at this location, where it then produced a *singular*—certainly charmed—transaction to happen between the individual's material *brain* and immaterial *mind*. Researchers, including Danial Dennett, view today's education on mind-brain relations; and no one is seriously certain if there is a physical center to the brain, a Cartesian bottleneck of dualism. There is no longer a character for a regional gateway, or certainly for any practical center to the brain. The pineal gland or any other physical feature is not the fax machine to the soul, nor is it the office of the brain. There is no such *observer gland inside the brain*. While studies *might* eliminate the anatomical gear of Descartes' dualism, it is harder to remove the idea of a *central processing* area of the *mind itself.*

There is a key finish line and frontier somewhere in the brain, design a place where the instruction of stimuli arrival equals the instruction of performance. Mind, consciousness is still the hard problem, despite the new century. If studies truly accomplish to explain consciousness as might as it will diminish us all, might turn us into simple protein machines. Hence, humans have a mind, and that might be explained by science one day. If evolution built them, they can be reverse-engineered. The *hard problem of consciousness* is the problem of *explaining* why and how humans have phenomenal experiences. Almost as if to say it is the problem of why individuals have personal, first-person experiences, often described as experiences that feel like something (subjective experience). In comparison, we assume there are no such experiences for nonliving things such as a table, a chair, a toaster, or a form of artificial intelligence.

The study and philosophy including David Chalmers, who familiarized the term "hard problem" of consciousness, differentiates this with the easy problems of explaining the physical organizations that give us and other animals the capability to distinguish, integrate information, report mental states, focus attention, and so forth. Easy problems are fairly easy since all that is essential for their explanation is to specify a mechanism that can accomplish the function. That is, even though we have yet to explain most of the easy problems (the understanding of the brain is still opening), these questions can perhaps ultimately be understood by trusting entirely on average scientific approaches.

However, once studies have solved such problems about the *brain* and *experience*, the hard problem will continue even when the presentation of all the applicable functions is enlightened. Furthermore, many philosophers reflect on experience to be the *essence* of *consciousness*. Experience can only fully be known from the inside *(interpersonal)* subjectively, yet if consciousness is subjective *(independent)* and not visible from the outside, why do the vast majority of people trust that other people are conscious and rocks and trees are not? This is called the problem of other minds *(mind between us or embedded)*. The problem of *other minds* is a philosophical problem conventionally detailed as the following epistemological question, meaning that I can only observe the behavior of others. How can I know that others have mind? It is a major issue of the philosophical idea known as solipsism (holds that knowledge of anything outside one's own mind is unsure; the external world and others' mind cannot be recognized or might not exist outside the mind).

It is particularly acute for people who trust in the option of philosophical zombies, that is, people who think it is likely in opinion to have an entity that is physically vague from a human being and acts like a human being in every way but absent consciousness. The most frequently given answer is that people characterize consciousness to other people since we see that they resemble us in appearance and behavior. Hence, individuals reason that if they look like us and act like us, they must be like us in other ways, for example, having experiences of the sort that we do (somehow similar to mirror neurons). There are, however, a variety of problems with that explanation. More broadly, philosophers who do not accept the possibility of zombies generally trust that consciousness is imitated in behavior and that individual trait the consciousness on the basis of behavior. Related issues have also been studied regarding the idea of *artificial intelligence*.

Likewise, the practice of founding equality, dignity, and human rights on the principles of the blank slate, the noble savage, and the *ghost in the machine* is a product of unclear thinking about both ethics and science. As we explored more on the mind-brain relation we viewed at the outset, these are stimulating times in the study of the human mind and in the national of human knowledge in general. From cognitive science, neuroscience, and behavioral and evolutionary psychology, we have the foundation to attain an understanding of human nature that will tie the last enduring gaps of information: between matter and mind and between biology and culture. This has potential to lead to a predominantly filling depth of understanding of our own kind, the earliest injunction to know thyself (self-identity). Other thinkers, like Darwin, showed how the amazing diversity of life and its universal signs of good design could arise from the physical procedure of *natural selection* between replicators.

Aside, how the replication itself could be understood in physical footings. Nonetheless, one vast gap remains in the landscape of human statistics. That is the story of nature needs nurture: biology versus culture, nature versus society, matter versus mind, and the sciences versus the arts and humanities survive as decent contrasts afterward and the other walls which isolating human understanding have fallen apart. Many thinkers have faith that there is a fundamental gap between human behavior and other physical events. Physical behavior has causes as individual behavior has reasons. Reflect how a person clarifies an everyday performance of behavior. For example, John gets on a school bus because he wants to, no one would appeal some physical push or pull John toward the bus nor the gust of wind.

Likewise, nor would anyone need to put John 's head in a brain scanner, etc. The most lucid clarification of John 's behavior demands in its place to his views and desires, such as that John wanted to go to his school. No explanation has as much predictive power as that one. For long periods, the gap between physical events, on the one hand, and meaning, content, thoughts, reasons on the other, has been understood as a border line between two fundamentally diverse kinds of clarification. From 1950s, the cognitive revolution, linguistics, computer science, and philosophy of mind with the help of a powerful new idea explains that mental life could be enlightened in physical relations through the philosophies of information, computation, and feedback.

To put it approximately, beliefs and memories are sources of information, residing in patterns of activity and structure in the brain. Thinking and planning are arrangements of alterations. The idea of the *computational theory* of mind similarly describes how intelligence and rationality can ascend from a simple physical procedure. If the transformations reflect rules of logic, possibility, or cause and effect in the world, they will produce precise forecasts from effective information in search of goals, which is a good period of intelligence. The other knowledge of science bridging mind and matter is neuroscience, particularly cognitive neuroscience, the education of the neural centers of thinking, perception, and emotion. The traditional and more aware origin of the mind is grounded on the soul, an immaterial being. In other explanations, the mind is what the brain does, specifically the information-processing system.

The biology of the mind might view that chemicals can send their way to the brain from the stomach, lungs, or veins and change an individual's awareness, mood, character, and judgments. Likewise, when a patch of brain tissue dies due to trauma, intoxication, infection, or absence of oxygen, a part of the individual is gone. The person may think, feel, or perform so differently as to become quite figuratively a different individual. Furthermore, the evolutionary psychology is the study of the phylogenetic history and adaptive purposes of the mind. *Evolutionary psychology* grips out the confidence of understanding the purpose of the mind, not in mystical or teleological intellect, but in the wisdom of the appearance of design or illusion of engineering that is universal in the natural world as to Darwin clarified by the theory of natural selection.

Though there are many disagreements within *biology*, what is not debated is that the philosophy of natural selection is vital to make intellect of a multifaceted organ such as the ears. The ears accuracy of engineering for the function of hearing and could not be the result of some huge accident in tissue development like the appearance of tumor that can lead to simpler traits. Evolutionary psychology spreads this kind of dispute to another part of the body. For all its delicate natural engineering, the ear is hopeless without the brain. Human body parts are an organ of information processing. Hence, it connects to complicated neural circuits that abstract information about the depths, colors, motions, and shapes of substances in the real world. Likewise, the aptitude to make sense of our experience, to attribute causes to events and to remember things.

Speaking of body relation to brain, recent research has shown aspects of the *psyche* that were formerly measured mysterious. For example, fears and phobias, family dynamics, and romantic love have a methodical evolutionary reason when analyzed like other biological organizations, organs, and tissues. How the mind works is the understanding of the mind and *human nature*. It is important to note that this understanding is not a substitute to more old-style clarifications in terms of education, experience, culture, and socialization. Somewhat it aims at a clarification of how those procedures are conceivable to initiate.

Culture has its possessions as of mental algorithms that attain the feat, that we know as learning. And learning can be powerful and useful only if it is designed to work in certain ways. Human conceptual and linguistic originality contains numerous mental abilities and involves the presence of mental organization. It depends on perceptual-articulatory organizations and conceptual-intentional schemes. The mind comprises a widespread group of innate components, one of which is language, which Chomsky mentioned well in his theory. Each component functions routinely, self-sufficiently of individual control, on the foundation of a separate, domain-precise set of instructions. Such take determinate inputs from some units and produce determinate productions for others. This work of operations is called *computations*.

The several modules network in multifaceted ways to produce a perception, a thought, and a large number of other cognitive products. By definition, *human nature* comprises the core characteristics (feelings, psychology, behaviors) shared by all individuals. Everyone has different experiences of the humans in their life, and this is where the understanding begins. The views of others are colored by the inspiration of the people we know and what the culture and subcultures tell us. The group you are born into will pass on its specific concepts about what makes humans human (nature and nurture—self-identity).

From the natural selection to our physical ear (our body) and from tongue-language *information* consists of energy that has figurative meaning which guides the brain to choices. Nonetheless, the whole word may have no symbolic reference if we don't speak Greek. The perception of *informational* boundary can help explain the relatives and relationships between the human mental behavior. Similar, this permits to clearly specify the relationship between the mind, mental behaviors, and the brain. Informational interface raises to the handover of information among organizations. Information processing reproductions contain a series of stages, or boxes, which represent stages of processing. For instance, *input* procedures are concerned with the examination of the stimuli.

Storage procedures contain everything that occurs to stimuli internally in the brain and can include coding and guidance of the stimuli. *Output* processes are accountable for formulating a suitable response to a stimulus. However, there are a number of assessing facts to bear in mind when reviewing these replicas, and the information processing method in general. These include the following: *Serial processing* successfully means one procedure has to be accomplished before the next begins. *Parallel processing* accepts some or all procedures intricate in a cognitive task(s) happening at the same time. There is an indication from dual-task trials that corresponding processing is conceivable. It is problematic to regulate whether a precise task is handled in a sequential or parallel manner as it perhaps depends (a) on the procedures obligated to solve a task and (b) the quantity of exercise on a task. Parallel dispensation is perhaps more common when someone is very expert. The equivalence between human cognition and computer functioning accepted by the information processing approach is limited. Computers can be viewed as information processing organizations as they combine information accessible with stowed information to deliver explanations to a diversity of problems.

Likewise, maximum computers have a central processor of limited volume, and it is typically supposed that dimension limitations mark the human attentional organization. Nonetheless, the human brain has the dimensions for widespread parallel processing and computers frequently depend on serial dispensation. Moreover, humans are inclined in their cognitions by a quantity of conflicting emotional and motivational influences. The indication for the philosophies of attention which come under the information processing method is mainly originated on trials under controlled, scientific circumstances.

In everyday life, cognitive processes are frequently accompanying a goal (Russ takes the school bus because he wants to go to school), while in the laboratory, the trials are approved out in separation from other cognitive and motivational features. While such laboratory trials are easy to infer, the information may not be appropriate to the actual world separate the laboratory. Attention has been studied mainly in seclusion from other cognitive processes, while obviously it functions as a dependent organization with the connected cognitive processes of perception and memory. The more successful a person becomes at the exploratory part of the cognitive scheme in isolation, the less the information is likely to tell us about cognition in everyday life. Even though it is approved that stimulus-driven (bottom-up) information in cognition is significant, what the individual carries to the task in relation to potentials and past experiences is similarly vital.

We can see the human mind by observing the informational interface occurring between the four domains of *human mental behavior.* To map the human mind generally, we ought to be considering the subsequent four domains: how different fragments of the human nervous scheme transfer messages and save information; how the brain-based information dispensation gives rise to and is inclined by individual conscious experience; how information flows from the nervous arrangement into the physiques to give rise to controlled, practical movements and determined actions.

Furthermore, how experiential consciousness and other neuro-information processes are interpreted into representative language that can then be joined straight with others. From such viewpoint, we can think of the human mind as a neuro-behavioral-experiential-linguistic informational interface arrangement. When individuals and animals are acting on the environment, they are involved in mental behavior; and in that sense, it is all part of the mind-brain organization. Language-based mental behavior is a particularly clear example. A discussion between two individuals is the straight flow of language *information,* an understandable domain of human mental performance.

By the same token, we can practice the perception of the mind to technically signify the information instantiated inside and processed by the nervous system. When distinct in such, we see that perceiving the mind straight, without interface with the additional domains, is complicated. In distinction, the physical written shopping list does exist outside the individual's mind, when separate this way. However, by the same token, writing the shopping list and reading it are human mental behaviors, and in that wisdom, they are obviously a fragment of the comprehensive sense of who we are mentioning to when speaking about the human mind.

There are a number of supplementary fragments that are required to completely explicate the dispute. For instance, there is much involved about the construction of the human mind as a *neuro-information processing* organization, about the numerous domains of human consciousness, and the insinuations of human language as a new system of information processing that progressed in the hominid line, and in what way that altered the informational interface calculation. Hence, as other information processing systems emerge, there may be openings for combining the information processing of the human mind with those classifications.

Certainly, one can willingly reason that a fifth domain of human mental behaviors is developing as a function of how they cross point with computational technologies. *The Future of the Mind* by the *physicist Michio Kaku* already specified the advances that are arising in several ranges. Besides, just as the informational interface perception would suggest, such developments actually are giving rise to a new form of mental behavioral sequence as they are permitting for fundamentally dissimilar categories of informational interface. *Information* accompanying education, and learning system, regardless of brain, mind, consciousness ground, yet everything there is need to know for contributing better life.

Despite its overwhelming statement on *how much information* or perhaps *intellect is good enough* for individuals (brain-memory storage) to conquer, unfortunately, it depends how considerable an individual wants to be which distinguishes the intellect level among species. Likewise, intellect and will are involved in an energetic, multifaceted interface, with manifold phases among an initial perception and cognition by the intellect to the concluding action of the will, with infrequent interruptions or overrides through the desires. These phases may happen in the twinkle of an eye or in a long-drawn-out development. At any phase the will can change the theme and request the intellect to think about something new. The entire picture greatly looks like the modern theater of consciousness model of Bernard Baars, with the will focusing or selectively leading the attention of the mind. In the Baars model of consciousness, there are six basic fundamentals to the theater metaphor—a phase, such as spotlights (which focus attention); actors (with their speeches); a spectator that frequently subsidizes comments about their own thoughts, goals, and knowledge centers (subconscious automatic level); a director (or executive function); and contexts.

Now, if we think of *contexts* as the current total contents of the *stream of consciousness*, it comprises numerous unconscious contributions in addition to all the current *perceptual information* that shapes the *interpretation* of the current *experience*. Context helps to answer to the question what's happening to me? The Baars enlightenment of the theater of consciousness was more like a theater metaphor for conscious experience. Conscious contents are partial to a radiantly lit mark of attention onstage, though the rest of the stage agrees to instant working memory. Behind the acts are executive processes, with a director, and a great variety of background operators that form conscious experience deprived of themselves becoming conscious. In the spectators is an enormous selection of intelligent unconscious instruments.

Some audience associates are involuntary procedures, like the brain mechanisms that guide eye movements, talking. Others include autobiographical memory, semantic networks representing our information of the world, asserting memory for principles (belief) and realities. Likewise, the implicit memories that preserve attitudes, skills, and social communication. Fundamentals of working memory—on stage, but not in the spotlight of attention—are also unconscious. Notice that different inputs to the stage can work together to place an actor in the conscious spotlight, a procedure of conjunction.

However, when on stage, conscious information diverges, as it is commonly distributed to associates of the audience. By far, the maximum comprehensive functions are approved on outside of awareness. All joint perceptions of cognition today comprise theater metaphors. The information-carrying volume of the conscious stream is very limited, yet the admission to information assemblies in the brain is actually enormous. Subsequently, individuals have no knowledge of *its information storage capacity*. The brain may have *access*, within *seconds*, to any of *its past experiences*. Intellect is the product of memory. Maybe one day 90 percent of human activities will be assigned to robots.

Human intellect is the function of memory and capability of physical activities that is not hard for technology to pass on. However, what cannot be implemented is *human identity*. Our DNA carries more memory than our entire brain. The skin individuals grow into still has the color of their great-great-ancestors, yet our memory can only be aware of where our car might be. Centuries ago, the philosopher Thomas Aquinas's idea about the will was a complex of three powers of the human soul. That can be designated as the intellect (perceptive, apprehensive, cognitive), the will (motive, appetitive, conative), and the passions or feelings (sensitive, emotive). However, other theories come to practice and view of human freedom with modern accounts of free will. For Aquinas, freedom is a possession of the whole human being, not a component part of a person. Similarly, the will is not independent of the intellect. Thus, how human understanding *self* is *partially* through the intellect level, means save the information into the storage what has played a role for this understanding was the memory. Then what self-identity might be? Identity has less to do with intellect or memory of understanding self, yet more interconnected to consciousness. However, the conscious mind, so to speak, tends to refer to many descriptions, such as awaken system or being aware.

Consciousness is where there is no memory or intellect level; it's pure identity of being self (self-aware). Human culture is a huge contributor to who persons generally think of themselves yet cannot identify well with materialistic lives. What gives a person meaning is not found through intellect or informative of knowledge but what resists with a person's true nature. When individuals creating boundaries on anything that gives its definition yet it loses its potential. Hence, what is beyond physical, what is infinite is human consciousness where there is the potential. How persons invest in consciousness is how humans reason. People come far better equipped with intellect and understanding of information and technology that guides into making sense of things which are reliable to learn more than school levels. The theory of everything is a future concept in the scientific community which positions that there is one all-encompassing system that proposes a framework of understanding all of physics, combining the quantum mechanics and classical physics into an integrated method which enlightens the laws of the universe.

While no one has actually been able to come up with such a theory nor is it mandatory to know it all, Stephen Hawking was able to explain a construction that unified quantum mechanics and classical physics as it relates to the description of black holes. Individual might think, so what is the big deal of know it all (or most of it)? The agreement is that while both classical and quantum mechanics define the world around us, one relating the motion of large bodies whereas the other describing the motion of small particles that make up large bodies. However, finding a unified explanation compatible with both branches of physics has been one of the greatest continuum challenges for scientists.

Hawking's possibly highest influence was the encounter of the Hawking radiation. Hawking radiation is black-body radiation that is predicted to be released by black holes, owed to quantum possessions close the black hole event horizon a theoretical argument for its existence in1974. The concept of the Hawking's encounter is resourceful in that it is simple but deeply creative. To understand the science behind the finding its better to start by understanding some basic concepts of physics and how they interplay. A black hole is distinct as a densely packed region of space. Humans can visualize it as a stress ball made up of matter.

Also, the gravitational pull is very strong which nothing can discharge out of it. Around such stress ball, there is a rounded district of space which encapsulates it. Besides the edge of this circle is acknowledged as the event horizon, which can be alleged of as a wall that splits what the reality, we can observe from that which inside the black hole, yet nothing viewable from hereafter. Furthermore, the second law of thermodynamics conditions that the quantity of entropy of a system will always increase. This means that entropy is a degree of disorder and the universe is continuously naturally moving toward a more chaotic state.

Nonetheless, anything that has entropy necessity similarly have a temperature that it should release energy. Though, the entire point of the black hole is that it reserves everything so securely that nothing gets out which makes hard to explain? The importance of information and interconnected system of whole individual might draw attention as far as black hole. The *quantum mind* or *quantum consciousness* is a group of theories suggesting that classical mechanics cannot explain consciousness. It suggests that quantum-mechanical phenomena, such as *entanglement* and *superposition*, may performance a significant share in the *brain's function and could explain consciousness*. Declarations that consciousness is someway quantum-mechanical can overlap with quantum mysticism, a pseudoscientific (consists of statements, beliefs) movement that allocates paranormal features to various quantum phenomena such as nonlocality and the observer effect.

Nonlocality is the measurement figures of a composite quantum system do not acknowledge an interpretation in terms of a local realistic theory. Quantum mechanics positions that what seems like an empty space, is actually not empty. It is active with energetic activity of simultaneous creation and destruction of energy on the subatomic scale. Particles and antiparticles are created in pairs, where one particle has positive energy and the other has negative energy. One particle is matter and the other is supposed of as anti-matter. Formerly they rapidly collapse back together in a procedure recognized as annihilation.

Consequently, that no new energy is shaped or demolished, in agreement with the first law of thermodynamics. Since this procedure occurs so fast, it is recommended that such particles are virtual as they have not been perceived. What the twentieth century and Stephen Hawking viewed was that if the particles are shaped very close to the event horizon, formerly they do not require to be annihilated collected as one of the particles can be sucked into the black hole. In addition, in command for the laws of conservation of energy to hold, the particle that goes back into the black hole requests to have negative energy.

Accordingly, if the black hole acknowledged negative energy, this is in consequence of it losing energy, and accordingly, losing mass. Through Einstein's equations energy and mass are interchangeable as $E = mc^2$. Consequently, that would show that the black hole is producing energy, and is getting smaller as a consequence. This is the bright knowledge that shows that black holes are not essentially all black and dark and that they do not last forever. What we have to comprehend is that even the very first living things, things like bacteria, were very complex and it was as if they had minds. They were very capable at remaining alive and replicating and what Darwin viewed has been confirmed one hundred times, one thousand times over ever then is that a totally natural, material, purposeless, procedure of *natural selection* has produced over billions of years, ever progressively multifaceted minds, brains. Besides, human beings are the *possessors* of the most *amazing minds of all*. In fact, human minds are exclusive in many different ways. Nonetheless, that doesn't make them supernatural.

They are natural parts of the natural world and the hard part is explaining how that can perhaps be so. Consciousness is certainly the highlight of the human *mind*; we can explain it all in terms of what's going on in brains or beyond and the things out in the world that those brains are responding to. Likewise, what distinguishes persons mind from the cat mind is that the cat got you might say, a simple brain, doesn't have much thinking tools. People, though, have been picking up thinking tools subsequently they were born.

Likewise, individual cant do much carpentry with bare hands, nor cant do much thinking with bare brain. For example, every word in the vocabulary is a thinking tool which people invented them. On the face of things, quantum mechanics and the biological sciences do not mix. Biology emphases on larger-scale procedures, from molecular interactions between proteins and DNA up to the behavior of organisms as a whole. Quantum mechanics defines the often-strange nature of electrons, protons, muons, and quarks—the smallest of the small. Many events in biology are measured upfront, with one response causing another in a linear, expectable way. By difference, quantum mechanics is unclear since when the world is observed at the subatomic scale, it is seeming that particles are also waves.

Research (and Hameroff) ventures that anesthetics interrupt a delicate quantum process within the neurons of the brain. Each neuron contains hundreds of long, cylindrical protein structures, called microtubules, that serve as scaffolding. Anesthetics, liquify inside tiny oily regions of the microtubules, affecting how some electrons inside these regions behave. Is consciousness an epiphenomenal coincidence of this particular universe, or does the very concept of a universe depend upon its presence? Does consciousness merely perceive reality, or vis versa? Did consciousness simply emerge as an effect of evolution? Or was it, in some sense, always out there in the world? Such questions and answers are continuum journey of brain-mind defining. We viewed a fraction of matters that has been a contributor to this book journey, to name a few, cosmological foundations of consciousness, origins of thought, evolution of consciousness, neuroscience of free will, quantum physics, and consciousness. Furthermore, it is relevant to conclude some of other topics such as out-of-body and near-death experiences, dreams and hallucinations, and how consciousness becomes the physical universe. What is an integrated approach to psychology (mind) and philosophy (thinking)? Can it be an enlightenment gap with psychology's metaphysics? Metaphysics is a recognized branch of philosophy, and this word is used less in everyday conversation that examines the fundamental nature of reality. This includes the relationship between mind and matter and substance and attribute and between potentiality and actuality.

The word "metaphysics" comes from two Greek words that, composed, factually mean after or behind the natural. Metaphysics education questions associated with what it is for something to exist and what types of existence there are. Metaphysics pursues to answer, in an intellectual and fully universal method, the questions "What is there? What is it like?" Metaphysics is also distinguished from other branches of philosophy, not by the aprioricity of its approaches but by the simplification of its concerns. Other divisions of philosophy deal with this or that feature of reality—with justice and well-being. For example, or with feeling and thought. Metaphysics, on the other hand, contracts with the maximum general characters of reality—with value, or mind. The perceptions of metaphysics are also illustrious by their transparency.

Generally speaking, a concept is transparent if there is no important gap among the concept and what it is a concept of. Therefore, there is an important opening between the concept water and the substance H_2O of which it is a perception but no significant gap between the perception identity and the identity relative of which it is a concept. The thought formerly is that the concepts of metaphysics are more parallel to the concept of identity than that of water. Metaphysics as consequently categorized might be a somewhat anemic discipline—there might be very little for it to do.

Nevertheless, it has also been assumed that metaphysics might play an significant foundational character. It is not simply one procedure of investigation among others but one that is accomplished by providing some kind of foundation or underpinning for other forms of examination. In some intellect that relics to be determined, claims from these other procedures of investigation have a foundation in the claims of metaphysics. There are possibly key ways in which metaphysics might assist as a foundation. One, which has established substantial consideration of late, is as a basis for the entire reality. As significant as this conception of metaphysics may be, there is, it seems, another conception that is even more dominant to a person's understanding of what metaphysics is, and that would continue.

Metaphysics, on this substitute conception, aids as a foundation, not for reality as such, but for the nature of reality. It delivers persons with the most elementary explanation, not of things (of how they are), but of the nature of things (of what they are). In command to comprehend this conception well, we need to get vibrant on the relata, on what is a groundwork for what, and on the relative, in what way the one relatum is a substance for the other. It might, on the one hand, be a declaration such as water is H_2O, which defines the nature of water, but includes no position (reference).

Moreover, obvious or understood, to the nature of water; or it might be a declaration of water is by its nature H_2O. That does include a position, either obvious or suggested. A slight answer to the second inquiry, concerning the *relation*, is that the metaphysical *eidetic* truths should deliver a rational foundation for the other eidetic truths; the concluding should shadow rationally from the base. One might want to maintain, of course, on something more than a reasonable foundation; it might be obligatory, for instance, that the eidetic facts of metaphysics must deliver some sort of clarification for the other eidetic facts.

Nevertheless, the concept of clarification here is slightly incomprehensible. Hence, the doubt is that, for all applied determinations, it will be adequate to maintain upon a logical foundation—that anyone who thrives in finding a logical foundation will also thrive in finding a clarification in so far as a clarification can be found. Consequently over, in difference to the preceding circumstance, there is no need, in making sense of the foundational originality, to demand to a typical form of clarification or base. Part of what has made the impression of an a priori substance for eidetic certainty appear striking is the alleged that there must be a priori link principles relating the noneidetic facts to the eidetic truths.

Consider, for instance, the earlier claim that water is by its nature H_2O. This is an eidetic privilege that does not fit metaphysics together as it is not a priori and since it is not satisfactorily general. Nevertheless, it might be occupied to be a significance of the succeeding two privileges: any matter with a given arrangement is by its nature of that arrangement; water is an element whose arrangement is H_2O. Before bearing in mind the inquiry of the *subject matter of metaphysics*, we can make some overall observations on subject matter. These remarks could be positioned within an even more general education of the nature of different arenas of examination and of how they are connected to each other. But then again this is not a feature of the question that intend to follow. Any arena of inquiry contracts with convinced intentions, those that lie inside its purview and whose truth it pursues to examine.

Consequently, mathematics contracts with mathematical intentions, logic with logical intentions, and so on. We might demand the customary of propositions with which an arena of inquiry contracts its domain of inquiry. Any intention has a convinced subject matter. Hence, the intention that Aristotle is a philosopher has as its subject matter the famous man Aristotle and the possessions of being a philosopher. We interpret the subject matter approximately so that the proposition that Aristotle is not a philosopher might likewise be engaged to have the process of denial as share of its subject matter, yet then again, we do not interpret it so generally that the intention that all philosopher is intelligent also has each individual philosopher as fragment of its subject matter. In accumulation to the possessions of being intelligent and the quantifier each philosopher.

On an organizational conception of intentions, we might take the subject matter of a proposition to be established by the constituents from which it is shaped. However, it might also be likely to come to at a beginning of the subject matter of propositions on a less advanced conception of what they are. The subject matter of a field, as we have distinct it, might be termed the comprehensive or overall subject matter. Nonetheless, there is similarly a finer concept of subject matter that might be distinct. For there seems to be a logic in which convinced elements of subject matter are characteristic to a field—a logic in which an element is characteristically mathematical, around, or characteristically metaphysical, or characteristically physical.

Proposition that two things are the identical every time they are fragments of one another. Its constituents are fragment, universality, unification, and individuality. Then only the first is characteristically metaphysical, the rest are logical. For example, reflect the physical proposition that $E = mc^2$ as most are aware. Its elements are energy, mass, the speed of light, product, square, and distinctiveness. Nonetheless, only the first three are characteristically bodily (physically). The next two are mathematical slightly over physical and the last is rational (logic). A component of subject matter characteristic to a given field in some way has its home in the field. It may look in the propositions of other fields still only as the consequence of having been transferred from its field.

Likewise, other fundamentals of subject matter may arise in the propositions of the agreed field yet only as the consequence of having been introduced from their ground. Hence, the general subject matter of a field will in general be comprehensive than its characteristic subject matter. Numerous elements will give the idea in the propositions of the field that are not characteristic to the field. What then is it for an element of subject matter to be characteristic to a given field? From between all of the elements that may befall in its proposals, how do we tell which are characteristic? Perhaps, one arena of investigation may presuppose or be constructed upon the subject matter from other fields.

In order hand to municipal the propositions of attention to the agreed field, we may obligate to make use of subject matter from these other arenas, even though firmly unnecessary to the field itself.

Going back to the example regarding water is typical in the respect, since element is overall than water and composition more general over the molecular form of composition intricate in H_2O. Thus, one might be confident that in the restrictions of eidetic clarification, the basics of subject matter will be of a high, and possibly even of a penultimate step of generalization. Once studies have attained the anticipated stage of generality, it is not hard to understand how we might protect eidetic transparency. For as a regulation, the supplementary general a component of subject matter—the additional cut off it is from the world—the easier it is to lock transparent position. Accordingly, it is that we have the logic of greater transparency as we move from dog to animal, roughly, or from animal to living thing. In conclusion, with the mixture of requirement and transparency originates the opportunity of a priori information. One key complication to accomplishing a priori information is removed, and possibly no other complication positions in its way. Therefore, if all goes well, eidetic clarification will dismiss in the general a priori truths of metaphysics.

If we look back to the question on the enlightenment gap and fixing the problem with *psychology's metaphysics*, we might travel as far as 1715 century, during Galileo's times. The Enlightenment is the age that treasured the power of reason. It was an age in which principal intellectuals claimed that we could comprehend the natural world using logic, math, and the scientific process. Definitely, the work of early scientists/natural philosophers like Galileo and Descartes placed main parts of the foundation.

Some claim that the Enlightenment had better be dated to the publication of Isaac Newton's *Principia* (*Mathematical Principles of Natural Philosophy*) in 1687, that is the sole most vital methodical publication in history. Isaac established a mathematical basis that defined matter in motion (classical mechanics). This essentially opened a mathematical theory of matter that was the substance of people understanding which continued nearly 225 years, till the progress of recent physics (which involved the development of general relativity and quantum mechanics). Consequently, the Enlightenment is the *age of reason* and is the opening of the contemporary age.

When psychology developed on the act, the primary psychologists did not have a metaphysical basis for learning evidently about what it was that they were studying. The absence of the required metaphysical edge gave rise to philosophical questions affecting whether psychology was about human's behavior or the mind, unconscious methods, or self-conscious replication, as well as questions affecting free will and determinism. The universe is an unfolding upsurge of energy-information system, the same description we give to the human brain. That can be designated in behavioral footings of objects, fields, and change and occurs in four different dimensions of complexity: matter, life, mind, and culture. These are distinguishable dimensions of complexity as the behaviors that take place at the stages above matter are facilitated through systems of information processing, precisely, genetic (life), neuronal (mind), and linguistic (culture).

The research point of education, the universe came into being 13.7 billion years ago and gave rise to the four fundamental forces: electromagnetic, strong, weak, and gravity, then the elementary particles, bosons, quarks, and leptons. These forces and particles molded into atoms and galaxies. Because of discrepancy concentrations of energy and matter, there has been a flow of energy across numerous segments of the universe, and this has caused the development of diverse arrangements of complexity. Energy flow on the exterior of planet Earth occasioned in the development of self-organizing, self-replicating organizations that we call *life*.

Human beings are a sole form of energy-information flow. They are sort of animal, and in the animal kingdom there arose self-organizing process facilitated by the nervous system which gave rise to experiential consciousness. Humans then developed full, open language capacities, which caused in them displaying exclusive behavior forms and having exclusive capacities for self-reflective information and for producing knowledge about the world. In terms of *cosmology*, the understand system of history, views of the Universe are that we can comprehend the universe as an energy matter space time grid that developed from a singularity at the big bang, about 13.8 billion years ago. In relationships of *ontology*, energy is the decisive substance mutual denominator.

The observable universe is *energy* in all its different forms, matter is break apart, frozen energy. The universe evolves kind of an unfolding wave of energy-information, which, steady with the history formulation, can be located on the scopes of time and complexity. Furthermore, many studies posit a general behavioral metaphysics. That is, the *ontological* essence of the universe can be well-designated as change in object-field associations over time. Likewise, such considered as the flow of energy-information.

Since the essence of the universe be present as an unfolding wave of energy-information, the knowledge stretches to an original interpretation of main categories in nature. Precisely, it maintains that there are four recognizable dimensions of intricacy that are described and characterized as matter, life, mind, and culture. These dimensions apprehension the behavior of objects, organisms, animals and humans. It suggests that such essential classes are distinguished since individually class acts in a fundamentally novel way. That is, living substances act qualitatively differently over nonliving objects. Animal objects perform qualitatively differently over other group of organisms.

Likewise, human objects behave differently over other animals. These fundamental separations occur as of the evolution of diverse systems of information processing. The storage and dispensation of information on the DNA molecule stretches to fundamentally dissimilar types and stages of self-organization, like that the workings of a cell are qualitatively different over the performance of organic molecules. The rise of a nervous organization in general and brain in specific contribute to another information dispensation scheme that caused in animal behavior and experiential consciousness. Hence, are qualitatively dissimilar behavior outlines over are understood at the level of the cell or molecule.

The mind, brain, and behavior sciences including behavioral neuroscience, computational-cognitive neuroscience, comparative psychology views such specific dimension of behavior. Likewise, the appearance of language associated human minds together in innovative way, giving rise to human culture and societal group establishments that are primarily dissimilar than is understood in the rest of the animal kingdom. Behavior is the relating of energy-information; hence, matter and life behave. Likewise, mental behaviors are the behaviors of the animal as a whole, interceded by the nervous system. In such a formulation, the mind raises to the functional information kept and administered by the nervous system.

It is largely identical with the comprehensive classification of cognition. Experiential consciousness is intellectualized as an embodied whole brain motion that gives rise to experiential responsiveness, and is well distinct and deliberate analytically by frameworks such as global neuronal workspace. Humans exhibit *mental behavior* like other animals, yet there is an additional dimension of intricacy. Human language associated human minds, considerable like the internet connects individual computers. Such consequences in a qualitative obstacle in behavioral complexity. Language, sideways with other technological progresses such as agriculture, historically make the step for enormous societal, cultural evolutionary deviations.

As society converted more and more compound, great scale belief/justification schemes arose, like religion, law, and science. This system is signified as Culture (with a capital *C*). Similarly, human *self-consciousness* is a second order form of consciousness in which the experiential conscious organization is imitated upon and described, either to one's self *(embodied-self-consciousness)* or to others *(embedded self-consciousness)*. The human self-consciousness organization functions to shape reasoning structures for one's actions in society. However, the subconscious mind is like a huge memory bank. Its capacity is virtually unlimited. It permanently stores everything that ever happens.

The function of your *subconscious mind* is to store and retrieve *information*. Its trade is to confirm that person respond precisely the way they are programmed. The subconscious mind makes everything person say and do fit a pattern dependable with persons *self-concept*. The subconscious mind—something that has a vast consequence on every action—nonetheless, is regularly ignored. As a substitute, the concentration is often on our conscious mind, which comprises the serious thought function of our brains. The subconscious is the powerful layer underneath. It involves the awareness of all things the conscious mind cannot identify. Once the subconscious is appointed into, this extraordinary part of the brain plays many different characters in persons everyday life. Subconscious mind is *subjective*, it does not think or reason independently, thus merely obeys the commands it receives from the conscious mind.

The conscious mind can be supposed of as the gardener, implanting seeds; and the subconscious mind can be supposed of as the fertile soil, in which the seeds develop to grow. Consequently, the conscious mind instructs, and the subconscious mind conforms. The subconscious mind is an absolute retainer. It works to make the behavior fit a pattern steady with the emotionalized thoughts and desires. Mostly all the habits of thinking and acting are stored in your subconscious mind. It has memorized all the comfort zones, and it works to keep you in them. The subconscious mind causes a person to feel emotionally and physically uncomfortable whenever a person attempts to do anything new or different since it goes against changing any of the person's established patterns of behavior.

The subconscious mind also practices homeostasis in a person's *mental* dominion. It keeps the person thinking and acting in a method dependable with what the person has done and said in the *past* (relationship, attachment, personal experience, etc.). Learning about the unconscious vs. the subconscious mind and how to manage minds subconsciously and unconsciously is key to daily mental function. There's much a person can acquire by understanding the meaning and concepts of the unconscious and subconscious. In the best performance of diversity and inclusion, it will advantage people when they understand how the mind typically work *deliberately, unconsciously,* and *subconsciously.* Psychologists believe individuals are intelligent to navigate the emotions and reactions well when they are able to comprehend the unconscious prejudice vs. subconscious prejudice.

Through the chapters, we distinguished that there are *three levels of the mind* model—*conscious, subconscious, and unconscious;*

briefly, *consciousness defines our thoughts, actions, and awareness.* The unconscious and subconscious are two dissimilar phenomena. The unconscious is a procedure that occurs *automatically* and is not *obtainable* for *introspection.* The *subconscious,* by difference, is a share of the consciousness procedure that is not *actively in principal awareness.* Persons can derive the subconscious through self-examination that they can likely recognize the *behavior subconsciously, motivation,* and *impulse.*

The unconscious can't be, for absence of a better word, summoned. It's not uncommon for some studies to use the method interchangeably because of their subtle differences. One of the informal ways to comprehend them is through visualization of an iceberg. What is observable is the conscious, though what lies below and more profound are the subconscious and unconscious. The *education* of the *human psyche* is stimulating. Considering the unconscious vs. subconscious can assist a person in circumnavigating their emotions and reactions better. Once individuals can find the anchor of how they think and behave to what the brain has experienced, it may permit people to have healthier consciousness.

Some studies (including that of Dr. Bruce Lipton) opened the position of psychology when working in the field of *epigenetics.* Epigenetics reasons that the choices persons make in their lives actually influence the genes and the cells more than the DNA. The information from epigenetics and how genes are controlled by signals don't come from the cell but come from *outside* of it that is a grounded decade of experience from cell biologist, as well as with quantum physics and deep understanding of the processing system of cells. The cell membrane, which is the outer layer of the cell, actually looks a lot like a computer chip. This makes it the brain of the cell. The environment outside the membrane operated through the membrane, and it controlled the behavior of the cell, turning cells on and off.

Our DNA and genes are not the ones that regulate our bodies, but our *DNA* is *controlled* from signals that come from *outside* the *cell,* and these are signals that come from the *energetic messages* from our *thoughts,* both positive and negative (embedded mind or collective consciousness). People *construct meaning* in a way that is compatible with the modern scientific understanding of how the brain functions. It examines the structure of systems of belief and the character those systems play in the guideline of emotion, using multiple academic arenas to show that connecting myths and beliefs with science is vital to fully understand how people make *meaning*. Why have people from different cultures and eras articulated myths and stories with alike constructions? What does this resemblance express to us about the mind, morality, and structure of the world itself? Most studies (including that of psychology professor Jordan B. Peterson) offer a provoking new theory that explores the connection between what modern neuropsychology tells us about the brain and what rituals, myths, and religious stories have long narrated. A cutting-edge work that brings together neuropsychology, cognitive science, and Freudian and Jungian methods to mythology and narrative.

What's making meaning presents a rich theory that makes the wisdom and meaning of myth accessible to the critical modern mind. Collective unconscious, raises to structures of the unconscious mind that are communal among beings of the same species. It is a period created by Carl Jung. Human collective unconscious is populated by instincts as well as by archetypes universal symbols (like Tree of life, water, The Great Mother). The collective unconscious to reinforce and surround the unconscious mind, distinguishing it from the personal unconscious of Freudian psychoanalysis.

The collective unconscious had philosophical influence on the lives of individuals, who lived out its symbols and clothed them in meaning through their experiences. In addition to our instant consciousness, which is of a methodically personal nature and which we believe to be the only empirical psyche (even if we tack on the personal unconscious as an adjunct), there is present a second psychic organization of a collective, universal, and impersonal nature which is undistinguishable in all individuals. This collective unconscious does not develop individually but is inherited. It consists of preexistent methods, the archetypes, which can only develop conscious secondarily and which give certain formula to convinced psychic contents. As modern humans go through their process of self-identity or individuation, moving out of the *collective unconscious* into *mature selves*. They create a personal identity which can be understood simply as that small portion of the collective psyche which they *embody, perform,* and *identify* with (interpersonal brain definition).

The collective unconscious employs overwhelming impact on the minds of individuals. These possessions of course vary widely, though, since they include virtually every emotion and situation. At times, the collective unconscious can frighten, nevertheless it can also heal. A Voyage to the heart of being human on earth is a thought-provoking exploration for studies and that offers a comprehensive, powerful definition of the mind-consciousness. Aside to understanding of the mind as a developing, self-organizing, embodied, and interpersonal development that adjusts the stream of energy and information.

Throughout much explanations, we understood the brain structure, mind relation, interpersonal experience, self-identity, behavior, mental health, the importance of relationship, attachment, communication, the importance of how to communicate, the effect of genes, evolutional development, nature and nurture, metaphysics, subconscious and the role of memory, universe . . . *a whole range of integration* and when, what, where, of who we are while emphasizing and explaining the brain-mind's competence and how to describe it precisely. Therefore, by relating a wide range of disciplines together, we cultured many aspects of the human mind and interpersonal procedure that regulates such energy and information. As a result, this view permits us to understand energy and information system as the fundamental element of an organization from which the mind arises. Such communication (integration) occurs both within the individual, including its brain, and in the distribution of information among an individual and others and the environment (earth) in which the people live.

The characteristics of such organization include that it is *open (open-ended system, definition)*, capable of being disordered, and nondirect. Thus, a small contribution principal to large and difficult to predict the results (that might be good or bad). Multifaceted organizations have developed properties that arise from the communication of the fundamentals of the system (as a processes of self-organization).

This explanation of the brain-mind as a self-organizing process enables us to ask the question, what is an ideal self-organization? The arithmetic of compound systems—those that have these developing self-organizing procedures—makes known that when features of the organization are differentiated and connected, when they are unified, they move in a way that is flexible, adaptive, comprehensible, animated, and steady. This movement originates when a complex scheme is participating—when it links distinguished fundamentals to each other. When integration is impassable, overall misunderstanding in individual life and health occurs, meaning, confusion, abnormal behaviors, lost of self-identity, disease, divorce, social-emotional concerns, and even death. That the best predictor of a wide range of measures of well-being is how interconnected the individual is—that is, how integrated the brain is.

By contribution of such explanation *(as a form of information flow)* to the mind-brain organization, we can perceive how the *reality* is both within us *(interpersonal brain definition)* and between us, within the body and the brain *(brain-mind structure of development)*, and within the *interpersonal networks* we have with *one another (relationship, attachment, interpersonal experience, embedded)*, and as far as the *universe (the elementary stage of development from matter to atoms to molecules to chemistry of life, etc.)*. With *consciousness*, a person can differentiate the *wisdom of knowing*, of a receptive awareness, from that which is known. Consciousness defines how people see the mind through insight, empathy, and integration.

When people misunderstand such, they do not sense the internal mental experience of themselves (self-identity, subjective experience, interpersonal experience) or *others* (the *we* aspect of themselves), and they consequently cannot deliberately generate integration *(sense of whole)*. The position of the brain as a process of *energy* and *information* procedure plays a role in the overall development. By the same token, it allows the *mind to stretch* as far as the *universe* and back. With *self-assurance of consciousness* comes down the wisdom of knowledge who we are as humans. What is our body made of? The first thought might be that it is made up of different organs—such as heart, lungs, and stomach, or many different types of cells—that work together to keep the body going. Nevertheless, at the furthermost elementary stage, the human body—and, in fact, all of life, as well as the *nonliving* world—is made up of *atoms*, often organized into *larger structures* termed *molecules*. Atoms and molecules trail the guidelines of chemistry and physics, even when they're part of a multifaceted, living, breathing being.

Likewise, approximately atoms incline to gain or lose electrons or form bonds with each other, such realities persist true contempt when the atoms or molecules are fragment of a living thing. In element, simple relations among atoms—played out many times and in many different combinations, in a single cell or a larger organism—are what make life conceivable. Consequently, as an extremely multifaceted being made up of roughly 7,000,000,000,000,000,000,000,000,000 atoms, its probably best to distinguish roughly elementary chemistry as we begin to explore the world of development in general. Tapping in to the memory box while carefully leaving room to compare and contrast as to what we have learned from school.

The term "matter" raises to anything that occupies space and has mass. All *matter* is made up of *substances* called *elements*, which have exact chemical and physical properties and cannot be broken down into other substances through ordinary chemical reactions. Each element is selected by its chemical representation, which is a single capital letter or, when the first letter is previously occupied by another element, a combination of two letters. Some elements follow the English method for the component, like C for carbon. Additional elements' chemical codes come from their Latin names. For instance, the symbol for sodium is Na, which is a short form of natrium, the Latin word for sodium.

The *four elements* mutual to *all living* organisms *(integration system of whole)* are *oxygen* (O), *carbon* (C), *hydrogen* (H), and *nitrogen* (N), which composed make up around 96 percent of the *human body*. In the nonliving world, elements are originated in dissimilar proportions, and some elements common to living organisms are comparatively infrequent on the earth as a whole. Altogether elements and the chemical responses among them follow the identical chemical and physical regulations, regardless of whether they are a *fragment* of the *living or nonliving* system *(metaphysic)*. Atom is the smallest component into which matter can be separated without the release of electrically charged particles. Or, an *atom* is the least unit of matter that holds all of the chemical possessions of an element. As such, the atom is the basic building block of chemistry (the chemistry of life).

Furthermore, an atom contains two sections. The small *atomic nucleus*, which is in the center of the atom and comprises positively charged particles named *protons* and neutral, uncharged, particles named *neutrons*. The second, considerably greater, area of the atom is a *cloud of electrons*, negatively charged particles that orbit around the nucleus. The magnetism among the positively charged protons and negatively charged electrons embraces the atom together. Most atoms encompass *all three* of these categories of *subatomic particles—protons, electrons, and neutrons*. Hydrogen (H) is an exclusion since it characteristically has one proton and one electron, but no neutrons. The number of protons in the nucleus regulates which element an atom is, though the number of electrons adjacent the nucleus regulates which type of responses the atom will experience. Protons and neutrons do not have the same charge. Nevertheless, they do have approximately similar mass.

Meanwhile grams are not a very expedient unit for measuring masses that small, scientists indicated to outline a substitute measure, the *atomic mass unit* (amu). A solitary neutron or proton has a mass very close to 1 amu. Electrons are far smaller in mass over protons, only about 1/1800 of an atomic mass unit. Accordingly, they do not subsidize ample to an element's general atomic physique. However, electrons do importantly disturb an atom's charge, as individually electron has a negative charge equal to the positive charge of a proton. In uncharged, neutral atoms, the number of electrons circling the nucleus is equivalent to the number of protons within the nucleus. The positive and negative charges cancel out, moving to an atom with no net charge.

Moreover, protons, neutrons, and electrons are much small, and maximum of the capacity of an atom—larger than 99 percent—is essentially *empty space*. With such notion of empty space, why alleged *solid objects* don't just pass through one another. The response is that the negatively charged electron clouds of the atoms will deter each other if they get close enough, subsequent in our insight of solidity. Because of the nature of *quantum mechanics*, no single image has been completely acceptable at visualizing the atom's numerous characteristics, which therefore forces physicists to use complementary images of the atom to clarify different possessions.

From atoms to life on planet Earth, the question, do our *minds have quantum structures* that give rise to consciousness? Human consciousness is one of the outstanding mysteries of our time on earth. Does the sense of being aware of self come from mind or is it the body that is creating it? What really happens when one enters an altered state of consciousness with the help of some chemical or plant? Are animals conscious? While we would think this basic mystery of our self-awareness would be at the forefront of scientific inquiry, science does not yet have strong answers to these questions. One way research think of consciousness is to perceive of it as a *by-product of numerous computations* that are happening in the brain.

The *integrated information* concept, created by neuroscientist suggests that conscious experience is an integration of a great of amount of information that comes into our brain, and that this *experience* is irreducible. The brain intertwines a sophisticated information network from sensory and cognitive contributions. Other neuroscientists view that maybe consciousness is simply the performance of *broadcasting information around the brain from a memory bank.* Nonetheless, there are some research reasons the efforts at understanding the nature of consciousness through neuroscience are condemned to fail except *quantum mechanics* is elaborated, like physicist Sir Roger Penrose, for one, thinks that consciousness has quantum origins.

Studies including Penrose trusts that consciousness is not computational. People awareness is not simply a mechanistic by-product, like something you can make a machine do. To understand consciousness, we need to revolutionize the understanding of the physical world. In precise, the answer to consciousness may lie in a deeper knowledge of quantum mechanics. *This quantum coherence takes place in protein structures termed microtubules. Such microtubules reside inside the neurons in our brains and can accumulate and develop information and memory. Microtubules are quantum devices that are composing the conscious awareness (embedded system).*

We studied mind and brain as more or less equivalent subjects, often unconfident how to fully *integrate* them. Thus far, the science of the *mind-brain relationship* has made enormous advances, assisted through new technologies such as sophisticated neuroimaging: neuroscientists are progressively solving the unknown of how perceptions, thought processes, and the subjective sense of self all develop from the immensely multifaceted relations of billions of neurons, individually with thousands of networks, establishing compound networks and feedback, formed through hundreds of millions of years of untraced *natural selection compressions*. The *complexity concept* delivers significant evidence to scientists concerning the form that an eventual philosophy of consciousness might take. The complexity system is now integral to neuroscientists' mission to comprehend *how information processing and circular control function in the brain's neural networks*. Those networks function as cybernetic loops, with no single region in complete control.

The human brain is the most *complex adaptive organization* known. Besides, consciousness as a phenomenon is the most fundamentally diverse from *physical matter* of all phenomena known to study. Nonetheless, the consciousness is not continuously rich and complex— it arises in degrees in dissimilar species and in different conditions of brain health in humans. There are numerous categories of minimal and simple conditions of consciousness. Other than consciousness, the next most fundamentally different phenomenon known to education that has developed from ordinary matter is life itself.

Living things are a superior group of *complex adaptive systems*. A dominant characteristic of complex adaptive systems is *organization*. Unusually, such classifications form by self-organization or a *process of spontaneous command*. They generate overall instruction from local communications among parts of an originally disordered organization. The procedure does not involve strategy or regulator through any exterior agent or any centralized regulator. The guidelines leading the communications of constituents of a complex adaptive system are typically basic and function at a local stage among the individual constituents.

In the circumstance of *living* organisms, the well-understood developments of *evolution by natural selection* and *sexual selection* perform an enormous character in additionally shaping the elaborate *complexity* people perceive in nature, significantly reinforcing the arrival of *intelligent design*. Nonetheless, the *self-organizing processes of complex adaptive systems* befall individualistically of evolution and smear to both *living and nonliving systems*. Undoubtedly, we come down to understanding of the brain is a phenomenon in which the *whole is greater than the sum of its parts*. Besides, its *product, the mind or subjective sense of self*, is fundamentally diverse qualitatively from its fragments—and developing property. *Self-organization raises* to varied outline development processes in the physical and biological world, from sand grains accumulating into rippled dunes to cells compounding to generate vastly organized tissues to individual insects working to produce sophisticated civilizations.

What these diverse systems grasp in mutual is the proximate resources through which they attain instruction and structure. In *self-organizing systems*, sequence at the global level arises merely from communications among lower-level mechanisms. Remarkably, even very multifaceted assemblies result from the repetition of astonishingly simple behaviors achieved by individuals trusting on solitary local information. Such outstanding inference proposes significant outlines of examination: To what degree is the environment relatively over individual involvedness accountable for group complexity? To what degree have extensively contradictory organisms implemented parallel, convergent approaches of pattern formation? And how, exactly, has *natural selection* strongminded the guidelines governing relations within biological systems?

Consequently, self-organization states to the emergence of an *overall order* in time and space of a given system that consequences from the *cooperative relations* of its individual mechanisms. *(the integration and relation system of whole organisms from bacteria to universe).* This notion has been broadly documented as a central principle in sequence formation for multi-component systems of the *physical, chemical and biological world*. It can be illustrious from *self-assembly* through the continual contribution of *energy obligatory* to continue order.

Hence, self-organization characteristically arises in nonequilibrium systems. Cells, with their continuous *energy consumption* and multitudes of local *communications* among distinct proteins, lipids, carbohydrates and nucleic acids, characterize the seamless ground for self-organization. Consequently, comes as no wonder that many properties and structures of self-organized systems, such as natural formation of patterns, nonlinear link of responses, bi-stable switches, waves and oscillations, are originate in all characteristics of contemporary cell biology.

At last, self-organization deceits at the heart of the robustness and adaptability originate in cellular and organismal organization, and hereafter establishes a fundamental foundation for *natural selection and evolution*. Fundamentally, we learned this is not just the circumstance for the *brain*, but for any complex adaptive organization. For example, individual organisms, systems within an organism like the immune system or brain, associations of social insects, bird flocking, herd migration, traffic flows, cities, the internet, ecosystems, and climates. Each is a *system* with a *network* of many negotiators/elements networking (relationship communication system of whole). Multifaceted adaptive systems that produce developing phenomena, are measured complex in that they are *self-motivated networks of interactions* among their fundamental fragments. They are measured *adaptive* in that they transform and self-organize in response to their altering environment.

Nonetheless, some philosophy states that perceptual experiences do not match or approximate properties of the objective world, yet as an alternative offer a basic, species-specific, user boundary to that world. Such study including Donald D. Hoffman reasons that conscious beings have not progressed to perceive the world as it essentially is yet have advanced to perceive the world in a way that maximizes suitability payoffs. The best example is the metaphor of a computer desktop and icons—the icons of a computer desktop deliver a practical edge so that the operator does not have to transact with the fundamental programming and microchip technology in order to use the computer efficiently.

Likewise, substances that a person perceives in time and space are metaphorical images which perform as our interface to the world and empower us to function as competently as possible deprived of having to contract with the irresistible amount of information underlying reality. Furthermore, conscious realism is designated as a nonphysicalist (monism) which grasps that consciousness is the principal reality and the physical world develops from that.

The objective world contains conscious agents and their experiences that cannot be resulting from physical *particles* and *fields*. What occurs in the objective world, self-governing of individual observations, is a world of conscious agents, not a world of unconscious particles and fields. Consciousness is fundamental. In such wisdom, the fitness for evolution may be advanced in entities that see some of reality or generate replicas of reality, over in those which understand more or all of reality. How the mind works and how psychology sits at the center of intellectual life is diverse. In one path, its appearance to the *biological sciences*, to neuroscience, to genetics, to evolution. Nonetheless in further, it seems to the *social sciences* and the *humanities*.

Civilizations are molded and take their form from the *social instincts*, the capacity to interconnect and collaborate. And the *humanities* are the knowledge of the products of the *human mind*, of the works of literature and music and art. Hence, psychology is developing, yet for much of its *history*, it was gloomy. *Perception* was fundamentally psychophysics, the education of the *relationship* among the *physical extent of stimulus* and of its *alleged scale*, aside from *illusions*. Social psychology was a group of research laboratory demonstration presentations that individuals could behave unwisely and be mindless conformists, but also without a suggestion of *theory explaining why*.

However, recently, in an exchange of ideas with other disciplines, psychology has activated to answer the *why questions. Cognitive science*, for instance, that *connects psychology* to linguistics, theoretical computer science, and philosophy of mind, has assisted in enlightening intelligence in relations of *information, computation*, and *feedback*.

With evolutionary thinking, it is obligatory to ask the why questions. Such questions like why does the mind work the way it does as an alternative of some other way in which it could have worked? Hence, such communication has made psychology more intellectually sustaining as opposed to it's just one damn phenomenon after another. There has been much description in history that requires answering two psychological questions. Why was there so considerable amount of violence in history, and what flock does the violence go down? For some studies, the pair of phenomena raised as a rationale of an idea principally that *human nature is complex.*

Hence, there is *no single method* that informs what makes people impulse, no wonder tissue, no magical multipurpose learning algorithm. The *mind* is a *system of mental organs* if person willing, and some of its mechanisms can lead a person to confusion, though others can constrain a person from disorder. What transformed over the decades is which parts of *human nature* are most involved. The idea that there are many *mechanisms* to human nature, some of which can lead to *cooperation* and *harmony.* Human nature states to a set of inherent characteristics which all humans share. Efforts to recognize and comprehend such characteristics go back to ancient times.

The matter of whether human nature is *biologically* hardwired or whether it is formed by *socialization* and *education* is highly controversial. In any circumstance, there are several decent explanations for trying to articulate an objective understanding of human nature, not the least of which is, in doing so, we somewhat express who we are as individuals. Nonetheless, in the twenty-first century, it has developed even further significantly important than ever for educated individual to comprehend human nature since human nature influences are regularly used to avoid accountability.

Some individual might have a wider description of human nature and say that everything humans do is in our nature. For example, love is in human nature and hate is in are nature. War is in are nature so as peace is in are nature. Likewise, reflection is definitely in human nature. If reflection is in are nature, then so is conclusion about are actions. And theorists declare that consciousness, reflection, and choice are where morality lies. In the 1800's Darwin's concept absorbed on humans' primate heritage and activated a new historical of inquiring. From such originated the modern scientific education of humans in grounds as varied as *biology, anatomy, physiology, genetics, psychology, sociology* and *anthropology*. Hereafter, from these grounds have come contemporary concepts of human nature. Primatology embraces human are strongminded in their deep brain structures, the instincts, and the physical make-up through the primate heritage.

History shows fears and anxieties were hardwired into human and prehuman species throughout millions of years when these species were susceptible target to wild creatures. Thus, human fears and anxieties of other (wild creatures), were later shifted to fear of other human beings. Through the view of *anthropology* six-million-year evolutionary track, about twelve species in the human family tree evolved *biologically* and *culturally*. The twelve species all extinctic and modern humans are the only surviving species of such evolutionary trail. Such study viewed; all of the prehuman species were bipedal. Walking upright led to hands becoming free to use tools. The use of utensils obligatory eye-hand coordination and attentiveness which led to an upsurge in brain size. The cumulative use of speech to name and label structures of the environment likewise directed to the growth of the brain. Sociability permitted for communal learning.

The growth of the brain and social communication in groups inspired the brain to an idea where species in the genus Homo progressed to being very conscious and intelligent. Hereafter, from modern anthropological concepts, it can be determined that due to 6 million years of evolution, humans emerged hardwired for tool use, speech use, sociability, and high levels of consciousness. Further into *Psychology* among the many different concepts and schools of psychology, a few stand out for their efforts to discover human nature. Freud viewed *aggression* was a key component of human nature which allows survival, yet which is sometimes convoyed through violence.

Carl Jung thought there was a *collective unconscious* which could infuse an enemy with hateful behaviors, characters which really initiated within oneself. Alfred Adler stated concepts about *interpersonal struggles* for social dominance. Harry Stack Sullivan thought humans have fears and anxieties resulting from repressed communication which instigated a tendency to strike out at those who are dissimilar. Erik Erikson thought social ambiguity in a society can crop misperception in individuals and an inclination to follow unwise significant. Irving Janis explored *group think* which originates from human beings' social nature. Although it is stimulating to travel the theme of human nature, it becomes a requirement in human times due to the misuse of the concept to endorse a philosophical and pessimistic viewpoint that prevents people from evolving ethically.

Human beings are much more than simply self-centered, aggressive, and competitive. Current inclinations to misuse the perception of human nature verify what individual has established he or she is master of everything—except his/her own nature. Hence, the human mind has evolved as a device for enhancing human survival and reproductive success giving to the ultra-Darwinian principles implemented through his new specialists. Moreover, it is best comprehended not as a single coherent unity, but as an interrelating community of diverse elements, individually specialized for a specific function. As it makes vibrant, neither idea is original; slightly they manufacture themes resulting from the past and present guides.

No biologist will have much trouble with the entitlement that humans, with all our characteristics—behavioral as well as physical—have been enhanced to our present form at least in good part by *natural selection*. For instance, if the mind is as a machine, we can apply the technique used by engineers to determine how a competing firm has constructed its equipment—so-called reverse engineering. The misfortune with reverse engineering the mind is that we have to settle what this vague term *means*. Unlike with any human artifact—once we have created a story on how the mind might have arisen, we have no way of challenging it out. Minds are intimately associated with brains, and biologists approaching many questions deliberating the structure, function and evolution of the brain, about which it is conceivable to acquire more experiential indication than can be discovered over just so reverse engineering.

However, the meaning of life is not that we are, evolutionary psychology reasons, simply the deterministically ambitious products of the genes and their sole interest, replication. Likewise, the biology of belief is a relevant work in the field of new biology. Medical professors and research scientists present many experiments, and those of other leading-edge scientists, who observe in great detail the mechanisms by which *cells receive* and *process information*. The insinuations of such study fundamentally change the understanding of life, observing that *genes and DNA do not control an individual's biology*. Hence, DNA is controlled by indications from *outside the cell*, including the energetic messages originating from our positive and negative thoughts (mind-body embedded system). This deeply positive integration of the modern and best examination in cell biology and quantum physics has been received as a major revolution, viewing that our bodies can be transformed as we retrain our thinking. The physical concepts of the human brain organ are open formations of the human mind, and other notions not, however it may seem, exceptionally determined by the external world.

The basic appetites of individual life, anger, love, dread, hate, optimism, and maximum inclusive divisions of the intelligent activity, to remember, expect, think, know, dream, feel, are the solitary pieces of evidence of a subjective demand. So far, we viewed it is a physical statistic that the brain encompasses neurons that fire to create mental states or reason behavior, and this happens self-governing of human *experience* and measurement. Thus, it is not a basic fact but that this neuronal activity can be straightforwardly classified as *automatic processing* or *controlled processing*. Moreover, some keys in the brain comprehend *cognitions* while others understand *emotion* or even that *the self,* or *goals,* or *memories* live in explicit parts of the brain.

Study, use categories to distinct ongoing mental activity into distinct mental states, like culture, anger, an attitude, a memory, etc., to organize a stream of physical movements into behaviors, like lying, theft, or to categorize parts of the physical environments as circumstances. These classes come from and found human experience. The group occasions are actual, yet they originate their certainty from the human mind and in the framework of other human minds. Mental activity is organized this way for explanations having to do with cooperative intentionality, *communication*, and even *self-regulation*, however not as this is the superlative way to recognize how the brain mechanistically generates the mind and behavior. Emotion and cognition make up the Western psychological and social reality. Thus, they can by necessity be explained by the natural detail of how the human brain works, yet emotion and cognition are not mechanisms that are certainly cherished by the human brain or groups that are essential by the human brain. Brain circumstances are *observer-independent* realities.

The presence of *mental conditions* is also an *observer-independent* detail. Hence, cognitions, emotions, memories, beliefs, and so on are not observer-dependent events. They are groupings that have been molded and termed by the human mind to signify and clarify the human mind. Psychological constructionist representations of the mind were established in early years of psychology and have appeared steadily through the history of the science. Even though they have inclined not to control, they are settled in the account that experienced psychological conditions are not the elemental components of the mind or the brain, for example, just as fire, water, air, and earth are not the elementary foundations of the universe. As an alternative, they are products that arise from the interaction of more elementary, all-purpose components.

Furthermore, the contemporary constructionist method that predicts for psychology in the twenty-first century is settled in a simple practical observation. Every minute of waking life the brain comprehends *mental conditions* and activities through a combination of three foundations of stimulation. This stimulus sensory inspiration is made available through and apprehended from the world *outside* the human skin, such as the exteroceptive sensory range of light, vibrations, and chemicals. Sensory signals apprehended from *inside* the body that grasps the brain (the internal milieu) and previous *experience* that the brain makes obtainable through the recurrence and re-inhibition of sensory and motor neurons. These three foundations—vibrations from the *world*, sensations from the *body*, and *prior experience (continuum-integration system of development)*—are repeatedly obtainable, and they form the three central characteristics of all mental life.

Different guidelines (integration and weights of these three components) produce the countless mental procedures that establish the mind. Reliant on the emphasis of attention and tendencies of the scientist, this stream of brain activity is explained into distinct psychological moments that we call by dissimilar titles of *feeling, thinking, remembering,* and so on, which each assessment is accurate in its own way. When the emphasis is working to comprehend what externally determined ambiences raise to in the civilization, mental activity is called *perception.* Scientists are inquiring how the brain creates predictions on what the meaning of the present sensory array from the world, tolerating to recognize the relative to the instant settings in a moment-to-moment way and performance consequently.

When the emphasis is working to comprehend how previous experiences are restored in the brain, mental activity is called *cognition.* When an individual experiences the performance of remembering, such mental activity is called *memory.* If they do not, it is called *thinking.* Moreover, when the mental activity states to the future, it is termed *imagining.* Hence, such mental activity delivers a sense of *self* that endures through time. When the emphasis is working to comprehend what inner sensations from the body stand for, the mental activity is called *emotion.* Emotions, like fear and love, are carried out by the limbic system, that is positioned in the temporal lobe. Although the limbic system is made up of numerous parts of the brain, the center of emotional processing is the *amygdala,* which obtains input from other brain purposes, like memory and attention.

Researchers who are interested in understanding emotion experience, for instance, how do I feel? Observe how sensory information from the world and theoretical information about emotion organized create a framework for what internal bodily sensations position for in psychological relations. Together, these three foundations of input generate the mental states called with emotion words. These conceptualized conditions are the mental tackles that the human brain practices to adjust itself and the body's internal state either straight or through substitute on the world. Such general explanation of mental life can be established into a psychological constructionist method that can contain these principles. At first, the mind is comprehended through the repeated relationship of more elementary primitives that can be designated in psychological terms. The elementary procedures that establish multifaceted psychological classes can be designated as psychologically primitive.

This means that they are psychologically complex and cannot be redescribed as something different psychological. These *psychological primitives* are the elements in a method that will produce an instance of a multifaceted psychological state—what we call an emotion, memory, or thought. Psychological primitives are the fundamental and complex fundamentals of the mind, mediating all biopsychosocial aspect stimuli on psychopathology. All psychological phenomena develop from these primitives.

Distinct the culturally comparative compound psychological classes that they comprehend, psychological primitives are widespread to all human beings. The primitive-constructed process does not disregard the character of biopsychosocial influences yet rather reorganizes them as indeterminate fundamental impacts on psychological primitives. In doing so, it reframes studies away from factor-constructed inquiries like which situations cause suicide, and toward primitive-constructed questions such as how are suicidality concepts shaped, transformed, triggered, and applied. This is a respected alteration since factor-constructed inquiries have indeterminate responses, such as countless circumstances could reason suicide, while primitive-constructed inquiries have definitive responses as there are detailed procedures that undergird all concepts.

Hence, studies might be possible to designate the operations that the brain is performing to create psychological primitives, yet such operations would be recognized in relations of the psychological primitives that they establish. Second, all mental conditions (yet characterized) can be causally abridged to these more elementary psychological primitives. Multifaceted psychological groups raise to the contents of the mind that can be redescribed as the psychological primitives which are the products of neuronal firing. Recent dealings of mind-brain communication that explicitly deliberate the necessity for a multilevel method, and it understood that each level of the ontology necessity position in relation to the other levels. Third, these elementary psychological primitives link closely to circulated networks in the brain.

In addition to ontology, multifaceted psychological groups, like anger, link to an assembly of brain conditions that can be brief as an approximately circulated neural reference space. A neural reference space, given to neuroscientists, raises to the neuronal workspace that implements the brain states that link to a class of mental actions. A precise instance of a group corresponds to a brain state inside this neural reference space. The distinct brain states surpass functional restrictions and are implied as a flexible, circulated network of neurons. Each mental state can be redescribed as an integration of psychological primitives. Hence, in such ontology, psychological primitives are practical concepts for brain networks that subsidize to the development of neuronal integration that creates each brain state. They are psychologically constructed, network-level accounts.

These networks are disseminated across brain extents. They are not certainly isolated; they can partly overlap. Each network is inside a framework of networks to other networks, all of which run in corresponding, each determining the movement in the others. All psychological conditions, including behaviors, arise from the relationship of networks that work collected, prompting and confining one another in a category of linking as they generate the mind. From case to case, networks may be differentially established, arranged, and employed. This resources that instances (case to case) of a multifaceted psychological group will be established as a dissimilar neuronal network inside an individual at different times.

Through such observation, we might ask that what if the psychological states be an emergent phenomenon which consequence from a complex system of dynamically networking neurons within the human brain at manifold stages of explanation? The scientific ontology future of such observation is likewise separate from other scientific ontologies in few central ways. Perhaps most significant, it contracts with the being of two realms of reality as subjective and objective, and their relation. It helps explain why diverse categories of behavioral tasks are connected with parallel outlines of neural activity. For instance, looking back into the brain anatomy and its *networking system*, the so-called *default network*, which includes the ventral medial prefrontal cortex, dorsomedial prefrontal cortex, posterior cingulate and retrosplenial cortex, and inferior parietal cortex.

In addition, medial temporal assemblies like the hippocampus and lateral temporal cortex. Such demonstrations amplified activity not only through the natural (spontaneous), associative mental action that is deprived of an exterior stimulus, yet similarly when one recalls the autobiographical past, predicts the future. Likewise, this can concludes mental states in others; through the self-referential system and ethical choice making; whereas visualization fabricated experiences through act structure and relative standard and through the experience and perception of our emotion. Many roles have been future for such explanation; therefore, one tactic is to inquire what all these responsibilities have in *common*. We might see they draw on (memory) *previous experience (interpersonal experience)* in the form of episodic projection likewise to *mental simulation that forms sensory information from the body and the world (embodied and embedded)*. Once we are working together as a functional *network (integration system)*, such circuitry's more overall drive may be to impart. This means the current sensory array based on past, episodic *experience*. They allow the brain to forecast what the present sensory information revenue founded on that last time somewhat like it was met and to express a suitable response. Hence, this psychological constructionist ontology likewise *integrates* a number of smaller scientific paradoxes with some explanation.

It helps the study to comprehend how *perceptual memory can impact declarative memory tasks* while implicit and explicit memory are theoretical to be mechanistically diverse. Aside how the identical *subjective sensation of remembering* (or mental descriptions) can be *shaped in diverse behaviors*. Hereafter, can study conclude that, the mind is more like a set of formulae than like a machine. And mental events are probabilistically, not mechanistically, fundamental. In the psychological constructionist ontology anticipated here, the image for the mind in the twenty-first century is not a machine, but a procedure.

Psychological primitives are not isolated, networking bits and parts of the mind that have no fundamental relation to each other such as the devices and engine of a machine. They are extra like the elementary components in any storage that can be cast-off to make any number of different formulae. This brand the mental conditions that individuals experience and give names to. The products of the numerous formulae are not general, while they are not extremely variable either. Thus, the process for anger will differ from instance to instance with a context inside an individual.

Even though if there is an average procedure, it might vary from individuals within a certain cultural background and across cultural circumstances. However, at the psychological level, the elements that make up the formulae might be general despite, how they role in combination with each other may not be. And as with all formulae, the amount of each element is only one aspect that is significant to making the *whole product* what it is. The *process of integrating elements* is likewise vital.

As a consequence, it is not sufficient to just classify what the influences are, yet likewise how they organize and form one another throughout the procedure of structure. The *process* of analogy similarly assists to comprehend the scientific utility of characteristic among multifaceted psychological classes, psychological primitives, and *neuronal firing.* Networks of neurons *(neuronal integration system)* understand psychological primitives that in turn are the elementary components of the *mind.* These elementary components construct instances of multifaceted psychological groups such as the *self, attitudes,* controlled processing, *emotion,* and so on.

For the *science* of the *mind,* psychology is organized with the capacity to analyze how being human touches the procedure of doing science. Study is in an improved ground than most to understand how scientists make inadvertently influenced explanations of the world and have the measurements to correct for this all-too-common error. Centuries ago, psychology has castoff phenomenological groups to ground the scientific inquiries into the mind and behavior. These groups impact the inquiries research ask, the trials they project, and the explanation of the statistics.

Education have spent the last century distinguishing between psychological phenomena, educating on the subject, and searching for the communication in the natural setting (world) or positions in the brain. In such respect education is in respectable development. As we cited throughout this journey, Aristotle supposed that fire, earth, air, and water were the basic foundations of matter since these are the ingredients that he knowledge. However, once modern physicists first viewed at the world to learn the building blocks of matter, they saw distinct particles, like *atoms*. Later education recognized parts of atoms, like electrons, protons, and neutrons. From here it was revealed that electrons were not actually physical particles at all yet that they are instead like probabilistic energy states.

Ultimately physicist future the presence of something smaller— particles. They could not see and had to generate new terms for like, quarks and leptons. Today, among much discussion, numerous physicists trust that the universe is established of little strings vibrating in several methods across eleven diverse dimensions. Furthermore, *time* and *space* are skilled as distinct phenomena and were once used by physicists to guide inquiries around the material universe. That is, till Einstein transformed the relationships of the inquiries completely with his *theory of relativity*. Education now distinguishes that time and space are not strictly independent groups—they are diverse ways of experiencing the same phenomenon. *Psychology*, of course, has studied *time* and *space as subjective experiences* for many years.

Knowledge about the human mind is accomplished from information captured through observing the natural world (e.g., neuronal firing), still not self-sufficiently of individual conceptual understanding of what such information *means* for a human living in large, compound groups of other humans. It might be easier to have a faith (open-minded) in that a *psychological phenomenon exists* and be real in a certain sense, make it so. There have been many functional imaging educations of the brain foundation of concept of mind (theory of mind) skills, yet the results are varied and associate functional areas as far apart as orbitofrontal cortex and the inferior parietal lobe.

The functional imaging studies are studied to regulate whether the varied findings are due to methodological influences. The educations are measured giving to the model employed the *mental state*(s) examined, and the *language* demands of the tasks. Methodological variability does not appear to explanation for the difference in results, while this inference may somewhat imitate the moderately small number of studies. Otherwise, numerous diverse brain sections may be triggered throughout theory of mind reasoning, creating an *integrated functional network*. The imaging results propose that there are numerous central regions in the network—including parts of the *prefrontal cortex* and *superior temporal sulcus*—though numerous extra peripheral districts may subsidize to theory of mind reasoning in a manner depending on moderately minor features of the theory of mind task.

Theory of mind (ToM)—the aptitude to think about mental states, like thoughts and beliefs, in oneself and others—*motivates social communication* and permits individuals to make sense of the behavior of others (communication to embedded mind). ToM is a multifaceted *cognitive function* that necessitates *integration of information* from numerous foundations. Some theories offer to enlighten the psychological procedures fundamental to ToM. The concept of such philosophy suggests that a set of *connecting acts* linking *exterior* states, *interior* states, and behaviors is used to construct concepts about the mental states of *others* (integrated system of whole). Likewise, the *simulation* concept submits that the mental conditions of others are simulated using the same mental mechanisms tangled in *experiencing each state oneself.*

Furthermore, it has been predicted that the simulation of mental states might be reinforced through *mirror neurons* that were first recognized in nonhuman primates. Hence, as with numerous cognitive functions, it is expected that ToM may likewise have a localized neurobiological foundation. On the foundation of information from sole neuron recordings in nonhuman primates, logical the orbitofrontal cortex (OFC), the superior temporal sulcus (STS), and the amygdala were keen—while not completely so—to primate social cognition, *forming a social brain*. Studies distinguish *social cognition* as the *processing of any information* that concludes in the precise insight of the dispositions and intents of other individuals.

This explanation might be a little more up-front over the traditional explanation of concept of the mind. Besides, it is limited to the insight of dispositions and intents, as only such perceptions are common to both human and nonhuman primates. Additionally, *social cognition* is distinct as the capability to understand an individual's behavior through the practice of signals like *facial expression*, eye gaze, body postures—including *gesture*—and *social linguistic* influences, like the social content of *speech*. Thus, the current explanation of concept of the mind is incorporated inside the term "social cognition." However, ToM is measured differently in that it states explicitly the persons' mental states. Even though facial expression and eye gaze might be used to lead *interpersonal relations*, they do not certainly contain the deliberation of mental states. Studies and imaging of naturally developing adults, retaining positron release tomography (PET) and functional magnetic resonance imaging (fMRI), have tried to categorize the neurobiological foundation of ToM.

Nonetheless, the findings are varied, associating districts as anatomically distant as orbitofrontal cortices and the inferior parietal lobe. However, an outline arises once stimulated anatomical regions are assembled (networking system). For example, the medial prefrontal (mPFC) and orbitofrontal (OFC) region was implicated in nearly most studies, leading education at some point to arrange that this region is critical for ToM. Steady with the concept of a social brain, the anterior temporal lobe—encompassing the amygdala—and superior temporal regions were somehow associated with ToM.

However, the varied methodology working in the ToM imaging educations raises the inquiry of whether disparity in the regions activated through ToM reasoning is payable to task variables, like the mental state(s) explored, and task language demands. There might be neither pattern type nor the verbal or nonverbal nature of the tasks suggestively affected the form of ToM-associated activity. However, there is initial indication that activity in at least partially different brain districts might be accompanied with individual mental states, like false belief and the discovery of deceit. Similarly, separable outlines of activity have been informed when representing the mental states of parallel and dissimilar others directing to another dissimilarity that might be drawn inside the wide-ranging perception of ToM. Multifaceted *cognitive functions* probably contain activity in several brain districts relatively (networking neurons system of communication) than being localized to a solitary critical section.

Despite the networking, the other three essential regions that establish the primate social brain are the OFC, the STS, and the amygdala. In many studies, the mPFC/OFC region and the STS emerge as *fundamental* areas activated through ToM tasks, yet the amygdala seems to be less steadily stimulated. The detailed nature of brain networks for complex *cognition* is not there yet. There is a growing harmony that *cognitive functions* are reliant on large-scale cognitive networks. Thus, such consist of spatially distinct computational components, that with its own established of relation specializations that collaborate broadly.

Hence, such networks are self-motivated *(self-organizing system)*, with relation rather than complete knowledge of individual network mechanisms. Not only can a brain district perform several cognitive purposes, yet the same cognitive function could be accomplished through numerous districts. While the detailed application of such function might differ from district to district. The connection of a district in a cognitive function would only be well-thought-out in the framework of the complete outline of brain activity.

Meaning, that is, inside the background of a *network*. Integration catalyzes flexibility, adaptability, rationality, energy and constancy. Thus, sustains differentiation whereas promoting linkage among network. Integration and networking are vital from brain relation to mind and stretches to universe. Newton's laws of motion, similarly stating the *relations* between the *forces acting* on a body and the motion of the form. Neuroplasticity increases with flexibility and adaptabilities since neuroplasticity similarly known as neural plasticity, or brain plasticity, that is, the ability of *neural networks* in the brain to change through growth and reorganization. These changes range from individual neuron pathways manufacturing new networks, to systematic adjustments such as cortical remapping.

Neuroplasticity embraces *circuit* and network changes that consequence from knowledge a new skill, environmental inspirations, repetition, and psychological tension. The mind progresses through *natural selection* and self-*organized system* (to most point) to solve problems that were life-and-death matters to our *ancestors*, not to commune with perfection. Nevertheless, self direction is an organism's amazing ability of *controlling* a stream of order on itself and hence escaping the decay into atomic chaos. Existing order displays the power of *maintaining* itself and manufacturing order procedures. Likewise, the *tree of life* or universal tree of life is a metaphor, model and research tool used to explain the *evolution of life* and describe the *relationships (integration system)* among *organisms*, both living and extinct.

To understanding the development of ToM, as well as individual and sex differences, it is some what strong that establishing whether reasoning about specific mental states is connected with different patterns of brain activity is a vital future goal. These different mental states can perhaps be greatest explored through developing a nonverbal pattern, to *avoid linguistic* confounds, in which dissimilar mental states are explored without changing any other probationary variables. Exploring the character of practical and structural networks among brain regions connected with ToM will be important for a comprehensive considerate of the alleged network. One can learn to increase the mind capacity for being aware so that person will be able to adjust the ratio of the experience of awareness itself to objective of persons awareness. This might call *cultivating consciousness*; might call it consolidation of the mind.

Studies make known that such process would be correct in even calling this *integrating* the brain growing the linkages among its different regions, strengthening the brain capability to adjust mental states like emotion, attention, thoughts, and behavior. From neurons to consciousness education, there are several views that explain how neuroscience is trying to link the gap among *phenomena* that people experience and how the physical brain regulates itself. In such efforts, education views connection work from either side of the water. For example, from the physical regulation side, if the study views how neurons demonstrate and, or, and not logic declarations, and so if the human presented as a computer. Then from the conscious side that we recognize of *existence*. This view might explain several concept deceptions through means of the similarly computational adjacent inhibition, opponent procedures, and habituation.

Nonetheless, even if the education given such clarifications, there is evidently still amply of missing bridge left to complete. Neuroscience and related grounds in general will need better *architecture* from which to accurately progress. However, throughout the mind-brain journey, we have distinguished several vital knowledge such as the *relationship* (how to communicate neurons); the *physical brain* in the form of *embodied system*, self-organized and self-regulated mechanism; mind as an emergent self-organizing process likewise is a system from and also regulating the process of energy and information within the body (embodied) and within relationships (embodied and embedded). In addition, the other important facets of mind are subjective experience, consciousness, information (information meaning also covering on *education*: knowledge, learning, evolution, data, history, universe, faith, beliefs, genes, mental health) in the self-organizing system.

The most important shared elements of the organization of the mind are *energy and information system*. As we overview, such *energy* (and knowledge, awareness) is not limited by the human skull nor skin. *When the brain makes maps (accumulates information to process), it structures itself. Furthermore, the information contained in the maps can be used nonconsciously to direct motor behavior effectively, a most desirable consequence considering which survival leaning on taking the correct action. Furthermore, when the brain designs (organizes) a map (neuron assembly), it is likewise creating pictures (the mental images or mindsight), hence the core currency of the minds. Consciousness agrees to experience the maps as descriptions (information), to operate such images, and to apply motive (action, energy) to them. Maps are structured (or neuron fires and wires) once individuals network with objects like people, a machine, a place, from the outside of the brain toward its interior (integration communication system).*

If we refer to such images as *mindsight,* then it is the way we can emphasize attention on the nature of the *internal world.* This is how a person emphasizes the awareness on self, so as the emotions, thoughts, and feelings, and it's how individuals are able to focus on the internal world of others. Consequently, it's how persons have insight into self *(through awareness and interpersonal experience to self-identity)* and empathy for others *(from relationship to integration).* With that said, mindsight *(mental image)* is more than just a thought. Mindsight stretches further, providing the tools to display the internal world with more simplicity and depth, adjusting the internal world with more influence and strength.

Consequently, in all such explanations, mindsight (mental image/ MI) is a concept that's greater than insight and mindfulness. It's fully not just about being present moment to moment, yet it's about being present (being aware) so persons *screen* what's going on but *then alter* what's happening *(process the information to apply the knowledge over observing alone/observe-absorb-release).* It's permitting the action-oriented system of unfolding the power of the *mind* to truly change the assembly (neuron networking) and *regulation* of the *brain.* It's more than the synaptic alone that knowledge had since individuals had these experiences that got shaped.

With mindsight/MI person can essentially modify the development of their life as they become awakened to the understanding of *attention* to really *integrate (how to communicate that's how neuron networking)* areas that weren't integrated before. Therefore, once individual alter the internal world, they can move it from disordered ways of being (not connected fully) to more tuneful (integrated) function. And as a result, person move the mind toward well-being is exactly what mindsight/MI allows us to do. It's a way of captivating the *mind* and awakening it to the notion that individuals aren't just a passive participant in life, yet can be an active captain of their skills (experience, evolution is *building blocks* of our development to *build* up on).

Once individual recognize that the mind can change the brain itself, they become empowered to truly alter their lives. And once we lead from a mindsight (mental image) point of view at how we can profoundly know what's processing in the brains like, when we can look very obviously at what's happening in are *relationships*, what happens is we're able to really understand patterns where we're miss-guide in life. Contrary to what education used to trust we now know that the brain is *open* to change throughout the life span *(open-ended brain definition)*. Today we know, not only can the brain change, yet we can study to use the effort of the mind to really shape the *connections (integration)* in the brain itself. Since the brain gets set up by the genes, for instance temperament, and likewise by just chance.

Nonetheless, the *experiences* truly form *synaptic connections* in the brain itself (experience-dependent brain). Yet here's the important: that once neurons *fire* person can get them to *rewire*. Then experience stimulates neurons, the basic cells of the brain, to fire in precise sequence. One system of *experience* (information-memory) that we now know forms neuronal firing, and also synaptic development—changes in the progress of the networks among the neurons—is how individual effort *attention*. Once individual gain to focus their attention on the nature of the mind itself, they truly can *rewire* vital portions of the brain that aid *regulate* how the entire nervous system functions. For example, how the body regulates itself, how stabile the emotions—and how to participate in relationships with others. This insightful capability of mental image (mindsight/MI), and it's how individual can learn to use the *emphasis* of their *attention* on the *mind* itself really *transform* the *networks* in the *brain*, to transfer the brain to a further *integrated system* of functioning. In addition, in the light of awareness-mindsight/MI method, the brain is not just limited to what's in the skull yet essentially stretched nervous system that is the mechanism through which energy and information streams. Hence, once we view at such network between mind, brain and relationships, we become empowered in fact to transfer to well-being. In the mindsight (mental image) or mindfulness approach what we do is recognize domains of integration, and absorb what are the ways networking can be endorsed.

Now, there's something termed the networking of consciousness aside from neural networking where individual develop the dimensions to sense the regulations of the mind with more simplicity and modify them with further strength. Further, bilateral integration is where individual connect the different purposes of the left side of the brain to that of the right. While vertical incorporation where allows the consciousness experience of the cortex at the top of the brain to be allied to the parts like the limbic area, the brain stem and the body itself.

From memory integration as we already explored, to what is memory, how does a person know who he or she is (interpersonal self-identity), how does a person remember what he or she experienced and generate the autobiographical records that individual has in mind? Then the connected one is narrative integration: how do people really pile the stories of their lives, since research has obviously shown that if people make sense of their life, their own life will have new energy to it, and the form they interrelate with others, including your lovers, your friends, family members, your own children. As a result, these *relationships* will be enhanced when they have made sense of their life. State incorporation *(networking all state as a whole)* is when realizing human have different states of being, and how such states link to each other.

Consequently, within one state person can feel very differed, and finding linkage within a state is vital. For example, a person has one state that wants to be draw self from others and another state that wants to be connected, social. Finding time and being mindful for such different states that person has that *constitute a self,* is a part of state integration where linkage all aspects plays role.

Interpersonal linkage *(interpersonal communication)* that is how individuals relate to one another in empathetic and caring ways. Further, temporal networking, which is how do people grip the sincere existential matters of ways in which persons struggle with wanting predictability yet life being indeterminate aside from wanting immortality, yet we face mortality. Such are what temporal combination holds. In addition, another realm emerges as transpiration linkage, where individual begin to have a prolonged wisdom of self. The feeling of being a part of a much larger whole, and the important part around that is that human begin to sense a profound insight of meaning in life.

That is the wisdom of knowing (energy and information stream within us, between us and beyond the mind) under the light consciousness of how to communicate (linking all aspect of life as a whole). Consideration, awareness, *love* and motivation is in this way used for how we feel another person's feelings, how person can feel felt by someone else. This is the most significant share of people relationships with one another. Understanding is how person has a mindsight record (mental image, insight), an image in the mind of what's going on inside the mind of others. Just like we learned on the *mirror neurons* absorbs in what people perceive in someone else, it resonates with inner bodily responses and emotional parts of the brain respond. It travels back up to the middle portion of the front most part of the brain cortex, the exterior part of the brain the prefrontal cortex which permits individual to produce an image of their own bodily state, and formerly envision what's going on in others.

Unfortunately, the human mind is a multifaceted phenomenon constructed on the physical scaffolding of the brain which neuroscientific investigation endures to observe in great detail. However, the nature of the relationship among the mind and the brain is far from understood. In our journey, we travel the recent advances in complex system structures. We examine what is past and presently known about the complexity of the brain and recent applications of complex network wisdom to the study of brain connectivity. We then discuss the logical concept of emergence as a possible framework for the examination of mind-brain mechanisms. We explain currently available exploratory tackles for the clarification of this matter, from physics, science, metaphysics, nature and nurture, genes, evolution, the universe, to qualitative metaphors, and deliberate their relative advantages and limits.

Similarly, we highlight crucial areas where further work is necessary to achieve progress or development, including both detailed modeling and large-scale theoretical contexts. The complex network concept from physics, mathematics, computer science, and the social sciences is to deliver a principled outline in which to study the complex systems that are composed of exclusive components and exhibition nontrivial component-to-component relations. Such background has been practical to systems as diverse as metabolic integration, food webs, gene–gene interactions, and social networks and recently the human brain.

The simplest application of the concept to such systems is in the use of the mathematical table concept to outline the statistical properties of the system's connectivity, which can provide central insights into fundamental organizational principles. Hence, the graphical possessions of schemes can be somehow linked to features of the system's function and to external constraints that might have formed the organization's development, progress, and process (mostly by the process over the products of chart information, as a form of reverse engineering).

Such outline reproductions can be extended to generate more complicated replicas in which simple connectivity maps are complemented with further information on the features of individual mechanisms, functional algorithms, and more. A supplementary significant path of review is the structure of reproductive replicas of network organization that can bring wisdom to the structural predictors of transformed function, for instance, in disease states. Such complex network concept is typically relevant to the education of the human brain—a complex system on numerous scales including space and time that can be decomposed into subcomponents and the relations among them.

Further into applicability, the outline is generalizable throughout neuroimaging modalities and delivers outcomes that can be instinctively understood relative to large bodies of former neuroscientific and academic work. Significantly, graphical possessions of human brain networks have been directly associated with system function through relationships with behavioral and cognitive variables as well as verbal fluency, IQ, and working memory precision. Studies have indicated that metabolic assets of the brain can be recorded to the network organization signifying energetic constraints on fundamental architecture.

We learned the physical restrictions on the anatomical organization of the human brain constrain its function. For instance, two regions of the brain that are logically active (functionally integrated) with one another are often linked through a straight white matter pathway. Multiscale networking is one notion of multifaceted organizations and offers the operational foundation for another major phenomenon; such is the system of *emergence* in which the behavior, function, and properties of the system like consciousness and subjective structures of consciousness are more than the sum of the system's parts at any particular level or across levels (whole system in the form of integration over its sum part). In detail, these system possessions can develop from complex patterns of fundamental subsystems.

Conceivably emergence—of consciousness or else—in the human brain can be thought of as describing the communication between two comprehensive stages: the mind and the physical brain. Even though *emergence* can be abstracted most generally as happening between the two stages of the mind and the brain, emergence might be a more *fundamental* possession of the human brain classification happening among several physical and functional stages. The *mind* is the set of abilities counting cognitive aspect such as consciousness, imagination, thinking, intelligence, judgment, language, and memory, as well as to noncognitive aspects such as people's emotions and instinct. Hence, such complex system has its location, within us, between us, among us.

Chapter 4

The Developing Consciousness

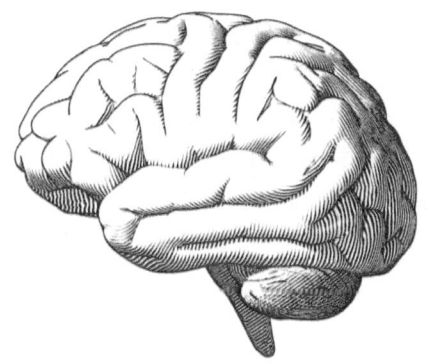

Consciousness, at its simplest, is awareness of internal and external existence. Sometimes the meanings of the two terms "conscience" and "consciousness" are confused and are misunderstood. Consciousness has many definitions aside from the mind-body problem. Consciousness is the function of the human mind that receives and processes information, forms it, and then stores it or rejects it with the help of the five senses, the reasoning ability of the mind, imagination, and emotion and memory. Individuals' five senses enable the mind to receive information before: imagination and emotion process it, motive judges it, and memory stores or rejects it.

Despite areas of studies, descriptions, explanations, and debates by philosophers and scientists, consciousness remains mystifying and debatable, being at once the most aware and most mysterious feature of our human life. Conceivably the main widely agreed notion about the topic is the *intuition* that it *exists*. Views differ about what exactly needs to be studied and explained as consciousness. Occasionally, it is identical with the mind, and at other times, an aspect of it. While consciousness has been observed widely in its different aspects, like in philosophy, psychiatry, neurophysiology, neuroplasticity, etc., philosophies though it is an equal significant aspect of the human existence, which remains a mysterious to a great degree as an almost inspirational aspect of as we mentioned as the human mind.

Conscience and consciousness are parts of a system of information that oversees a person's experience and decision-making process. In the ancient times, it was one's *inner life*, the world of introspection, of private thought, imagination. Nowadays, it often includes experience, cognation, feelings, and perception. It may be awareness, awareness of awareness, or self-awareness. In some views, the particular parts of the human brain where those functions take place are theoretically distinct by neurophysiology. A vital remark is that the more information one is able to accumulate and produce, the better aware and the better conscious one develops concerning one's internal and external world. Characteristically, awareness and wakefulness characterize the two main mechanisms of consciousness.

Awareness is distinct through the content of consciousness, and arousal is distinct through the degree of consciousness. Awareness encompasses self-awareness that observes the interior world of thoughts, reflection, imagination, emotions, and daydreaming. Likewise, external awareness that observes the outside world is with the assistance of the five senses. Further into neurological conception, consciousness encompasses a range of states that vary from physiological states to states of weakened consciousness that are observed through exact principles comprised in the Glasgow Coma Scale but also contains altered states either through self-training or by drug consumption.

Neuroanatomical education discovered several structures engaged (linked) in the consciousness on the multidimensional concept of consciousness. An indispensable structure that intermediates the arousal is the ascending reticular activating system that encompasses neurotransmitter-precise fibers from the reticular nuclei of the brain stem that are associated with the cortex via thalamic and extra-thalamic pathways and projecting to the hypothalamus and basal forebrain. Other important structures in consciousness are the *amygdala*, which controls memory, attention, emotion and higher cognitive functions, aside the cerebellum, that controls executive function, cognition and emotion.

Through brain structure we viewed, both the prefrontal cortex and precuneus seem to be linked with self-perception and *metacognition*. Moreover, the precuneus and prefrontal cortex along with the temporoparietal intersection and anterior cingulate gyrus signify parts occupied in the default mode of brain regulation throughout the conscious inactive (resting) state. Frontoparietal integration and the thalamus are measured the most significant *neural associates of consciousness*. This linkage is occupied in sustaining awareness, in attention and in behavioral assortment of received and deposited information.

The *thalamus* is the concluding relay station for perceptual statistics prior reaching the cortex. It likewise acting an important character through modulating cortical activity. The thalamus and cortex are linked in a reciprocal method and this integration appears accountable for advanced cognitive procedures. Furthermore, the thalamic reticular nucleus seems to regulate thalamocortical harmonisation.

A very diverse concept from that of a neural correlate of consciousness that adopts that consciousness is a solitary integrated unit, is the concept of multiple consciousnesses with three classified stages like, micro-consciousness, macro-consciousness, and the unified consciousness. One of the numerous concepts of micro-consciousness reflects that the practical element of consciousness contains a triangular *neuronal formation*. The integration of such is free through conventional anatomical borders. These integrations differ in scope from one instant to the next, with each instant being linked with dissimilar steps of consciousness.

The difficulty and measurement of these integration rest on the synchronicity of their synapses, the forte of the activate that pledges their transient synchrony, and on the accessibility of neurotransmitters. Past the neurological accounts of consciousness that reflect that consciousness is produced at the neuronal level is the quantum physics method, overseen through traditional physics, that discusses an extra dynamical visualization yet which similarly stretches to numerous debates. The *quantum physics* view, consciousness rest on self-observation.

It is unceasingly self-creating through unconscious procedures that are continuously coming into life by self-awareness, like the performance of observing an electron which concretizes that electron through collapsing the wave function. This copy of consciousness permits for the cohabitation of numerous, half-formed concepts, all skimming under the edge of *awareness* at the same time waiting for the self-perceiving procedure to end this superposition and to concretize a particular knowledge. This dynamical concept indicates an incessant alteration in the brain's organization.

Neuroplasticity and consciousness are bidirectionally linked. Meaning, with consciousness, on the one hand, being the consequence of the rising difficulty of the integration of some activity and, on the other side, restructuring brain networks thro learning activities. The conscious brain is in a continuous state of learning. It learns how to explain and redefine its own action to itself, emerging complex systems of metarepresentations. Likewise, the self-motivated influence of consciousness upon brain integration remains past wakefulness, with dreaming similarly having a significant effect upon neuronal integration.

Alternative vital feature of neuroplasticity in consciousness is characterized through the altered state of consciousness throughout mindfulness procedure. The neuroscience points of assessment, directing attention exercise produces calculable variations in spontaneous brain activity through growing gamma frequencies. Such electromagnetic variations are validated through imaging educations that established both dynamic white matter changes like amplified myelination and connectivity and enlarged cortical thickness.

The question might come to mind is, how does the brain become *aware of information?* In this book we learned scientific theories, practice of what consciousness might be and how the brain could construct it. We went over the history of the human evolution, brain base structure, integration of mind and how our facts fit in to this large context. Would consciousness be the result of electrical signals in our brain oscillate? The brain is self-possessed of neurons which pass the information flow among each other.

Likewise, we know the information efficiently associated from neurons to neurons that maintain for short periods, if the electrical signals of neurons oscillate in synchrony. This electrical activity of many neurons oscillate together could origin consciousness? However, the hard problem is to comprehend, how we become aware of all these patterns scientifically inside our head or not, as awareness is metaphysic.

We also explored the natural selection from Darwinian discovery, still might not be convenient answer to many and scientists of today. Looking at the brain stimulation, we can tell brain uses *attention* when emphasis its processing for handling information stream. While brain is electric to emphasis on giving information, it uses its internal integration of interpersonal experience as forms of statistics assembly. When brain normalizes such integration within its organization and among subjective experiences through consideration (attention) is another vital technique of awareness. Through which brain is aware of itself, it's account of information and the *witness of paying attention to this integration.* This observing of integration can be among the awareness of self (interpersonal experience) others (mind between others and universe) as infinite opportunities.

As we read through the mind and brain integration system, we traveled many possibilities for the mind isn't enskulled, embodied, nor has barrier between self and others. In this instance, consciousness is that nature that is indispensable for awareness to all these interconnectedness organization of the whole. I might refer to this action of consciousness as signals or the modern *Wi-Fi* of the brain. Individuals are well equipped with a modern, scientifically essential human brain that can no longer hide its physical infinite mind network nor its consciousness that is capable of witnessing this infinite awareness. (When a mother breastfeeds her baby, for that milk production, only a crying of its baby is good enough. There are many times when the mother is miles away from the infant and feeling her breast getting hard—full of milk, because at that moment, her infant was hungry and searching her mother.)

The brain structure—stimulation throughout the body, mind integration between self and others—universe and awareness from consciousness made it sound simpler. From the brain integration system, we conclude this one aspect (cerebral cortex) of our brain becomes active when we are socially involved—thinking, especially the superior temporal sulcus in addition to temporoparietal junctions.

Would it be possible for individuals who have less experience in self or other awareness or any health condition in the cerebral cortex might have placed this for disabilities? Might be. However, the mind is helpful in mirroring this attention to be not the only explanation. For instance, we are paying attention to others; and while we are not paying attention to ourselves, others make us realize it, which requires no words.

Education notes that the regularly held view that brain activity causes conscious experience has, so far, proved to be intractable in terms of scientific explanation. A study proposes a solution to the hard problem of consciousness by implementing the converse interpretation that consciousness reasons brain activity and, in fact, generates all objects and properties of the physical world. To this end, we might view the combined two concepts: scheme of perception and conscious realism. Perceptual experiences do not compete or estimate possessions of the objective world but in its place deliver a basic, class-precise, user boundary to that world. The conscious beings have not advanced to observe the world as it truly is yet have progressed to perceive the world in a way that exploits fitness payoffs.

Such study is as we already shed light on to include the Hoffman's practices, the metaphor of a computer desktop and icons—the icons of a computer desktop deliver a practical boundary consequently that the user does not have to contract with the fundamental software design and electronics in command to use the computer proficiently. Likewise, substances that people perceive in time and space are metaphorical icons which perform as the edge to the world and permit individuals to function as resourcefully as conceivable without having to contract with the irresistible quantity of information's original reality.

Conscious realism is designated as a nonphysicalist which embraces that consciousness is the key reality and the physical world arises from that.

The objective world contains conscious agents and their experiences that cannot be resulting from physical particles and fields. Those particles and fields are icons in the of conscious agents, yet are not themselves fundamental inhabitants of the objective world. Hence, consciousness is fundamental. The mechanisms of consciousness are multifaceted and complex, while the workings of conscience are considerably simple.

The perception of conscience, as generally used in its moral sense, is the integral capability of every healthy individual to observe what is right and what is wrong and, on the forte of such insight, to regulate, screen, estimate, and perform their actions. Such ethics as right or wrong, good or bad, and fair or unfair have existed during our history yet are similarly formed through a person's cultural and economic environment.

The closer our internal state of conscience recognizes with the developed perception of these perceptions, such as good, right, just or fair, the advanced our level of conscience, and less physical pressure is knowledge if person sense that he performs conferring to such concepts. It can be said that conscience is the step of integrity and honesty of each person since it screens and controls the value of one's actions. One who performances with a pure conscience has the benefit of feeling internal peace, which is a sensation that moderates the opposing physiological effects experienced in periods of pressure.

Conscience is the maximum specialist and assesses information to regulate the excellence of an act either good or evil, fair or unfair. *Conscience* is a *cognitive process* that produces emotion and rational links founded on an individual's moral viewpoint or value system. Conscience positions in difference to provoked emotion or thought due to relations based (integration system of whole) on instant sensory insights and automatic replies, as in sympathetic central nervous system CNS responses. In mutual relationships, conscience is regularly viewed as principal to feelings of remorse when a person obligates an act that conflicts with their moral standards.

An individual's moral values and their disagreement with familial, social, cultural and historical understandings of moral attitude are measured in the examination of cultural dependence in both the practice and study of psychology. Subsequently, conscience positions advanced in are *consciousness*, in count, has the aptitude and the specialist to resolve how information will be used. Nevertheless, conscience is typically inclined through and adapted in its results through the natural instincts of individuals for survival and perpetuation.

This whole procedure of information-consciousness-awareness-conscience must be understood in its whole as a complex, incessant and integrated established of functions in all healthy individual. If any part of these regulation is substandard the whole system will breakdown. This establishes the integration, consistency and steadiness of the are brain's structure, and it means that, even though we hypothetically can differentiate among functions for the determinations of research and considerate, these functions in detail work as a *universal whole* with a complete linkage between the parts (embedded mind and consciousness).

As we already participate on viewing human consciousness from many angles including Penrose output on consciousness is nonalgorithmic, and therefore is not proficient of being demonstrated through a conventional Turing machine type of digital computer. Further, quantum mechanics plays a crucial character in the understanding of human consciousness precisely, the microtubules within neurons sustenance quantum superpositions. The objective collapse of the quantum wavefunction of the microtubules is critical for consciousness. The collapse in inquiry is physical behavior that is nonalgorithmic and surpasses the restrictions of computability. The human mind has capabilities that no Turing machine could hold because of this mechanism of noncomputable physics.

If we think of *contexts* as the whole contents of the flow of consciousness, it includes numerous unconscious contributions aside from all the existing perceptual pieces of information that form the interpretation of the present experience. Context services to response to the inquiry such as what's happening to me? The hard problem of consciousness is the problem of *explaining* why and how individuals have phenomenal experiences. That is to say, it is the problem of why people have particular, first-person experiences (interpersonal experience) often designated as experiences that feel like something.

By *contrast*, persons assume there is no such experiences for nonliving things such as a table, a chair, a car, a computer, or a sophisticated form of reproduction intelligence. The academic who presented such notion of hard problem of consciousness differentiates this with the easy problems of *explaining* the physical classifications that give human and other animals the aptitude to favor, integrate information, account mental states, emphasize attention, and so on. Easy problems are comparatively easy since all that is obligated for their explanation is to require a mechanism that can achieve the function. That is, even though we have yet to explain most of the easy problems, such inquiries can perhaps finally be understood through trusting completely on typical scientific methods.

However, once individuals have resolved such problems about the *brain and experience (interpersonal neurobiology)*, the hard problem will continue even when the presentation of all the relevant functions is explained. As we explored, the existence of a hard problem is controversial. It has been acknowledged by philosophers of the mind and cognitive neuroscientists. However, its existence is disputed by philosophers of mind and cognitive neuroscientists. The hard problem might be remain for the question of *how experience arises* out of nonsentient matter.

Some studies framed the problem as facing up to the problem of consciousness and prolonged upon knowledge while some have shown rigor and impeccable clarity. Others trust that hard problem is actually more of an assembly of easy problems and will be resolved through further analysis of the *brain and behavior*. Consciousness remains an ambiguous term. Hence, it is used to mean self-consciousness, awareness, the state of being awake, and so forth, as well as the feeling of what it is like to be something. Consciousness, in this logic, is synonymous with experience.

Even when education has clarified the performance of all the cognitive and behavioral functions in the locality of experience—perceptual insight, classification, inner access, verbal account—there may still endure an additional unrequited inquiry, like why is the presentation of such functions convoyed through experience? Challenging the hard problem of consciousness, the problem might be these problems, the easy problems, and the hard problem.

The easy problems may comprise how sensory organizations function, how such information is administered in the brain, how such information stimuli behavior or verbal intelligences, the neural foundation of thought and emotion, and so on. The hard problem might be the problem of why and how are those procedures convoyed through experience? Similarly, why are these progressions convoyed through that specific experience relatively than another experience (how to communicate or how to experience as part of an integration system)?

The easy problems are open to reductive review. They are a logical consequence of lower-level pieces of evidence about the world, parallel to how a car's ability to drive is a logical consequence of its carwork and its mechanic structure, or a snowstorm is a logical consequence of the structures and functions of firm weather forms. A car, a snowstorm, and the easy problems are all the sum of their integrated parts. Additionally, experience is further than the sum of its parts. Unlike a car, a snowstorm, or the easy problems, clarification of constructions and functions leave something out of the depiction.

These functions and assemblies could possibly exist in the absence of experience. Otherwise, they could exist together with a diverse set of experiences. It is reasonably possible for a perfect replica of to have no experience at all. Alternatively, it is reasonably imaginable for the replica to have a dissimilar customary of experiences, like an inverted observable range. The same cannot be said about car, snowstorm, or the easy problems. A perfect replica of a car is a car, a perfect replica of a snowstorm is a snowstorm, and a perfect replica of a behavior is that behavior. The alteration might be that experience is not rationally necessitated through lower order structures and functions; it is not the sum of its physical parts. This means that experience is resistant to reductive examination, and consequently positions a hard problem.

Other constructions of the hard problem of consciousness might include: How is it that some organisms are subjects of experience? Why does consciousness of sensory information exist? Why do qualia exist? Why is there a subjective element to experience? And why aren't people philosophical zombies? Some philosopher argued in that the hard problem is, in element, linked with two descriptive goals, namely, physical processing stretches to experiences with a phenomenal appeal. Individual phenomenal potentials are hence and therefore. The first notion concerns the *relationship* among the *physical* and the *phenomenal* while the second issue the very nature of the phenomenal itself, meaning, what does the felt notion feel like? Philosophical zombies are a thought trial commonly used in deliberations of the hard problem. They are theoretical beings physically matching to person yet lack conscious experience.

Many philosophers take zombies as *impossible* inside the limits of nature yet likely within the limits of logic. This would suggest that pieces of evidence about experience are not rationally involved through the physical pieces of evidence. Consequently, consciousness is complex. The knowledge dispute likewise known as Mary's Room is additional communal thought trial. It centers around a hypothetical neuroscientist named Mary. She has lived her all life in a black-and-white room and has never seen a different color. She similarly occurs to distinguish everything there is to know about the brain and color insight.

The philosopher trusts that if Mary were to see the color red for the first time, she would advance new knowledge of the world. That means information of the what red appearances like is different from the understanding of the brain or visual system. Meaning words comprehension of what red appearances like *is* complicated to understanding of the brain or nervous system; consequently, experience is complex to the regulation of the brain or nervous system.

Other philosopher disagrees, saying the same could be said about Mary understanding everything there is to know about swimming, or driving at the first time, etc. While others, has put forward a hypothetical suggestion of developing a language that could enlighten to an individual blind from birth what it is like to see. If such a language is possible then the force of the knowledge argument may be undercut. Through our journey, we explored the physical brain and its integrated structure and the brain directs our body's internal functions.

It also *integrates sensory instincts and information to form perceptions, thoughts, and memories*. The brain gives person self-awareness and the aptitude to speak and move around. Its four key districts make this conceivable are, the *cerebrum*, with its cerebral cortex, gives person conscious control of their actions. The *diencephalon* arbitrates feelings, accomplishes emotions, and instructions whole interior systems. The *cerebellum* adjusts body activities, speech coordination, and balance, though the *brain stem* communicates signals from the spinal cord and guides elementary interior functions and reflexes. The cerebrum is the major brain assembly aside from being part of the forebrain.

The cerebral cortex, not only procedures sensory and motor information yet permits *consciousness*, our aptitude to consider ourselves, others and the outside world *(mind-brain-consciousness system of whole through understanding of information and knowledge)*. It is what most individuals think of when they perceive the term "gray matter." The cortex tissue contains mostly of neuron cell bodies, and its folds and fissures (recognized as gyri and sulci) pass the cerebrum its symbol rumpled surface. Likewise, the cerebral cortex has a left and a right hemisphere, each hemisphere can be separated into four lobes. Thus, the frontal lobe, temporal lobe, occipital lobe, and parietal lobe. Each lobe are functional sections; they specify in numerous parts of *thought and memory, of planning and decision-making, and of speech and sense perception.*

Further, the thalamus intercedes sensory information and relays signals to the Conscious Brain. The diencephalon is a region of the forebrain, associated with both the midbrain (share of the brain stem) and the cerebrum. The thalamus procedures most of the diencephalon which contains two symmetrical egg-formed masses, with neurons that release out by the cerebral cortex. Sensory information deluges into the thalamus from the brain stem, along with emotional, visceral, and other data from dissimilar parts of the brain. The thalamus communicates such messages to the suitable parts of the cerebral cortex. It regulates which signals need conscious awareness, and which should be obtainable for learning and memory.

Meanwhile 1990, researchers including the molecular biologist and the neuroscientist have made substantial development toward classifying which *neurobiological* proceedings happen parallel (integrated) to the *experience of subjective consciousness*. These hypothesised proceedings are raised to as *neural correlates of consciousness* (NCCs). Though, such study debatably reports the question of which neurobiological mechanisms are integrated to consciousness yet not the inquiry of why they must stretch to consciousness at all. Thus, integrated information theory, advanced by the neuroscientist and psychiatrist in 2004. The theory recommends an identity among consciousness and integrated information, with the latter item distinct mathematically and therefore in code measurable.

Hereafter, *global workspace theory* come to live and is a cognitive architecture and theory of consciousness proposed by the cognitive psychologist in 1988. Study including Baars clarifies the concept with the metaphor of a *theater*, with conscious procedures signified by an illuminated stage. This theater integrates inputs from a diversity of unconscious and or else independent networks in the brain and formerly transmissions them to unconscious networks. In this particular, GWT provided a hopeful explanation of how information in the brain could become globally available, yet reasoned that now the question stands up in a dissimilar form such as why would global accessibility stretch to conscious experience? Similarly, others point of view with GWT on the grounds that it offers, at best, an explanation of the cognitive function of consciousness, and miss the mark to clarify its experiential feature.

By difference, while GWT does not address the hard problem, specifically, the very nature of consciousness, it pressures any concept that challenges to do so and offers significant insights into the relative concept between consciousness and cognition. Hence, there is no hard problem of amplification qualia over and above the problem of explaining fundamental functions, as qualia are necessitated by neural activity and themselves fundamental.

Many studies excluded the concept of qualia and reasoned that easy problems of consciousness are essentially the hard problems, and the hard problem is grounded only upon less explained perceptions that are frequently instable as understanding progresses. However, when individuals' instincts are educated by cognitive neuroscience and computer simulations, the hard problem might fade.

The hypothetical impression of qualia, pure mental experience, disconnected from any information-processing role, could be viewed as a peculiar knowledge of the prescientific age. Further into the relation of consciousness, a science of consciousness necessarily explains the precise relationship among subjective mental conditions and brain conditions, the nature of the relationship between the conscious mind, and the electrochemical communications in the body.

Progress in neuropsychology and neurophilosophy somehow has come from concentrating on the body rather than the mind. In such scenario, the neuronal integration of consciousness may be observed as its reasons, and consciousness may be alleged as a state reliant on possessions of some indeterminate compound, adaptive, and vastly *interconnected biological system*. Determining and describing neural integration might not offer a philosophy of consciousness that can enlighten how specific organizations experience anything at all or how and why they are connected with consciousness.

Nonetheless, considering the NCC may be a step toward such a philosophy. The study of some other neurobiologists might be less clear that the variables giving rise to consciousness are to be found at the neuronal level, overseen by classical physics or quantum consciousness based on quantum mechanics. The quantum mind or quantum consciousness is an assembly of theories suggesting that classical mechanics cannot enlighten consciousness.

It theorizes that quantum-mechanical phenomena, such as entanglement and superposition, might perform a significant share in the brain's function and could clarify consciousness. Quantum theory and relativity are viewed as contradictory, which implies a supplementary fundamental level in the universe. Quantum theory and relativity pointed to this more profound concept, which is expressed as quantum field theory. This extra fundamental level theory was feature to signify an undivided unity (the integration of the whole system) and an implicated order from which arises the explicated order of the universe as we experience it.

Study of such (Davis Bohm) feature *implicate order applies* both to matter and to consciousness that it could explain the relationship between them. It shows the mind and matter as forecasts into individuals explicate order from the fundamental implicate order. This idea appealed that when we look at matter, we see nothing that helps us to understand consciousness. Hence, such views the feeling of movement and change that make up the experience of music originate from the field the instant past and the present in the brain together. The musical records from the past are alterations over than memories. The records that were implicate in the instant past develop explicate in the present which views this as consciousness evolving from the implicate order. This movement, change or flow, and the coherence of experiences, such as listening to music, is viewed as a manifestation of the implicate order. Studies claimed to derive evidence for this from Jean Piaget's work on infants.

These studies show that young children learn about time and space since they have a hardwired consideration of movement as a fragment of the implicate order and associated this hard-wiring to Chomsky's concept that grammar is hardwired into human brains. Likewise, quantum entanglement is a physical phenomenon that occurs when a group of particles is, produced, network, or share spatial in a way such that the quantum state of each particle of the assembly cannot be designated individualistically of the state of the others, including when the particles are divided by a great distance. The theme of quantum entanglement is at the heart of the disparity among classical and quantum physics. Entanglement is a main feature of quantum mechanics absent in classical mechanics.

Declarations that consciousness is somehow quantum mechanical can overlap with quantum mysticism, a pseudoscientific drive that allocates supernatural features to numerous quantum phenomena like nonlocality and the observer effect. There is great deceptive redundancy and correspondence in neural integration, so though activity in one assembly of neurons may associate with a percept in one circumstance, a dissimilar population might facilitate an associated percept if the previous population is lost or deactivated. It may be that each phenomenal, subjective state has a neural integrated.

Where the neural correlates of consciousness (NCC) can be encouraged theatrically, the subject might experience the linked percept, though inactivating the district of integration for a precise percept will reason it to vanish, giving a cause-effect relationship from the neural section to the nature of the perception. What demonstrates the correlates of consciousness? What is the integration perhaps among the NCC for seeing or hearing? Will the NCC contain all the pyramidal neurons (type of multipolar neurons found in areas of the brain including the cerebral cortex, the hippocampus, and the amygdala) in the cortex at any given point in time? Or is it the only subdivision of long-range forecast cells in the frontal lobes that project to the sensory cortices in the back?

Neurons that fire in a recurring or synchronous manner? Such neurons are some of the suggestions that have been progressive over the centuries. The growing capability of neuroscientists to operate neurons using approaches from molecular biology in blend with visual tools is contingent on the concurrent development of suitable behavioral assesses and typical organisms amenable to large-scale genomic examination and operation. It is the integration of such fine-grained neuronal examination in animals with ever more delicate psychophysical and brain imaging methods in humans, supplemented by the development of a healthy theoretical prognostic outline, that will hopefully useful to a rational consideration of consciousness, one of the dominant mysteries of human life.

There are two mutual yet different dimensions of the term "consciousness": one linking arousal and states of consciousness and the other linking content of consciousness and conscious conditions. Further, to be conscious of anything, the brain should be in a comparatively high state of arousal whether in wakefulness or REM sleep, intensely experienced in dreams while typically not remembered.

High arousal states are integrated with conscious states that have precise content, seeing, hearing, and memorising something. Diverse stages or states of consciousness are integrated with diverse types of conscious experiences. For example, the awake state is relatively different from the dreaming state and from the state of deep sleep. However, in all three states, the basic physiology of the brain is affected, as it likewise is in transformed states of consciousness, especially after taking drugs when conscious perception and insight may be improved compared to the usual wakeful state.

Studies talk about impaired states of consciousness as in the comatose state, the persistent vegetative state, and the minimally conscious state. Here, state raises to dissimilar quantities of external/physical consciousness, from a total absence in coma, persistent vegetative state, and general anesthesia, to a shifting and partial form of conscious impression in a slightly conscious state such as sleep walking. The range of conscious states or experiences available to a patient in a slightly conscious state is reasonably partial.

In brain death, there is no arousal, yet it is indefinite whether the subjectivity of experience has been intermittent, somewhat than its noticeable relationship with the organism. Practical neuroimaging has shown that fragments of the cortex are still energetic in vegetative patients that are alleged to be unconscious. Nevertheless, such parts seem to be functionally detached from integrative cortical parts whose movement is needed for awareness.

The possible fortune of conscious experience seems to rise from deep sleep to drowsiness to full wakefulness. Similarly, this might be computed, using ideas from the complexity concept that integrate both the dimensionality and the granularity of conscious experience to give an integrated-information academic explanation of consciousness. As behavioral arousal upsurges, so do the variety and difficulty of conceivable behavior. Yet in REM sleep, there is a distinguishing atonia, low motor arousal, and the individual is hard to wake up; yet there is still high metabolic and electric brain activity and intense perception.

Many nuclei with separate chemical signs in the thalamus, midbrain, and pons necessarily function for a focus to be in an adequate state of brain arousal to experience anything at all. These nuclei consequently belong to the allowing influences for consciousness.

Contrariwise, it is possible that the precise satisfaction of any specific conscious feeling is arbitrated by specific neurons in the cortex and their integration satellite assemblies, with the amygdala, thalamus, claustrum, and basal ganglia. Unfortunately, trauma, death, and treats are between unconscious driving energy behind people's most serious conclusions and choices. Death has existed as a key idea which carries individuals' most activities unconsciously. The brain is progressively getting better with daily denial which expels these feelings from people's consciousness mind.

Therefore, individuals learn death can be imaginable and, at some point, impossible. It evaporates the idea behind conscious and unconscious. If this can be an additional significance from death (unconscious) to life (conscious), it will donate additional to the biological fitness of humans over other animals. Likewise, denying the reality is a fundamental human characteristic. Other educational studies on consciousness including Ken Wilber's integral theory have identified several structures of an individual's consciousness. For example, on cognition, what one is aware of; on values, what one considers most important; and on self-identity, what one identifies with.

Other inputs, perhaps Wilber's most well-known model of human development or spectrum of consciousness, are rather simple, grounded as they are on three different levels: prepersonal, personal, and transpersonal. The prepersonal stage is typically described by traditional developmental thinkers like Piaget, Freud, Erickson, and Kohlberg. The personal phase is commonly labeled by ego psychologists like Jane Loevinger aside from humanistic psychologists such as Abraham Maslow.

Captivating the unique characteristics of an individual is a trial in any clinical encounter. By considering the mind as a self-organizing development, we can understand that chaos would be the consequence of an organization that is not *integrated*. In this way, disorder or confusion (mental health issues) can be evaluated in an individual's life to brighten how some *domain of integration* may be impaired for the well-being of people. Such person-specific domain valuation can remain to actions that are strategically planned to address this person's forms of impassable integration.

Education is information and energy flow like blood with us, through us, between us, and among us. This typical concept delivers a way of understanding the comprehensive spectrum of life's challenges and assists the clinician to perceive each individual as exclusive, to have conducts that do further than merely decrease symptoms, yet likewise transfer the individual to positions of well-being. As an alternative of being clinicians to aim only to decrease symptoms, this context permits people to explain the mind and mental health and aim treatment toward well-being through *endorsing integration*.

Thinking with an educated mind prior to meditating is a first solution to integration and linking all the domains of life step by step. Likewise, this understanding allows us to truly be mental health professionals as we promote health directly. With this typical system: of *the centrality of interconnectedness life and integration in health, energy, and information flow* in viewing the heart and the location of mind, we will integrate the research and recommend that consciousness is in need of continuum upgrade with the exciting findings and annually new information, and new technology, and new research (formally and unformal). I have confident that with human brain neuroplasticity we will *integrate consciousness*.

Integration or interconnectedness is a continuum linkage of differentiated aspects of all systems there are. With mind-brain-consciousness through updated information and energy flow, we can differentiate the wisdom of knowing, of a receptive awareness, from that which is known. Information (knowing) on brain development, interconnected neurons (embedded), and interpersonal neurobiology (embodied) enable humans to learn about the mind as well as create more clarity and *regulation of the mind* through this process of *continuum-integrating (open definition of interpersonal brain).*

The findings consequently far have reinforced the concept that this repetition strengthens the mind by improving the two aspects of mind as a regulatory development, namely, monitoring and modulation. With continuum practice, the emphasis of attention is steadied (reprograms the subconscious via neuroplasticity). Therefore, that energy and information system is recognized with supplementary wisdom and element, and the people likewise absorb straight how to moderate that process toward integration.

Through linking a wide range of disciplines (science, evolution, physic, history, biology, theories, research, technology, medicine, psychology, culture, belief, and faith system) together, we offer the *explanation* of some aspect of the mind as the emergent, self-organizing, embodied, embedded, interconnected, and relational procedure that adjusts the daily activity of energy and information. Such interpretation permits education to actually teach such continuum up-to-date energy and information movement as the *fundamental element of a system* from which the mind arises and our life stabilizes up on.

The characteristics of integrated system include that it is *continually open*, capable of being successful, chaotic, and nonlinear, meaning that any inputs principal to great or difficult to foresee consequences. Complex organizations have developing properties that arise from the *communication of the elements of the system*. Hence, one of such feature processes is the self-organization system. Constructivism is a philosophical viewpoint about the *nature of knowledge*. Specifically, it signifies an epistemological posture. There are many directions of constructivism, yet one example of a prominent theorist known for constructivist views is Jean Piaget, who studied on *how humans make meaning in relation to the interaction between their experiences and their ideas.*

Many studies (continuum journey of development/CJOD) tended to focus on human development in many relations aside from what is occurring with an individual as opposed to development that is influenced by other humans. Hence, there might only be a dead end if any study comes up with a single framework at any time now. For life and beyond human understanding (including education) is the *process over the products*; it is of simplifying our knowledge enough to move forward at our best.

I can trust enough to conclude the brain's hierarchy of needs begins prior to birth (developmentally appropriate biology and practice). Hereafter, for a well-developed brain, the hierarchy banks on *integration and "the continuum story of nature needs nurture."* Consequently, the *brain's definition* at any point of time remains "open-ended." ...

A New Century (Neurocentury)
Neurobiology (Neweurobiology)
The Interconnected Lives . . .

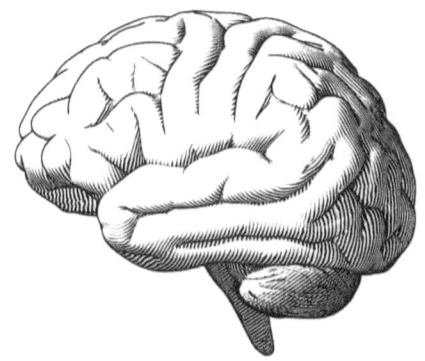